Myopia: Diagnosis and Management

Myopia: Diagnosis and Management

Maia Russell

AMERICAN
MEDICAL PUBLISHERS
www.americanmedicalpublishers.com

AMERICAN
MEDICAL PUBLISHERS
www.americanmedicalpublishers.com

Cataloging-in-publication Data

Myopia : diagnosis and management / Maia Russell.
p. cm.
Includes bibliographical references and index.
ISBN 979-8-88740-286-4
1. Myopia. 2. Myopia--Diagnosis. 3. Myopia--Treatment. 4. Eye--Refractive errors.
5. Ophthalmology. I. Russell, Maia.
RE938 .M96 2023
617.755--dc23

American Medical Publishers,
41 Flatbush Avenue,
1st Floor, New York,
NY 11217, USA

ISBN 979-8-88740-286-4 (Hardback)

Contents

Preface

Myopia, often known as near-sightedness or short-sightedness, is a vision disorder in which the image of the object is created in front of the retina rather than on it. As a result, the faraway objects appear hazy, while the close objects appear normal. Common symptoms of myopia include blurred vision when looking at distant objects, headache, eye strain, difficulty in driving (specifically during night hours), etc. It is an inheritable condition, and genome-wide association studies have identified some of the genes that play a role. From a clinical perspective, controlling myopia in children is critical for reducing the burden of pathological myopia when they enter adulthood. The diagnosis of this disorder requires carrying out the initial objective assessment of the refractive status of each eye and it is administered by an optometrist or ophthalmologist. The treatment of this eye condition is usually done with the help of glasses and contact lenses, surgery, LASIK, vision therapy, and eye exercises. This book discusses the diagnosis as well as management of myopia. It will help the readers in keeping pace with the rapid advancements in the study of this medical condition.

This book is a comprehensive compilation of works of different researchers from varied parts of the world. It includes valuable experiences of the researchers with the sole objective of providing the readers (learners) with a proper knowledge of the concerned field. This book will be beneficial in evoking inspiration and enhancing the knowledge of the interested readers.

In the end, I would like to extend my heartiest thanks to the authors who worked with great determination on their chapters. I also appreciate the publisher's support in the course of the book. I would also like to deeply acknowledge my family who stood by me as a source of inspiration during the project.

Maia Russell

1

Understanding Myopia

Chee Wai Wong, Noel Brennan, and Marcus Ang

Key Points

- Myopia is a significant global public health and socioeconomic problem.
- Pathologic myopia has become a major cause of blindness or visual impairment in both Asian and Western populations.
- Myopia may be a highly heritable trait, with environmental influences such as outdoor activity playing important roles in its development and progression.
- Control of myopia in children is important, and various strategies including pharmacologic and lens-related interventions have proven efficacy.
- Imaging is important to detect complications of pathologic myopia, and both medical and surgical interventions may be useful for their management.

C. W. Wong · M. Ang (✉)
Singapore National Eye Centre, Singapore Eye Research Institute, Singapore, Singapore

Duke-NUS Medical School, Singapore, Singapore
e-mail: marcus.ang@snec.com.sg

N. Brennan
R&D, Johnson & Johnson Vision Care, Inc, Jacksonville, FL, USA

1.1 Global Epidemiology

Myopia has become a significant global public health and socioeconomic problem [1–4]. East Asia, and other parts of the world to a lesser extent, has been faced with an increasing prevalence of myopia [5, 6]. The prevalence of myopia and high myopia (HM) (the definition of myopia and HM is spherical equivalence (SE) of −0.50 diopters (D) or less and SE −5.00 D or −6.00 D, respectively) in young adults in urban areas of East Asian countries has risen to 80–90% and around 20%, respectively [7, 8]. According to a summary of 145 studies regarding the global prevalence of myopia and HM, there are approximately 1950 million with myopia (28.3% of the global population) and 277 million with HM (4.0% of the global population), and these numbers are predicted to increase to 4758 million (49.8% of the global population) for myopia, and 938 million (9.8% of the global population) for HM by 2050 [9].

The prevalence of childhood myopia is substantially higher in urban East Asian countries (49.7–62.0% among 12-year-old children) [7, 10] compared with other countries (6.0–20.0% among 12-year-old children) [9]. Similarly, in teenagers and young adults, the prevalence of myopia is higher in East Asian countries (65.5–96.5%) [8] compared with other countries (12.8–35.0%) [9]. However, the geographic difference of myopia prevalence in older populations is less than that in younger populations. The prevalence rates of myopia in adults in urban East Asian countries are only slightly higher than in Western countries.

The prevalence of myopia has remained consistently high among Chinese children in urban settings, but the evidence does not support the idea that it is caused by purely genetic difference [10]. The association of an urbanized setting with high myopia rates is likely to be influenced by possible modifiable risk factors such as near work and outdoor time.

Despite the relatively low prevalence in the general population, pathologic myopia (PM) is a major cause of blindness or visual impairment in both Asian and Western populations. One study has shown that the prevalence of PM was 28.7% among high myopes and 65% of those with HM and were over 70 years old had PM [11]. Based on the global prediction of HM on 2050, PM may increase to over 200 million in future [9]. Treatment strategies against PM have not been effective [12].

Generational differences in prevalence are seen with the highest rates in young adults (myopia 65.5–96.5% and HM 6.8–21.6%) and the lowest rates in older adults (myopia 25.0–40.0% and HM 2.4–8.2%). The disease progression pattern of HM and subsequent development of PM may be different between young adults and older adults due to generational differences, or changes in the lifestyle factors such as the education system, near work, and outdoor time exposure in rapidly developing urban Asian countries.

1.2 Pathogenesis of Myopia

Ocular Biometric Changes in Human Myopia The axial length of the eye or, more precisely, the vitreous chamber depth is the primary individual biometric contributor to refractive error in children, young adults, and the elderly [13–15], with the vitreous chamber depth accounting for over 50% of the observed variation in spherical equivalent refractive error (SER), followed by the cornea (~15%) and crystalline lens (~1%) [15]. However, the dimensions, curvature, and refractive index of each individual ocular structure contribute to the final refractive state. The choroid is typically thinner in myopic compared to non-myopic eyes (most pronounced at the fovea [16, 17]) and thins with increasing myopia and axial length in both adults [18–25] and children [26–28]. Significant choroidal thinning is also observed in eyes with posterior staphyloma [29], and has been associated with the presence of lacquer cracks [30], choroidal neovascularization [31], and reduced visual acuity [32]. The choroid also appears to be a biomarker of ocular processes regulating eye growth given that the central macular choroid thins during the initial development and progression of myopia [33–35] and thickens in response to imposed peripheral myopic retinal image defocus [36, 37], topical anti-muscarinic agents [38, 39], and increased light exposure [40]; clinical interventions associated with a slowing of eye growth in children.

Visual Environment, Emmetropization, and Myopia Much of the knowledge on vision-dependent changes in ocular growth has emanated from animal experiments in which either the quality of image formed on the retina is degraded (known as form deprivation [FD]), or the focal point of the image is altered with respect to the retinal plane (known as lens defocus). Both FD and lens defocus result in abnormal eye growth and development of refractive errors.

Monochromatic Higher-Order Aberrations as a Myopigenic Stimulus Myopia may develop due to the eye's emmetropization response to inherent ocular aberrations that degrade retinal image quality and trigger axial elongation [41]. Evidence concerning the relationship between higher order abberation (HOAs) during distance viewing and refractive error from cross-sectional studies is conflicting [41, 42]. However, during or following near-work tasks, adult myopic eyes tend to display a transient increase in corneal and total ocular HOAs, suggesting a potential role for near-work-induced retinal image degradation in myopia development [43, 44]. Longitudinal studies of myopic children also indicate that eyes with greater positive spherical aberration demonstrate slower eye growth [45, 46].

Accommodation Given the association between near work and the development and progression of childhood myopia [47], numerous studies have compared various characteristics of accommodation between refractive error groups. Typically, this involves the accuracy of the accommodation response, since lag of accommodation (hyperopic retinal defocus) may stimulate axial elongation as observed in some animal models. The slowing of myopia progression during childhood with progressive addition or bifocal lenses, designed to improve accommodation accuracy and minimize lag of accommodation, adds some weight to the role of accommodation in myopia development and progression [48, 49]. However, the exact underlying mechanism of myopia control with such lenses may be related to imposed peripheral retinal defocus or a reduction in the near vergence demand [50]. Certainly, elevations in measured lag observed in myopes arise after rather than before onset [51].

1.3 Key Environmental Factors on Myopia

Near work and education: Many studies have established a strong link between myopia and education [52–57]. Moreover, Mountjoy et al. have shown that exposure to longer duration of education was a causal risk factor for myopia [53]. The exact mechanism linking increased education with myopia is unclear. Although it is possible that optical [43, 58] or biomechanical [59, 60] ocular changes associated with near work could potentially promote myopic eye growth in those with higher levels of education (and hence near-work demands), population studies examining the link between near-work activities and myopia have been conflicting, with some studies suggesting an association between near work and myopia [47, 61], and others indicating no significant effects [62]. The relatively inconsistent findings linking near work with myopia development suggests a potential role for other factors in the association between education and myopia.

Outdoor Activity A number of recent studies report that the time children spend engaged in outdoor activities is negatively associated with their risk of myopia [62–68]. Both cross-sectional and longitudinal studies indicate that greater time spent outdoors is associated with a significantly lower myopia prevalence and reduced risk of myopia onset in childhood. Although some studies report significant associations between myopia progression and outdoor activity [66, 68], this is not a consistent finding across all longitudinal studies [69]. A recent meta-analysis of studies examining the relationship between outdoor time and myopia indicated that there was a 2% reduction in the odds of having myopia for each additional hour per week spent outdoors [70].

Duration of Outdoor Activity and Myopia In a large longitudinal study, Jones and colleagues [62] reported that children who engaged in outdoor activities for 14 h per week or more exhibited the lowest odds of developing myopia. A number of recent randomized controlled trials have reported that interventions that increase children's outdoor time (by 40–80 min a day) significantly reduce the onset of myopia in childhood [71–73]. In the "Role of outdoor activity in myopia study" [74], children who were habitually exposed to low ambient light levels (on average less than 60 min exposure to outdoor light per day) had significantly faster axial eye growth compared to children habitually exposed to moderate and high light. These findings from human studies suggest that children who are exposed to less than 60 min a day of bright outdoor light are at an increased risk of more rapid eye growth and myopia development, and that approximately 2 h or more of outdoor exposure each day is required to provide protection against myopia development in the human eye.

1.4 Genetics of Myopia

Myopia is highly heritable; genes explain up to 80% of the variance in refractive error in twin studies. For the last decade, genome-wide association study (GWAS) approaches have revealed that myopia is a complex trait, with many genetic variants of small effect influencing retinal signaling, eye growth, and the normal process of emmetropization. Particularly notable are genes encoding extracellular matrix-related proteins (COL1A1, COL2A1 [75, 76], and MMP1, MMP2, MMP3, MMP9, MMP10 [77, 78]). For candidates such as PAX6 and TGFB1, the results were replicated in multiple independent extreme/high myopia studies and validated in a large GWAS meta-analysis in 2018, respectively [79, 80]. However, the genetic architecture and its molecular mechanisms are still to be clarified, and while genetic risk score prediction models are improving, this knowledge must be expanded to have impact on clinical practice.

Gene–environment (GxE) interaction analysis has focused primarily on education. An early study in North American samples examined GxE for myopia and the matrix metalloproteinases genes (MMP1–MMP10): a subset of single nucleotide polymorphism (SNPs) was only associated with refraction in the lower education level [78, 81]. A subsequent study in five Singapore cohorts found variants in DNAH9, GJD2, and ZMAT4, which had a larger effect on myopia in a high education subset [82]. Subsequent efforts to examine GxE considered the aggregate effects of many SNPs together. A study in Europeans found that a genetic risk score comprising 26 genetic variants was most strongly associated with myopia in individuals with a university level education [83]. A study examining GxE in children considered near work and time outdoors in association with 39 SNPs and found weak evidence for an interaction with near work [83, 84]. Finally, a Consortium for Refractive Error and Myopia (CREAM) study was able to identify additional myopia risk loci by allowing for a GxE approach [85].

Mendelian randomization (MR) offers a better assessment of causality than that available from observational studies [86, 87]. Two MR studies found a causal effect of education on the development of myopia [53, 80]. Both found a larger effect through MR than that estimated from observational studies suggesting that confounding in observational studies may have been obscuring the true relationship [55, 79]. As expected, there was little evidence of myopia affecting education (−0.008 years/diopter, $P = 0.6$). Another study focused on the causality of low vitamin D on myopia found only a small estimated effect on refractive error [88] suggesting that previous observational findings were likely confounded by the effects of time spent outdoors.

Due to the high polygenicity of myopia and low explained phenotypic variance by genetic factors (7.8%), clinical applications derived from genetic analyses of myopia are currently limited. Risk predictions for myopia in children are based on family history, education level of the parents, the amount of outdoor exposure, and the easily measurable refractive error and axial length. Currently, we are able to make a distinction between high myopes and high hyperopes based on the polygenic risk scores derived from CREAM studies: persons in the highest decile for the polygenic risk score had a 40-fold greater risk of myopia relative to those in the lowest decile. A prediction model, including age, sex, and polygenic risk score, achieved an area under curve (AUC) of 0.77 (95% CI = 0.75–0.79) for myopia versus hyperopia in adults (Rotterdam Study I–III) [80]. To date, one study has assessed both environmental and genetic factors together and showed that modeling both genes and environment improved prediction accuracy [89].

1.5 Prevention of the Onset of Myopia

The vast majority of literature suggests that most cases of myopia develop during the school-going age in children. After the age of 6 years, the prevalence of myopia starts to rise [90–94]. The highest annual incidence of myopia is reported among school children from urban mainland China [92] and Taiwan [95], ranging from 20% to 30% through ages 7–14 years, with earlier onset of myopia also being identified [94]. A study in Japan showed that while the prevalence of myopia has been increasing from 1984 to 1996, the prevalence among children aged 6 or younger has remained unchanged. This suggests that the majority of increased myopia onset is secondary to increased educational intensity [94].

Rates of progression increase dramatically with the year of onset and this has been suggested by spherical equivalent refraction and axial length [96]. Myopic refractions tend to stabilize in late adolescent but can remain progressive until adulthood. The mean age at myopia stabilization is 15.6 years but this can vary among children of different ethnicities [97].

Several factors have been found to be associated with the development of incident myopia in school. Asian ethnicity [93, 98], parental history of myopia [62, 99], reduced time outdoors [62], and level of near-work activity [47, 100] are risk factors for incident myopia, although the evidence can be seen as controversial in some instances.

Evidence of time spent outdoors as a risk factor for myopia progression was first presented in a 3-year follow-up study of myopia in school children, showing that those who spent more time outdoors were less likely to progress [64]. Consistent results were reported in various studies, such as the Sydney Myopia Study, Orinda Study, as well as the Singapore Cohort Study of Risk Factors for Myopia [63, 65, 101]. This led to the commencement of several clinical trials which confirmed the protective effect and indicated a dose-dependent effect, among them, the randomized clinical trial in Guangzhou which reported that an additional 40 min of outdoor activity can reduce the incidence of myopia by 23% [63]. Additionally, the trial in Taiwan suggested that an extra 80 min may further reduce incidence by 50% [72, 73].

Near-work activity as a risk factor for myopia has not been entirely consistent. A meta-analysis reported a modest, but statistically significant, association between time spent performing near work and myopia (odds ratio, 1.14) [47]. Core techniques to implementing interventions of near-work activities include effective measures of near-work-related parameters, real-time data analyses, and alert systems. Wearable devices that possess these techniques have emerged in the last decade.

It has been estimated that without any effective controls or interventions the proportion of myopes in the population will reach up to 50% and 10% for high myopes by 2050 [9]. Approaches that have produced a reduction of at least 50% in incidence, such as time outdoors, lead to delayed onset and have the potential to make a significant difference on the impending myopia epidemic.

Another critical issue is the need to balance educational achievement and interventions to prevent myopia progression in East Asia. This balance can be seen in Australia [102], with not only some of the highest educational ranks in the world but also high levels of outdoor activity and light intensity. Preventing the onset of myopia is certainly challenging in the East Asian population and requires a collaborative effort among clinics, schools, parents, and the entire society.

1.6 Understanding Pathologic Myopia

Pathologic myopia (PM) is a major cause of blindness in the world, especially in East Asian countries [103–107]. The cause of blindness in patients with PM includes myopic maculopathy with or without posterior staphyloma, myopic macular retinoschisis, and glaucoma or glaucoma-like optic neuropathy. The term "pathologic myopia" describes the situation of pathologic consequences of a myopic axial elongation. According to a recent consensus article by Ohno-Matsui et al. [108], pathologic myopia was defined by a myopic chorioretinal atrophy equal to or more serious than diffuse atrophy (by Meta-analysis for pathologic myopia (META-PM) study group classification [109]) and/or the presence of posterior staphylomas.

A posterior staphyloma is an outpouching of a circumscribed area of the posterior fundus, where the radius of curvature is less than the curvature radius of the surrounding eye wall [110], and can be associated with, or lead to, vision-threatening complications such as myopic maculopathy [109, 111–114] and myopic optic neuropathy/glaucoma [115, 116]. Based upon and modifying Curtin's [117] classical categorization of posterior staphylomas, with types I–V as primary staphylomas and types VI–X as compound staphylomas, Ohno-Matsui [118] used 3D-magnetic resonance imaging (3D-MRI) and wide-field fundus imaging to re-classify staphylomas into six types: wide macular, narrow macular, peripapillary, nasal, inferior, and others.

In the META-PM classification [109], myopic maculopathy lesions have been categorized into five categories from "no myopic retinal lesions" (category 0), "tessellated fundus only" (category 1), "diffuse chorioretinal atrophy" (category 2), "patchy chorioretinal atrophy" (category 3), to "macular atrophy" (category 4). These categories were defined based on long-term clinical observations that showed the progression patterns and associated factors of the development of myopic choroidal neovascularization (CNV) for each stage. Three additional features were added to these categories and were included as "plus signs": (1) lacquer cracks, (2) fuch spot and (3) myopic CNV.

Myopic CNV is a major sight-threatening complication of pathologic myopia. It is the most common cause of CNV in individuals younger than 50 years, and it is the second most common cause of CNV overall [119, 120]. Anti-vascular endothelial growth factor (anti-VEGF) therapy is the first-line treatment for myopic CNV, as shown by the RADIANCE study [121] and the MYRROR study [122].

Panozzo and Mercanti proposed the term "myopic traction maculopathy (MTM)" to encompass various findings characterized by a traction as visualized by optical coherence tomography (OCT) in highly myopic eyes [123]. A dome-shaped macula (DSM) is an inward protrusion of the macula as visualized by OCT [124–126]. Imamura, Spaide, and coworkers reported that a DSM was associated with, and caused by, a local thickening of the subfoveal sclera [127]. It was postulated that the local thickening of the subfoveal sclera was an adaptive or compensatory response to the defocus of the image on the fovea in highly myopic eyes.

1.7 Imaging in Myopia

Imaging the myopic eye can be challenging due to various structural changes (abnormal eye elongation, scleral and corneal curvature irregularities, cataracts leading to poor clarity; or retinal thinning causing abnormal projections of the final image [128, 129]).

Optic disc imaging can also be used to predict the development of glaucoma, where visualization of myopic tilting of the optic disc with peripapillary atrophy (PPA) and pitting of the optic disc [130] is a possible predisposing factor [131, 132]. Serial imaging investigative measures can therefore be utilized for monitoring the development of open-angle, normal-tension glaucoma [133]. Features such as optic disc tilt, PPA, and abnormally large or small optic discs are the earliest known structural alterations that potentially predict the development of pathological myopia and can be observed even in young highly myopic adults. Unfortunately, these features (some also with associations to glaucoma) also interfere with the visualization of optic disc margins [134, 135] and are also not easy to discern in highly myopic eyes [136]. There is also added difficulty in eyes with myopic maculopathy, where visual field defects result in further interference [137]. As such, the answer to these challenges may lie in imaging deep optic nerve head structures (such as parapapillary sclera, scleral wall, and lamina cribosa) [138] in highly myopic eyes for more precise diagnoses of glaucoma.

The ability to view distinct retinal layers with OCT has enhanced visualization of myopic traction maculopathy (MTM). Examples of features that can be seen include inner or outer retinal schisis, foveal detachment, lamellar or full-thickness macular hole, and/or macular detachment [139, 140]. Non-stereoscopic fundus photographs are inadequate for detailed studies of posterior staphylomas as the change in contour at the staphyloma edge is not always discernible. The OCT overcomes this limitation because of its excellent depth resolution [141, 142].

The OCT itself has its shortcomings; the sclera cannot be visualized using the OCT. These limitations also extend to the use of OCT angiography (OCTA). There is currently no standard protocol for segmentation; the outcome parameters for OCTA have not been clearly defined either. Although some authors have tried to use analysis of flow voids or signal voids in the choriocapillaris to quantify the area taken up by the microvasculature [143, 144], the data pertaining to myopic patients are but insufficient [145]. Looking into the future, there is, however, incipient research suggesting that the comprehension of blood supply and changes in vasculature from the anterior to the posterior segment of the myopic eye is crucial to the understanding of the disease [146–149].

Photoacoustic imaging has shown promise recently to fill the gaps between OCT and ultrasound in terms of penetration depth [150]. This modality has been used before to image the posterior pole of the eye in vitro and in animal models *in vivo*. This can also be used in concurrence with angiography, measuring oxygen saturation and pigment imaging [151]. However, there are some limitations pertaining to this modality notwithstanding moderate depth resolution, pure optical absorption sensing, need for contact detection with ultrasound sensor, and a relatively long acquisition time. In view of these limitations, we are yet to receive tangible results from photoacoustic imaging for posterior pole imaging in humans.

1.8 Glaucoma in Myopia

Axial myopization leads to marked changes of the optic nerve head: (1) an enlargement of all three layers of the optic disc (i.e., optic disc Bruch's membrane opening, optic disc choroidal opening, optic disc scleral opening) with the development of a secondary macrodisc, (2) an enlargement and shallowing of the cup, (3) an elongation and thinning of the lamina cribrosa with a secondary reduction in the distance between the intraocular space with the intraocular pressure (IOP) and the retro-lamina compartment with the orbital cerebrospinal fluid pressure, (4) a direct exposure of the peripheral posterior lamina cribrosa surface to the orbital cerebrospinal fluid space, (5) an elongation and thinning of the peripapillary scleral flange with development and enlargement of the parapapillary gamma zone and delta zone, (6) an elongation and thinning of the peripapillary border tissue of the choroid, and (7) a rotation of the optic disc around the vertical axis, and less often and to a minor degree around the horizontal axis und the sagittal axis. These changes make it more difficult to differentiate between myopic changes and (additional) glaucoma-associated changes such as a loss of neuroretinal rim and thinning of the retinal nerve fiber layer, and these changes may make the optic nerve head more vulnerable, potentially explaining the increased prevalence of glaucomatous optic neuropathy in highly myopic eyes.

Population-based investigations and hospital-based studies have shown that the prevalence of glaucomatous optic neuropathy (GON) was higher in highly myopic eyes than in emmetropic eyes [152–166]. A previous study revealed that at a given IOP in patients with chronic open-angle glaucoma, the amount of optic nerve damage was more marked in highly myopic eyes with large optic discs than in non-highly myopic eyes [165].

Highly myopic glaucomatous eyes as compared with non-highly myopic glaucomatous eyes may have a markedly lower IOP threshold to develop optic nerve damage. It could indicate that an IOP of perhaps lower than 10 mmHg might be necessary to prevent the development of GON in these highly myopic eyes, and that in highly myopic eyes with axial elongation-associated enlargement and stretching of the optic disc and parapapillary region as the main risk factors for GON in high myopia a normal IOP may be sufficient to lead to GON [136].

Although it has not yet been firmly proven that GON in high myopia is dependent on IOP, most researchers recommend lowering IOP in highly myopic patients with glaucoma. Based on the morphological findings described above, the target pressure in highly myopic glaucoma may be lower than in non-highly myopic glaucoma. Due to the peculiar anatomy of the optic nerve head in highly myopic eyes, most diagnostic procedures fail in precisely assessing the status of the optic nerve in highly myopic eyes with glaucoma. It includes factors such as a decreased spatial and color contrast between the neuroretinal rim and the optic cup making a delineation of both structures more difficult; a peripapillary retinoschisis leading to an incorrect segmentation of the retinal nerve fiber layer upon optical coherence tomography; a large gamma zone (and delta zone) which makes using the end of Bruch's membrane as reference point for the measurement of the neuroretinal rim useless; and macular Bruch's membrane defects and other reasons for non-glaucomatous visual field defects which reduces the diagnostic precision of perimetry for the detection of presence and progression of GON.

1.9 Management of Myopic Choroidal Neovascularization

Myopic choroidal neovascularization (myopic CNV) is the second most common cause of CNV after age-related macular degeneration (AMD) [167, 168]. It is one of the most sight-threatening complications of pathological myopia [119, 169] and is the most common cause of CNV in those 50 years or younger [167], with significant social and economic burden. The prevalence of myopic CNV is between 5.2% and 11.3% in individuals with pathological myopia [12], with female preponderance seen in most studies [167–170]. The long-term outcome of CNV is poor if left untreated. In a 10-year follow-up study of 25 patients with myopic CNV, visual acuity deteriorated to 20/200 or worse in 89% and 96% of eyes in 5 years and 10 years, respectively [168].

On slit-lamp biomicroscopy, myopic CNV manifests as a small, flat, grayish subretinal lesion adjacent to or beneath the fovea [109, 168, 169, 171]. On SD-OCT, myopic CNV presents as a hyper-reflective material above the retinal pigment epithelium band (type 2 CNV), with variable amount of subretinal fluid. Clinical diagnosis is confirmed by fundus fluorescein angiography (FFA). Most myopic CNVs are type 2 neovascularization and present with a "classic" pattern on FA. OCT angiography (OCTA) was able to detect flow within myopic CNV vascular complexes and hence delineate vascular networks in these myopic neovascular membranes that lie above the retinal pigment epithelium (RPE) where flow signals are spared from attenuation [172].

Prior to the advent of anti-VEGF therapy, the main treatment options for myopic CNV were limited to thermal laser photocoagulation [173], photodynamic therapy with verteporfin (vPDT) [174, 175]. These treatments had limited efficacy in improving vision significantly and have now largely been relegated to the annals of history by anti-vascular endothelial growth factor (anti-VEGF) therapy [176]. Once active myopic CNV is diagnosed, prompt treatment with intravitreal anti-VEGF therapy should be administered as soon as possible [121, 177]. Current evidence suggests a pro-re-nata (PRN) regimen without a loading phase can be considered in most patients. Patients should be monitored monthly with OCT and treatment administered until cessation of disease activity on OCT or visual stabilization.

1.10 Management of Myopia-Related Retinal Complications

Myopic traction maculopathy (MTM) [123] is estimated to occur in approximately 8–34% in individuals with high myopia [178–180] and encompasses retinal thickening, macular retinoschisis, foveal detachment, lamellar macular hole with or without epiretinal membrane and/or vitreomacular traction [123], and/or full-thickness macular hole (HM) with or without retinal detachment. Central to the pathogenesis of MTM is traction, which was postulated to arise from one or more of the following mechanisms [181]: vitreomacular traction associated with perifoveal posterior vitreous detachment (PVD) [182–184]; relative incompliance of the internal limiting membrane (ILM) [185–189], epiretinal membrane (ERM) [180, 182, 190–192], and cortical vitreous remnant after PVD [193] to the outer retina which conforms to the shape of the posterior staphyloma; and traction exerted by retinal arterioles [188, 194, 195]. Not all patients with MTM require interventions [184, 196, 197]. There are numerous reported interventions for MTM. The principles of the treatment are: (1) to relieve traction, mainly achieved through pars plana vitrectomy (PPV) with or without ILM peeling; (2) to minimize surgical damage to the weakened macula through technique modifications in order to prevent the formation of postoperative MH; and (3) in the presence of full-thickness MH, to maximize the chance of hole closure through the use of various surgical adjuncts.

1.10.1 Proposed Adjuncts to Improve Outcome of Macular Hole Surgery

Inverted Internal Limiting Membrane Flap This technique involves leaving a hinge of ILM flap at the edge of MH during ILM peeling. This ILM flap is then inverted upside-down to cover or fill the MH [198].

Autologous Internal Limiting Membrane Transplantation In eyes where ILM around the macula hole has already been removed, an appropriately sized ILM can be peeled off from a distant site and placed as a free flap onto the persistent MH [199, 200].

Autologous Blood In order to prevent subretinal migration of dye and the resultant retinal toxicity associated with vital stains, it was proposed to use autologous blood to cover the MH before injection of brilliant blue dye. It has been demonstrated that compared to conventional method, the use of pre-staining autologous blood led to better visual acuity outcomes and continuity of ellipsoid zone at all post-operative time points [201].

Lens Capsular Flap Transplantation Chen et al. demonstrated a 100% MH closure rate with anterior capsular transplantation among patients with refractory MH,

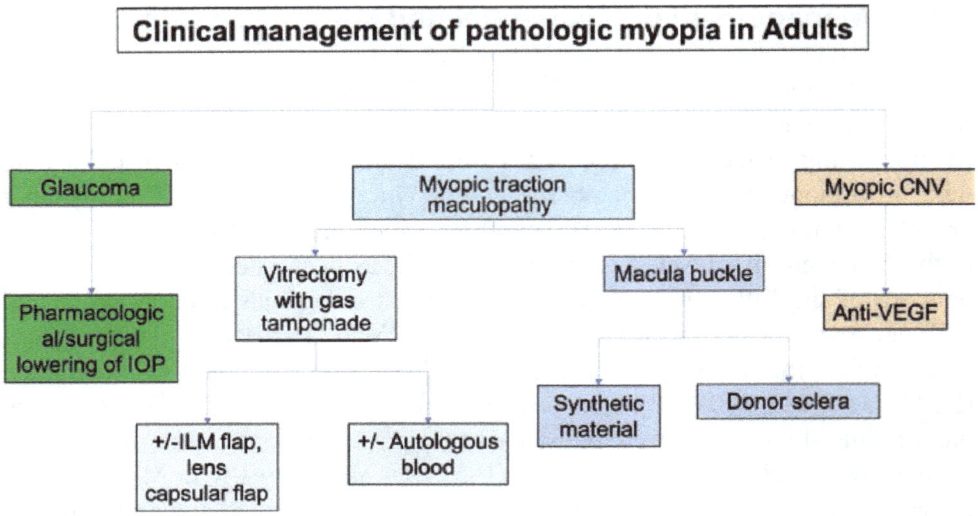

Fig. 1.1 Summary of the clinical management of pathologic myopia in adults

whereas the complete closure rate of MH after posterior capsular transplantation was only 50% and with another 30% enjoyed partial MH closure [202].

Macular Buckle Macular buckles have been used to shorten the axial length of myopic eyeballs in conditions such as macular hole retinal detachment (MHRD), myopic foveoschisis with or without foveal detachment, and MH with foveoschisis. There are many types of macular buckle, including scleral sponge, T-shaped or L-shaped buckle, Ando Plombe, wire-strengthened sponge exoplant, and even donor sclera and suprachoroidal injectable long-acting hyaluronic acid [203].

Autologous Neurosensory Retinal Transplantation The technique involves bimanually harvesting a free flap of neurosensory retina superior to the superotemporal arcade, with the harvest site first secured by endolaser barricade and endodiathermy. The free flap was translocated in its correct orientation over the macular hole and perfluoro-*n*-octane heavy liquid (PFC) was instilled over it, followed by direct PFC–silicone oil exchange [204].

Figure 1.1 presents an overview of the management of myopia-related complications in adults.

1.11 Management and Control of Myopia in Children

Currently, there are many types of interventions to slow myopia progression in children, including spectacle lenses, contact lenses, pharmaceuticals, and environmental or behavioral modification. However, none of these myopia control methods have been proven to stop the development or progression of myopia completely and each method has their own limitations.

Spectacle Lenses Under-correction of myopia in clinical trials has shown conflicting results and small, clinically insignificant effect on slowing myopia progression [205–207]. In view of these conflicting results, there is no convincing evidence to indicate that under-correction should be used to slow myopia progression.

Bifocal or Multifocal Spectacles Most studies showed that progressive addition lenses (PALs) have an insignificant effect on slowing myopia progression rate (less than 0.2 D per year) overall [48, 208–214]. In contrast, a randomized, controlled trial showed that executive bifocal lenses slowed myopia progression in Chinese-Canadian children aged 8–13 years by 39% and up to 51% with base-in prisms incorporated over 3 years [215]. More recently, the Defocus Incorporated Multiple Segments (DIMS) spectacle lens enabled clear vision and myopic defocus simultaneously for the wearer [216]. Hong Kong Chinese children aged 8–13 years wearing DIMS lenses had approximately 60% less myopia progression and axial elongation when compared with children wearing single vision spectacle lenses over 2 years. Moreover, about 20% of the DIMS lens wearers had no myopia progression during the study period.

Peripheral Myopic Defocus Glasses In 2010, Sankaridurg et al. published their results of three novel peripheral defocus spectacle lens. Unfortunately, there was no significant effect on myopic progression with all three designs [217]. In a recent randomized controlled trial (RCT) conducted in Japanese children with peripheral defocus lenses, no difference in myopia reduction was found [218].

Rigid Gas Permeable Contact Lenses Two randomized clinical trials [219, 220] showed that rigid gas permeable (RGP) contact lenses did not retard axial eye growth. However, Walline et al. [219] reported significant slower myopia progression in the group of RGP lenses compared with soft contact lenses, despite that no differences were found in axial elongation between the groups. The proposed reason for a treatment effect on refraction may be due to the changes in corneal curvature.

Orthokeratology Orthokeratology (Ortho-K) lenses are specially designed RGP contact lenses that are worn overnight to reshape the cornea and thereby temporarily correct low-to-moderate myopia. Various clinical studies have demonstrated the effectiveness of inhibiting myopic progression with Ortho-K. Individual studies and meta-analyses have shown a 32–63% reduction in the rate of axial elongation in East Asian children initially aged from 7 to 16 years and followed for up to 5 years [221–227]. Efficacy may decrease over time [224, 228], with a potential "rebound" after discontinuation, especially in children under 14 years [229]. There is also a potential non-response rate of 7–12% [223]. Interestingly, a recent study in Japan [230] showed that the combination of Ortho-K and low-concentration atropine (0.01%) eyedrops was more effective in slowing axial elongation over 12 months than Ortho-K treatment alone in myopic children. The risk of infective keratitis remains [231].

Soft Bifocal and Multifocal Contact Lenses These lenses are worn during the daytime. Compared to spectacles, contact lenses are more cosmetically acceptable, more easily handled, and are more convenient for daily activities of some children, especially during sports [232, 233]. For most of eye-care practitioners, the fitting procedures of soft bifocal contact lenses are relatively simpler than Ortho-K. Overall, soft bifocal and multifocal contact lenses slow the progression of myopia in children by an amount comparable to that of Ortho-K lenses. Studies exploring the effect of these bifocal soft contact lenses indicate slowing of myopia progression by 25–50% and axial length by 27–32% in children aged 8–16 of various ethnicities over a period of 24 months [234, 235].

Atropine The initial high doses of atropine (i.e., 0.5% or 1.0%) slowed myopia progression by more than 70% in Asian children aged 6–13 years over 1–2 years [229, 236–238]. However, lower doses (0.1% or less) can also slow refractive progression by 30–60% with less side effects (pupil dilation, glare, or blur) [238]. The Atropine Treatment of Myopia (ATOM) studies showed that there was a myopic rebound if atropine was stopped suddenly, especially at higher doses and in younger children [239, 240].

Time Spent Outdoors In the Sydney Myopia Study, exposure to more than 2 h of outdoor activity per day decreased the odds of myopia and countered the effects of near work [65]. Interventions involving increasing time outdoors appeared to reduce the onset of myopia and also its progression in myopic children [71]. A meta-analysis has suggested a 2% reduced odds of myopia per additional hour of time spent outdoors per week [70].

Environmental Interventions Based on new evidence, the advice has shifted from spending at least 2 h per day outdoors in addition to avoiding excessive near work. This has changed health and school messaging in many East Asian countries [71].

Higher Light Intensities and Dopamine Potential reasons why time outdoors may be protective include higher light intensities [241], differences in chromatic composition [242], the reduction in dioptric accommodative focus and psychometric influences encountered outdoors [243]. The role of chromaticity (red and blue) and ultraviolet (UV) light is still uncertain [244], while that of higher vitamin D levels has been debunked [88].

Figure 1.2 presents an overview of the management and prevention of myopia in children.

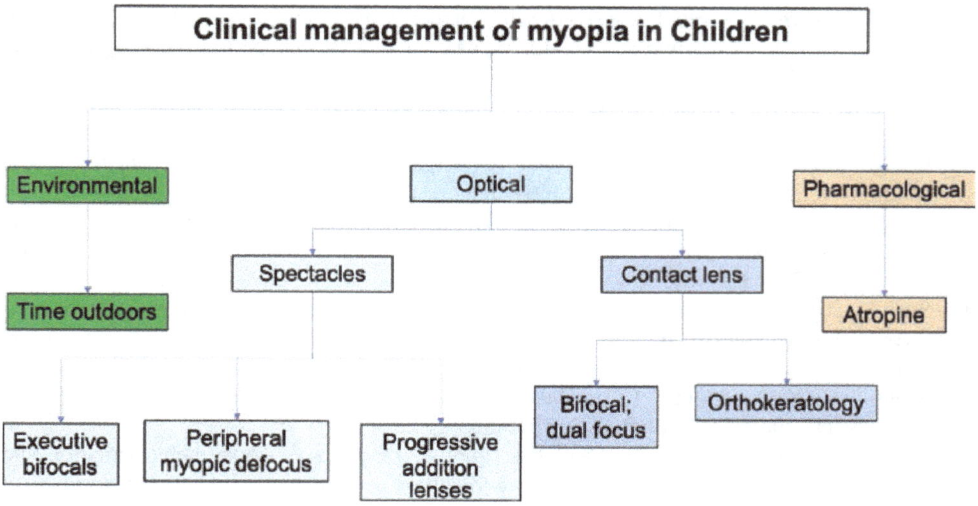

Fig. 1.2 Summary of the clinical management of myopia in children

References

1. Dolgin E. The myopia boom. Nature. 2015;519(7543):276–8.
2. Vitale S, Cotch MF, Sperduto RD. Prevalence of visual impairment in the United States. JAMA. 2006;295(18):2158–63.
3. Zheng YF, Pan CW, Chay J, Wong TY, Finkelstein E, Saw SM. The economic cost of myopia in adults aged over 40 years in Singapore. Invest Ophthalmol Vis Sci. 2013;54(12):7532–7.
4. Liang YB, Wong TY, Sun LP, et al. Refractive errors in a rural Chinese adult population the Handan eye study. Ophthalmology. 2009;116(11):2119–27.
5. Morgan IG, Ohno-Matsui K, Saw S-M. Myopia. Lancet. 2012;379(9827):1739–48.
6. Morgan IG. What public policies should be developed to deal with the epidemic of myopia? Optom Vis Sci. 2016;93(9):1058–60.
7. Lin LL, Shih YF, Hsiao CK, Chen CJ. Prevalence of myopia in Taiwanese school children: 1983 to 2000. Ann Acad Med Singap. 2004;33(1):27–33.
8. Jung SK, Lee JH, Kakizaki H, Jee D. Prevalence of myopia and its association with body stature and educational level in 19-year-old male conscripts in Seoul, South Korea. Invest Ophthalmol Vis Sci. 2012;53(9):5579–83.
9. Holden BA, Fricke TR, Wilson DA, et al. Global prevalence of myopia and high myopia and temporal trends from 2000 through 2050. Ophthalmology. 2016;123(5):1036–42.
10. Ding BY, Shih YF, Lin LLK, Hsiao CK, Wang IJ. Myopia among school children in East Asia and Singapore. Surv Ophthalmol. 2017;62(5):677–97.
11. Wong YL, Sabanayagam C, Ding Y, et al. Prevalence, risk factors, and impact of myopic macular degeneration on visual impairment and functioning among adults in Singapore. Invest Ophthalmol Vis Sci. 2018;59(11):4603–13.

12. Wong TY, Ferreira A, Hughes R, Carter G, Mitchell P. Epidemiology and disease burden of pathologic myopia and myopic choroidal neovascularization: an evidence-based systematic review. Am J Ophthalmol. 2014;157(1):9–25 e12.
13. Xie R, Zhou XT, Lu F, et al. Correlation between myopia and major biometric parameters of the eye: a retrospective clinical study. Optom Vis Sci. 2009;86(5):E503–8.
14. Li SM, Li SY, Kang MT, et al. Distribution of ocular biometry in 7- and 14-year-old Chinese children. Optom Vis Sci. 2015;92(5):566–72.
15. Richter GM, Wang M, Jiang X, et al. Ocular determinants of refractive error and its age- and sex-related variations in the Chinese American eye study. JAMA Ophthalmol. 2017;135(7):724–32.
16. Read SA, Collins MJ, Vincent SJ, Alonso-Caneiro D. Choroidal thickness in myopic and non-myopic children assessed with enhanced depth imaging optical coherence tomography. Invest Ophthalmol Vis Sci. 2013;54(12):7578–86.
17. Xiong S, He X, Deng J, et al. Choroidal thickness in 3001 Chinese children aged 6 to 19 years using swept-source OCT. Sci Rep. 2017;7:45059.
18. Chen FK, Yeoh J, Rahman W, Patel PJ, Tufail A, Da Cruz L. Topographic variation and interocular symmetry of macular choroidal thickness using enhanced depth imaging optical coherence tomography. Invest Ophthalmol Vis Sci. 2012;53(2):975–85.
19. Esmaeelpour M, Povazay B, Hermann B, et al. Three-dimensional 1060-nm OCT: choroidal thickness maps in normal subjects and improved posterior segment visualization in cataract patients. Invest Ophthalmol Vis Sci. 2010;51(10):5260–6.
20. Gupta P, Jing T, Marziliano P, et al. Distribution and determinants of choroidal thickness and volume using automated segmentation software in a population-based study. Am J Ophthalmol. 2015;159(2):293–301.e293.
21. Li XQ, Munkholm A, Larsen M, Munch IC. Choroidal thickness in relation to birth parameters in 11- to 12-year-old children: the Copenhagen child cohort 2000 eye study. Invest Ophthalmol Vis Sci. 2014;56(1):617–24.
22. Ouyang Y, Heussen FM, Mokwa N, et al. Spatial distribution of posterior pole choroidal thickness by spectral domain optical coherence tomography. Invest Ophthalmol Vis Sci. 2011;52(9):7019–26.
23. Tan CS, Cheong KX. Macular choroidal thicknesses in healthy adults--relationship with ocular and demographic factors. Invest Ophthalmol Vis Sci. 2014;55(10):6452–8.
24. Wei WB, Xu L, Jonas JB, et al. Subfoveal choroidal thickness: the Beijing eye study. Ophthalmology. 2013;120(1):175–80.
25. Sanchez-Cano A, Orduna E, Segura F, et al. Choroidal thickness and volume in healthy young white adults and the relationships between them and axial length, ammetropy and sex. Am J Ophthalmol. 2014;158(3):574–583.e571.
26. He X, Jin P, Zou H, et al. Choroidal thickness in healthy Chinese children aged 6 to 12: the Shanghai children eye study. Retina. 2017;37(2):368–75.
27. Jin P, Zou H, Zhu J, et al. Choroidal and retinal thickness in children with different refractive status measured by swept-source optical coherence tomography. Am J Ophthalmol. 2016;168:164–76.
28. Zhang JM, Wu JF, Chen JH, et al. Macular choroidal thickness in children: the Shandong children eye study. Invest Ophthalmol Vis Sci. 2015;56(13):7646–52.
29. Zhou LX, Shao L, Xu L, Wei WB, Wang YX, You QS. The relationship between scleral staphyloma and choroidal thinning in highly myopic eyes: the Beijing eye study. Sci Rep. 2017;7(1):9825.
30. Wang NK, Lai CC, Chou CL, et al. Choroidal thickness and biometric markers for the screening of lacquer cracks in patients with high myopia. PLoS One. 2013;8(1):e53660.
31. Ikuno Y, Jo Y, Hamasaki T, Tano Y. Ocular risk factors for choroidal neovascularization in pathologic myopia. Invest Ophthalmol Vis Sci. 2010;51(7):3721–5.
32. Nishida Y, Fujiwara T, Imamura Y, Lima LH, Kurosaka D, Spaide RF. Choroidal thickness and visual acuity in highly myopic eyes. Retina. 2012;32(7):1229–36.

33. Read SA, Alonso-Caneiro D, Vincent SJ, Collins MJ. Longitudinal changes in choroidal thickness and eye growth in childhood. Invest Ophthalmol Vis Sci. 2015;56(5):3103–12.
34. Fontaine M, Gaucher D, Sauer A, Speeg-Schatz C. Choroidal thickness and ametropia in children: a longitudinal study. Eur J Ophthalmol. 2017;27:730–4.
35. Jin P, Zou H, Xu X, et al. Longitudinal changes in choroidal and retinal thicknesses in children with myopic shift. Retina. 2018. https://doi.org/10.1097/IAE.0000000000002090.
36. Chen Z, Xue F, Zhou J, Qu X, Zhou X. Effects of orthokeratology on choroidal thickness and axial length. Optom Vis Sci. 2016;93(9):1064–71.
37. Li Z, Cui D, Hu Y, Ao S, Zeng J, Yang X. Choroidal thickness and axial length changes in myopic children treated with orthokeratology. Cont Lens Anterior Eye. 2017;40(6): 417–23.
38. Sander BP, Collins MJ, Read SA. The effect of topical adrenergic and anticholinergic agents on the choroidal thickness of young healthy adults. Exp Eye Res. 2014;128:181–9.
39. Zhang Z, Zhou Y, Xie Z, et al. The effect of topical atropine on the choroidal thickness of healthy children. Sci Rep. 2016;6:34936.
40. Read SA. Ocular and environmental factors associated with eye growth in childhood. Optom Vis Sci. 2016;93(9):1031–41.
41. Charman WN. Aberrations and myopia. Ophthalmic Physiol Opt. 2005;25(4):285–301.
42. Little JA, McCullough SJ, Breslin KM, Saunders KJ. Higher order ocular aberrations and their relation to refractive error and ocular biometry in children. Invest Ophthalmol Vis Sci. 2014;55(8):4791–800.
43. Buehren T, Collins MJ, Carney LG. Near work induced wavefront aberrations in myopia. Vis Res. 2005;45(10):1297–312.
44. Vincent SJ, Collins MJ, Read SA, Carney LG, Yap MK. Corneal changes following near work in myopic anisometropia. Ophthalmic Physiol Opt. 2013;33(1):15–25.
45. Lau JK, Vincent SJ, Collins MJ, Cheung SW, Cho P. Ocular higher-order aberrations and axial eye growth in young Hong Kong children. Sci Rep. 2018;8(1):6726.
46. Hiraoka T, Kotsuka J, Kakita T, Okamoto F, Oshika T. Relationship between higher-order wavefront aberrations and natural progression of myopia in schoolchildren. Sci Rep. 2017;7(1):7876.
47. Huang HM, Chang DS, Wu PC. The association between near work activities and myopia in children-a systematic review and meta-analysis. PLoS One. 2015;10(10):e0140419.
48. Gwiazda J, Hyman L, Hussein M, et al. A randomized clinical trial of progressive addition lenses versus single vision lenses on the progression of myopia in children. Invest Ophthalmol Vis Sci. 2003;44(4):1492–500.
49. Cheng D, Schmid KL, Woo GC, Drobe B. Randomized trial of effect of bifocal and prismatic bifocal spectacles on myopic progression: two-year results. Arch Ophthalmol. 2010;128(1):12–9.
50. Berntsen DA, Barr CD, Mutti DO, Zadnik K. Peripheral defocus and myopia progression in myopic children randomly assigned to wear single vision and progressive addition lenses. Invest Ophthalmol Vis Sci. 2013;54(8):5761–70.
51. Mutti DO, Mitchell GL, Hayes JR, et al. Accommodative lag before and after the onset of myopia. Invest Ophthalmol Vis Sci. 2006;47(3):837–46.
52. Nickels S, Hopf S, Pfeiffer N, Schuster AK. Myopia is associated with education: results from NHANES 1999-2008. PLoS One. 2019;14(1):e0211196.
53. Mountjoy E, Davies NM, Plotnikov D, et al. Education and myopia: assessing the direction of causality by mendelian randomisation. BMJ. 2018;361:k2022.
54. Morgan IG, French AN, Ashby RS, et al. The epidemics of myopia: aetiology and prevention. Prog Retin Eye Res. 2018;62:134–49.
55. Cuellar-Partida G, Lu Y, Kho PF, et al. Assessing the genetic predisposition of education on myopia: a mendelian randomization study. Genet Epidemiol. 2016;40(1):66–72.
56. Williams KM, Bertelsen G, Cumberland P, et al. Increasing prevalence of myopia in Europe and the impact of education. Ophthalmology. 2015;122(7):1489–97.

57. Han SB, Jang J, Yang HK, Hwang JM, Park SK. Prevalence and risk factors of myopia in adult Korean population: Korea national health and nutrition examination survey 2013-2014 (KNHANES VI). PLoS One. 2019;14(1):e0211204.
58. Gwiazda J, Thorn F, Bauer J, Held R. Myopic children show insufficient accommodative response to blur. Invest Ophthalmol Vis Sci. 1993;34(3):690–4.
59. Read SA, Collins MJ, Woodman EC, Cheong SH. Axial length changes during accommodation in myopes and emmetropes. Optom Vis Sci. 2010;87(9):656–62.
60. Woodman-Pieterse EC, Read SA, Collins MJ, Alonso-Caneiro D. Regional changes in choroidal thickness associated with accommodation. Invest Ophthalmol Vis Sci. 2015;56(11):6414–22.
61. Hepsen IF, Evereklioglu C, Bayramlar H. The effect of reading and near-work on the development of myopia in emmetropic boys: a prospective, controlled, three-year follow-up study. Vis Res. 2001;41(19):2511–20.
62. Jones LA, Sinnott LT, Mutti DO, Mitchell GL, Moeschberger ML, Zadnik K. Parental history of myopia, sports and outdoor activities, and future myopia. Invest Ophthalmol Vis Sci. 2007;48(8):3524–32.
63. Mutti DO, Mitchell GL, Moeschberger ML, Jones LA, Zadnik K. Parental myopia, near work, school achievement, and children's refractive error. Invest Ophthalmol Vis Sci. 2002;43(12):3633–40.
64. Parssinen O, Lyyra AL. Myopia and myopic progression among school children: a three-year follow-up study. Invest Ophthalmol Vis Sci. 1993;34(9):2794–802.
65. Rose KA, Morgan IG, Ip J, et al. Outdoor activity reduces the prevalence of myopia in children. Ophthalmology. 2008;115(8):1279–85.
66. Guo Y, Liu LJ, Tang P, et al. Outdoor activity and myopia progression in 4-year follow-up of Chinese primary school children: The Beijing Children Eye Study. PLoS One. 2017;12(4):e0175921.
67. Guggenheim JA, Northstone K, McMahon G, et al. Time outdoors and physical activity as predictors of incident myopia in childhood: a prospective cohort study. Invest Ophthalmol Vis Sci. 2012;53(6):2856–65.
68. Parssinen O, Kauppinen M, Viljanen A. The progression of myopia from its onset at age 8-12 to adulthood and the influence of heredity and external factors on myopic progression. A 23-year follow-up study. Acta Ophthalmol. 2014;92(8):730–9.
69. Jones-Jordan LA, Sinnott LT, Cotter SA, et al. Time outdoors, visual activity, and myopia progression in juvenile-onset myopes. Invest Ophthalmol Vis Sci. 2012;53(11):7169–75.
70. Sherwin JC, Reacher MH, Keogh RH, Khawaja AP, Mackey DA, Foster PJ. The association between time spent outdoors and myopia in children and adolescents: a systematic review and meta-analysis. Ophthalmology. 2012;119(10):2141–51.
71. Wu PC, Chen CT, Lin KK, et al. Myopia prevention and outdoor light intensity in a school-based cluster randomized trial. Ophthalmology. 2018;125:1239–50.
72. He M, Xiang F, Zeng Y, et al. Effect of time spent outdoors at school on the development of myopia among children in China: a randomized clinical trial. JAMA. 2015;314(11):1142–8.
73. Wu PC, Tsai CL, Wu HL, Yang YH, Kuo HK. Outdoor activity during class recess reduces myopia onset and progression in school children. Ophthalmology. 2013;120(5):1080–5.
74. Read SA, Collins MJ, Vincent SJ. Light exposure and eye growth in childhood. Invest Ophthalmol Vis Sci. 2015;56(11):6779–87.
75. Metlapally R, Li YJ, Tran-Viet KN, et al. COL1A1 and COL2A1 genes and myopia susceptibility: evidence of association and suggestive linkage to the COL2A1 locus. Invest Ophthalmol Vis Sci. 2009;50(9):4080–6.
76. Mutti DO, Cooper ME, O'Brien S, et al. Candidate gene and locus analysis of myopia. Mol Vis. 2007;13:1012–9.
77. Hall NF, Gale CR, Ye S, Martyn CN. Myopia and polymorphisms in genes for matrix metalloproteinases. Invest Ophthalmol Vis Sci. 2009;50(6):2632–6.
78. Wojciechowski R, Yee SS, Simpson CL, Bailey-Wilson JE, Stambolian D. Matrix metalloproteinases and educational attainment in refractive error: evidence of gene-environment interactions in the age-related eye disease study. Ophthalmology. 2013;120(2):298–305.

79. Tang SM, Rong SS, Young AL, Tam PO, Pang CP, Chen LJ. PAX6 gene associated with high myopia: a meta-analysis. Optom Vis Sci. 2014;91(4):419–29.
80. Tedja MS, Wojciechowski R, Hysi PG, et al. Genome-wide association meta-analysis highlights light-induced signaling as a driver for refractive error. Nat Genet. 2018;50(6):834–48.
81. Wojciechowski R, Bailey-Wilson JE, Stambolian D. Association of matrix metalloproteinase gene polymorphisms with refractive error in Amish and Ashkenazi families. Invest Ophthalmol Vis Sci. 2010;51(10):4989–95.
82. Fan Q, Wojciechowski R, Kamran Ikram M, et al. Education influences the association between genetic variants and refractive error: a meta-analysis of five Singapore studies. Hum Mol Genet. 2014;23(2):546–54.
83. Verhoeven VJ, Buitendijk GH, Consortium for Refractive E, et al. Education influences the role of genetics in myopia. Eur J Epidemiol. 2013;28(12):973–80.
84. Fan Q, Guo X, Tideman JW, et al. Childhood gene-environment interactions and age-dependent effects of genetic variants associated with refractive error and myopia: The CREAM Consortium. Sci Rep. 2016;6:25853.
85. Fan Q, Verhoeven VJ, Wojciechowski R, et al. Meta-analysis of gene-environment-wide association scans accounting for education level identifies additional loci for refractive error. Nat Commun. 2016;7:11008.
86. Ebrahim S, Davey Smith G. Mendelian randomization: can genetic epidemiology help redress the failures of observational epidemiology? Hum Genet. 2008;123(1):15–33.
87. Smith GD, Ebrahim S. Mendelian randomization: prospects, potentials, and limitations. Int J Epidemiol. 2004;33(1):30–42.
88. Cuellar-Partida G, Williams KM, Yazar S, et al. Genetically low vitamin D concentrations and myopic refractive error: a Mendelian randomization study. Int J Epidemiol. 2017;46(6):1882–90.
89. Ghorbani Mojarrad N, Williams C, Guggenheim JA. A genetic risk score and number of myopic parents independently predict myopia. Ophthalmic Physiol Opt. 2018;38(5):492–502.
90. Zhao J, Mao J, Luo R, Li F, Munoz SR, Ellwein LB. The progression of refractive error in school-age children: Shunyi district, China. Am J Ophthalmol. 2002;134(5):735–43.
91. Xiang F, He M, Zeng Y, Mai J, Rose KA, Morgan IG. Increases in the prevalence of reduced visual acuity and myopia in Chinese children in Guangzhou over the past 20 years. Eye. 2013;27(12):1353–8.
92. Wang SK, Guo Y, Liao C, et al. Incidence of and factors associated with myopia and high myopia in Chinese children, based on refraction without cycloplegia. JAMA Ophthalmol. 2018;136(9):1017–24.
93. Saw SM, Tong L, Chua WH, et al. Incidence and progression of myopia in Singaporean school children. Invest Ophthalmol Vis Sci. 2005;46(1):51–7.
94. Matsumura H, Hirai H. Prevalence of myopia and refractive changes in students from 3 to 17 years of age. Surv Ophthalmol. 1999;44(Suppl 1):S109–15.
95. Tsai DC, Fang SY, Huang N, et al. Myopia development among young school children: the myopia investigation study in Taipei. Invest Ophthalmol Vis Sci. 2016;57(15):6852–60.
96. Xiang F, He M, Morgan IG. Annual changes in refractive errors and ocular components before and after the onset of myopia in Chinese children. Ophthalmology. 2012;119(7):1478–84.
97. COMET Group. Myopia stabilization and associated factors among participants in the Correction of Myopia Evaluation Trial (COMET). Invest Ophthalmol Vis Sci. 2013;54(13):7871–84.
98. French AN, Morgan IG, Burlutsky G, Mitchell P, Rose KA. Prevalence and 5- to 6-year incidence and progression of myopia and hyperopia in Australian schoolchildren. Ophthalmology. 2013;120(7):1482–91.
99. Jones-Jordan LA, Sinnott LT, Manny RE, et al. Early childhood refractive error and parental history of myopia as predictors of myopia. Invest Ophthalmol Vis Sci. 2010;51(1):115–21.
100. Williams C, Miller LL, Gazzard G, Saw SM. A comparison of measures of reading and intelligence as risk factors for the development of myopia in a UK cohort of children. Br J Ophthalmol. 2008;92(8):1117–21.

101. Dirani M, Tong L, Gazzard G, et al. Outdoor activity and myopia in Singapore teenage children. Br J Ophthalmol. 2009;93(8):997.
102. Morgan IG. New perspectives on the prevention of myopia. Eye Sci. 2011;26(1):3.
103. Iwase A, Araie M, Tomidokoro A, et al. Prevalence and causes of low vision and blindness in a Japanese adult population: the Tajimi Study. Ophthalmology. 2006;113(8):1354–62.
104. Xu L, Wang Y, Li Y, Cui T, Li J, Jonas JB. Causes of blindness and visual impairment in urban and rural areas in Beijing: the Beijing Eye Study. Ophthalmology. 2006;113(7):1134 e1131–11.
105. You QS, Xu L, Yang H, Wang YX, Jonas JB. Five-year incidence of visual impairment and blindness in adult Chinese the Beijing Eye Study. Ophthalmology. 2011;118(6):1069–75.
106. Yamada M, Hiratsuka Y, Roberts CB, et al. Prevalence of visual impairment in the adult Japanese population by cause and severity and future projections. Ophthalmic Epidemiol. 2010;17(1):50–7.
107. Hsu WM, Cheng CY, Liu JH, Tsai SY, Chou P. Prevalence and causes of visual impairment in an elderly Chinese population in Taiwan: the Shihpai Eye Study. Ophthalmology. 2004;111(1):62–9.
108. Ohno-Matsui K, Lai TYY, Cheung CMG, Lai CC. Updates of pathologic myopia. Prog Retin Eye Res. 2016;52(5):156–87.
109. Ohno-Matsui K, Kawasaki R, Jonas JB, et al. International photographic classification and grading system for myopic maculopathy. Am J Ophthalmol. 2015;159(5):877–883 e877.
110. Spaide RF. Staphyloma: part 1. New York: Springer; 2014.
111. Fang Y, Yokoi T, Nagaoka N, et al. Progression of myopic maculopathy during 18-year follow-up. Ophthalmology. 2018;125:863–77.
112. Hayashi K, Ohno-Matsui K, Shimada N, et al. Long-term pattern of progression of myopic maculopathy: a natural history study. Ophthalmology. 2010;117(8):1595–611.
113. Yan YN, Wang YX, Yang Y, et al. Ten-year progression of myopic maculopathy: The Beijing Eye Study 2001-2011. Ophthalmology. 2018;125:1253–63.
114. Vongphanit J, Mitchell P, Wang JJ. Prevalence and progression of myopic retinopathy in an older population. Ophthalmology. 2002;109(4):704–11.
115. Xu L, Wang Y, Wang S, Jonas JB. High myopia and glaucoma susceptibility the Beijing Eye Study. Ophthalmology. 2007;114(2):216–20.
116. Nagaoka N, Jonas JB, Morohoshi K, et al. Glaucomatous-type optic discs in high myopia. PLoS One. 2015;10(10):e0138825.
117. Curtin BJ. The posterior staphyloma of pathologic myopia. Trans Am Ophthalmol Soc. 1977;75:67–86.
118. Ohno-Matsui K. Proposed classification of posterior staphylomas based on analyses of eye shape by three-dimensional magnetic resonance imaging. Ophthalmology. 2014;121(9):1798–809.
119. Neelam K, Cheung CM, Ohno-Matsui K, Lai TY, Wong TY. Choroidal neovascularization in pathological myopia. Prog Retin Eye Res. 2012;31(5):495–525.
120. Ohno-Matsui K, Yoshida T, Futagami S, et al. Patchy atrophy and lacquer cracks predispose to the development of choroidal neovascularisation in pathological myopia. Br J Ophthalmol. 2003;87(5):570–3.
121. Wolf S, Balciuniene VJ, Laganovska G, et al. RADIANCE: a randomized controlled study of ranibizumab in patients with choroidal neovascularization secondary to pathologic myopia. Ophthalmology. 2014;121(3):682–92.
122. Ikuno Y, Ohno-Matsui K, Wong TY, et al. Intravitreal aflibercept injection in patients with myopic choroidal neovascularization: The MYRROR Study. Ophthalmology. 2015;122(6):1220–7.
123. Panozzo G, Mercanti A. Optical coherence tomography findings in myopic traction maculopathy. Arch Ophthalmol. 2004;122(10):1455–60.
124. Gaucher D, Erginay A, Lecleire-Collet A, et al. Dome-shaped macula in eyes with myopic posterior staphyloma. Am J Ophthalmol. 2008;145(5):909–14.

125. Caillaux V, Gaucher D, Gualino V, Massin P, Tadayoni R, Gaudric A. Morphologic characterization of dome-shaped macula in myopic eyes with serous macular detachment. Am J Ophthalmol. 2013;156(5):958–67.
126. Ellabban AA, Tsujikawa A, Matsumoto A, et al. Three-dimensional tomographic features of dome-shaped macula by swept-source optical coherence tomography. Am J Ophthalmol. 2012;3(12):578.
127. Imamura Y, Iida T, Maruko I, Zweifel SA, Spaide RF. Enhanced depth imaging optical coherence tomography of the sclera in dome-shaped macula. Am J Ophthalmol. 2011;151(2):297–302.
128. Pope JM, Verkicharla PK, Sepehrband F, Suheimat M, Schmid KL, Atchison DA. Three-dimensional MRI study of the relationship between eye dimensions, retinal shape and myopia. Biomed Opt Express. 2017;8(5):2386–95.
129. Kuo AN, Verkicharla PK, McNabb RP, et al. Posterior eye shape measurement with retinal OCT compared to MRI. Invest Ophthalmol Vis Sci. 2016;57(9):196–203.
130. Samarawickrama C, Mitchell P, Tong L, et al. Myopia-related optic disc and retinal changes in adolescent children from singapore. Ophthalmology. 2011;118(10):2050–7.
131. Jonas JB, Jonas SB, Jonas RA, Holbach L, Panda-Jonas S. Histology of the parapapillary region in high myopia. Am J Ophthalmol. 2011;152(6):1021–9.
132. Park HY, Lee K, Park CK. Optic disc torsion direction predicts the location of glaucomatous damage in normal-tension glaucoma patients with myopia. Ophthalmology. 2012;119(9):1844–51.
133. Marcus MW, de Vries MM, Junoy Montolio FG, Jansonius NM. Myopia as a risk factor for open-angle glaucoma: a systematic review and meta-analysis. Ophthalmology. 2011;118(10):1989–1994.e1982.
134. Chang RT, Singh K. Myopia and glaucoma: diagnostic and therapeutic challenges. Curr Opin Ophthalmol. 2013;24(2):96–101.
135. Jonas JB, Gusek GC, Naumann GO. Optic disk morphometry in high myopia. Graefes Arch Clin Exp Ophthalmol. 1988;226(6):587–90.
136. Jonas JB, Nagaoka N, Fang YX, Weber P, Ohno-Matsui K. Intraocular pressure and glaucomatous optic neuropathy in high myopia. Invest Ophthalmol Vis Sci. 2017;58(13):5897–906.
137. Ohno-Matsui K, Shimada N, Yasuzumi K, et al. Long-term development of significant visual field defects in highly myopic eyes. Am J Ophthalmol. 2011;152(2):256–265 e251.
138. Han JC, Lee EJ, Kim SB, Kee C. The Characteristics of deep optic nerve head morphology in myopic normal tension glaucoma. Invest Ophthalmol Vis Sci. 2017;58(5):2695–704.
139. Johnson MW. Myopic traction maculopathy: pathogenic mechanisms and surgical treatment. Retina. 2012;32(Suppl 2):S205–10.
140. Wong CW, Phua V, Lee SY, Wong TY, Cheung CM. Is Choroidal or scleral thickness related to myopic macular degeneration? Invest Ophthalmol Vis Sci. 2017;58(2):907–13.
141. Ohno-Matsui K, Akiba M, Modegi T, et al. Association between shape of sclera and myopic retinochoroidal lesions in patients with pathologic myopia. Invest Ophthalmol Vis Sci. 2012;53(10):6046–61.
142. Shinohara K, Moriyama M, Shimada N, Yoshida T, Ohno-Matsui K. Characteristics of peripapillary staphylomas associated with high myopia determined by swept-source optical coherence tomography. Am J Ophthalmol. 2016;169:138–44.
143. Spaide RF. Choriocapillaris flow features follow a power law distribution: implications for characterization and mechanisms of disease progression. Am J Ophthalmol. 2016;170:58–67.
144. Zhang Q, Zheng F, Motulsky EH, et al. A novel strategy for quantifying choriocapillaris flow voids using swept-source OCT angiography. Invest Ophthalmol Vis Sci. 2018;59(1):203–11.
145. Al-Sheikh M, Phasukkijwatana N, Dolz-Marco R, et al. Quantitative OCT angiography of the retinal microvasculature and the choriocapillaris in myopic eyes. Invest Ophthalmol Vis Sci. 2017;58(4):2063–9.
146. Ang M, Devarajan K, Das S, et al. Comparison of anterior segment optical coherence tomography angiography systems for corneal vascularisation. Br J Ophthalmol. 2018;102(7):873–7.

147. Cai Y, Alio Del Barrio JL, Wilkins MR, Ang M. Serial optical coherence tomography angiography for corneal vascularization. Graefes Arch Clin Exp Ophthalmol. 2017;255(1):135–9.
148. Ang M, Cai Y, Shahipasand S, et al. En face optical coherence tomography angiography for corneal neovascularisation. Br J Ophthalmol. 2016;100(5):616–21.
149. Grudzinska E, Modrzejewska M. Modern diagnostic techniques for the assessment of ocular blood flow in myopia: current state of knowledge. J Ophthalmol. 2018;2018:8.
150. Silverman RH, Cannata J, Shung KK, et al. 75 MHz ultrasound biomicroscopy of anterior segment of eye. Ultrason Imaging. 2006;28(3):179–88.
151. Xie D, Li Q, Gao Q, Song W, Zhang HF, Yuan X. In vivo blind-deconvolution photoacoustic ophthalmoscopy with total variation regularization. J Biophotonics. 2018;11(9):e201700360.
152. Xu L, Wang Y, Wang S, Wang Y, Jonas JB. High myopia and glaucoma susceptibility the Beijing Eye Study. Ophthalmology. 2007;114(2):216–20.
153. Podos SM, Becker B, Morton WR. High myopia and primary open-angle glaucoma. Am J Ophthalmol. 1966;62(6):1038–43.
154. Greve EL, Furuno F. Myopia and glaucoma. Albrecht Von Graefes Arch Klin Exp Ophthalmol. 1980;213(1):33–41.
155. Daubs JG, Crick RP. Effect of refractive error on the risk of ocular hypertension and open angle glaucoma. Trans Ophthalmol Soc Aust. 1981;101(1):121–6.
156. Phelps CD. Effect of myopia on prognosis in treated primary open-angle glaucoma. Am J Ophthalmol. 1982;93(5):622–8.
157. Perkins ES, Phelps CD. Open angle glaucoma, ocular hypertension, low-tension glaucoma, and refraction. Arch Ophthalmol. 1982;100(9):1464–7.
158. Leske MC, Connell AM, Wu SY, Hyman LG, Schachat AP. Risk factors for open-angle glaucoma. The Barbados Eye Study. Arch Ophthalmol. 1995;113(7):918–24.
159. Chihara E, Liu X, Dong J, et al. Severe myopia as a risk factor for progressive visual field loss in primary open-angle glaucoma. Ophthalmologica. 1997;211(2):66–71.
160. Mitchell P, Hourihan F, Sandbach J, Wang JJ. The relationship between glaucoma and myopia: the Blue Mountains Eye Study. Ophthalmology. 1999;106(10):2010–5.
161. Grodum K, Heijl A, Bengtsson B. Refractive error and glaucoma. Acta Ophthalmol Scand. 2001;79(6):560–6.
162. Jonas JB, Martus P, Budde WM. Anisometropia and degree of optic nerve damage in chronic open-angle glaucoma. Am J Ophthalmol. 2002;134(4):547–51.
163. Wong TY, Klein BE, Klein R, Knudtson M, Lee KE. Refractive errors, intraocular pressure, and glaucoma in a white population. Ophthalmology. 2003;110(1):211–7.
164. Leske MC, Heijl A, Hussein M, et al. Factors for glaucoma progression and the effect of treatment: the early manifest glaucoma trial. Arch Ophthalmol. 2003;121(1):48–56.
165. Jonas JB, Budde WM. Optic nerve damage in highly myopic eyes with chronic open-angle glaucoma. Eur J Ophthalmol. 2005;15(1):41–7.
166. Kuzin AA, Varma R, Reddy HS, Torres M, Azen SP, Los Angeles Latino Eye Study G. Ocular biometry and open-angle glaucoma: the Los Angeles Latino Eye Study. Ophthalmology. 2010;117(9):1713–9.
167. Cohen SY, Laroche A, Leguen Y, Soubrane G, Coscas GJ. Etiology of choroidal neovascularization in young patients. Ophthalmology. 1996;103(8):1241–4.
168. Yoshida T, Ohno-Matsui K, Yasuzumi K, et al. Myopic choroidal neovascularization: a 10-year follow-up. Ophthalmology. 2003;110(7):1297–305.
169. Avila MP, Weiter JJ, Jalkh AE, Trempe CL, Pruett RC, Schepens CL. Natural history of choroidal neovascularization in degenerative myopia. Ophthalmology. 1984;91(12):1573–81.
170. Curtin BJ, Karlin DB. Axial length measurements and fundus changes of the myopic eye. I. The posterior fundus. Trans Am Ophthalmol Soc. 1970;68:312–34.
171. Lai TY, Cheung CM. Myopic choroidal neovascularization: diagnosis and treatment. Retina. 2016;36(9):1614–21.
172. Jia Y, Bailey ST, Wilson DJ, et al. Quantitative optical coherence tomography angiography of choroidal neovascularization in age-related macular degeneration. Ophthalmology. 2014;121(7):1435–44.

173. Virgili G, Menchini F. Laser photocoagulation for choroidal neovascularisation in pathologic myopia. Cochrane Database Syst Rev. 2005;4:CD004765.
174. Blinder KJ, Blumenkranz MS, Bressler NM, et al. Verteporfin therapy of subfoveal choroidal neovascularization in pathologic myopia: 2-year results of a randomized clinical trial--VIP report no. 3. Ophthalmology. 2003;110(4):667–73.
175. Verteporfin in Photodynamic Therapy Study G. Photodynamic therapy of subfoveal choroidal neovascularization in pathologic myopia with verteporfin. 1-year results of a randomized clinical trial--VIP report no. 1. Ophthalmology. 2001;108(5):841–52.
176. Chen Y, Sharma T, Li X, et al. Ranibizumab versus verteporfin photodynamic therapy in Asian patients with myopic choroidal neovascularization: brilliance, a 12-month, randomized, double-masked study. Retina. 2018. https://doi.org/10.1097/IAE.0000000000002292.
177. Tufail A, Narendran N, Patel PJ, et al. Ranibizumab in myopic choroidal neovascularization: the 12-month results from the REPAIR study. Ophthalmology. 2013;120(9):1944–1945. e1941.
178. Wu PC, Chen YJ, Chen YH, et al. Factors associated with foveoschisis and foveal detachment without macular hole in high myopia. Eye. 2009;23(2):356–61.
179. Baba T, Ohno-Matsui K, Futagami S, et al. Prevalence and characteristics of foveal retinal detachment without macular hole in high myopia. Am J Ophthalmol. 2003;135(3):338–42.
180. Fang X, Weng Y, Xu S, et al. Optical coherence tomographic characteristics and surgical outcome of eyes with myopic foveoschisis. Eye. 2009;23(6):1336–42.
181. VanderBeek BL, Johnson MW. The diversity of traction mechanisms in myopic traction maculopathy. Am J Ophthalmol. 2012;153(1):93–102.
182. Yeh SI, Chang WC, Chen LJ. Vitrectomy without internal limiting membrane peeling for macular retinoschisis and foveal detachment in highly myopic eyes. Acta Ophthalmol. 2008;86(2):219–24.
183. Smiddy WE, Kim SS, Lujan BJ, Gregori G. Myopic traction maculopathy: spectral domain optical coherence tomographic imaging and a hypothesized mechanism. Ophthalmic Surg Lasers Imaging. 2009;40(2):169–73.
184. Gaucher D, Haouchine B, Tadayoni R, et al. Long-term follow-up of high myopic foveoschisis: natural course and surgical outcome. Am J Ophthalmol. 2007;143(3):455–62.
185. Ikuno Y, Sayanagi K, Soga K, Oshima Y, Ohji M, Tano Y. Foveal anatomical status and surgical results in vitrectomy for myopic foveoschisis. Jpn J Ophthalmol. 2008;52(4):269–76.
186. Ikuno Y, Sayanagi K, Ohji M, et al. Vitrectomy and internal limiting membrane peeling for myopic foveoschisis. Am J Ophthalmol. 2004;137(4):719–24.
187. Kuhn F. Internal limiting membrane removal for macular detachment in highly myopic eyes. Am J Ophthalmol. 2003;135(4):547–9.
188. Panozzo G, Mercanti A. Vitrectomy for myopic traction maculopathy. Arch Ophthalmol. 2007;125(6):767–72.
189. Kumagai K, Furukawa M, Ogino N, Larson E. Factors correlated with postoperative visual acuity after vitrectomy and internal limiting membrane peeling for myopic foveoschisis. Retina. 2010;30(6):874–80.
190. Kwok AK, Lai TY, Yip WW. Vitrectomy and gas tamponade without internal limiting membrane peeling for myopic foveoschisis. Br J Ophthalmol. 2005;89(9):1180–3.
191. Tang J, Rivers MB, Moshfeghi AA, Flynn HW, Chan CC. Pathology of macular foveoschisis associated with degenerative myopia. J Ophthalmol. 2010;2010:175613.
192. Sayanagi K, Morimoto Y, Ikuno Y, Tano Y. Spectral-domain optical coherence tomographic findings in myopic foveoschisis. Retina. 2010;30(4):623–8.
193. Spaide RF, Fisher Y. Removal of adherent cortical vitreous plaques without removing the internal limiting membrane in the repair of macular detachments in highly myopic eyes. Retina. 2005;25(3):290–5.
194. Ikuno Y, Gomi F, Tano Y. Potent retinal arteriolar traction as a possible cause of myopic foveoschisis. Am J Ophthalmol. 2005;139(3):462–7.
195. Sayanagi K, Ikuno Y, Gomi F, Tano Y. Retinal vascular microfolds in highly myopic eyes. Am J Ophthalmol. 2005;139(4):658–63.

196. Benhamou N, Massin P, Haouchine B, Erginay A, Gaudric A. Macular retinoschisis in highly myopic eyes. Am J Ophthalmol. 2002;133(6):794–800.
197. Ripandelli G, Rossi T, Scarinci F, Scassa C, Parisi V, Stirpe M. Macular vitreoretinal interface abnormalities in highly myopic eyes with posterior staphyloma: 5-year follow-up. Retina. 2012;32(8):1531–8.
198. Michalewska Z, Michalewski J, Adelman RA, Nawrocki J. Inverted internal limiting membrane flap technique for large macular holes. Ophthalmology. 2010;117(10):2018–25.
199. Morizane Y, Shiraga F, Kimura S, et al. Autologous transplantation of the internal limiting membrane for refractory macular holes. Am J Ophthalmol. 2014;157(4):861–869 e861.
200. Leisser C, Hirnschall N, Doller B, et al. Internal limiting membrane flap transposition for surgical repair of macular holes in primary surgery and in persistent macular holes. Eur J Ophthalmol. 2018;28(2):225–8.
201. Ghosh B, Arora S, Goel N, et al. Comparative evaluation of sequential intraoperative use of whole blood followed by brilliant blue versus conventional brilliant blue staining of internal limiting membrane in macular hole surgery. Retina. 2016;36(8):1463–8.
202. Chen SN, Yang CM. Lens capsular flap transplantation in the management of refractory macular hole from multiple etiologies. Retina. 2016;36(1):163–70.
203. Alkabes M, Mateo C. Macular buckle technique in myopic traction maculopathy: a 16-year review of the literature and a comparison with vitreous surgery. Graefes Arch Clin Exp Ophthalmol. 2018;256(5):863–77.
204. Grewal DS, Mahmoud TH. Autologous neurosensory retinal free flap for closure of refractory myopic macular holes. JAMA Ophthalmol. 2016;134(2):229–30.
205. Chung K, Mohidin N, O'Leary DJ. Undercorrection of myopia enhances rather than inhibits myopia progression. Vis Res. 2002;42(22):2555–9.
206. Adler D, Millodot M. The possible effect of undercorrection on myopic progression in children. Clin Exp Optom. 2006;89(5):315–21.
207. Sun YY, Li SM, Li SY, et al. Effect of uncorrection versus full correction on myopia progression in 12-year-old children. Graefes Arch Clin Exp Ophthalmol. 2017;255(1):189–95.
208. Edwards MH, Li RW, Lam CS, Lew JK, Yu BS. The Hong Kong progressive lens myopia control study: study design and main findings. Invest Ophthalmol Vis Sci. 2002;43(9):2852–8.
209. Yang Z, Lan W, Ge J, et al. The effectiveness of progressive addition lenses on the progression of myopia in Chinese children. Ophthalmic Physiol Opt. 2009;29(1):41–8.
210. Correction of Myopia Evaluation Trial 2 Study Group for the Pediatric Eye Disease Investigator Group. Progressive-addition lenses versus single-vision lenses for slowing progression of myopia in children with high accommodative lag and near esophoria. Invest Ophthalmol Vis Sci. 2011;52(5):2749–57.
211. Berntsen DA, Sinnott LT, Mutti DO, Zadnik K. A randomized trial using progressive addition lenses to evaluate theories of myopia progression in children with a high lag of accommodation. Invest Ophthalmol Vis Sci. 2012;53(2):640–9.
212. Hasebe S, Jun J, Varnas SR. Myopia control with positively aspherized progressive addition lenses: a 2-year, multicenter, randomized, controlled trial. Invest Ophthalmol Vis Sci. 2014;55(11):7177–88.
213. Walline JJ, Lindsley K, Vedula SS, Cotter SA, Mutti DO, Twelker JD. Interventions to slow progression of myopia in children. Cochrane Database Syst Rev. 2011;12:CD004916.
214. Hasebe S, Ohtsuki H, Nonaka T, et al. Effect of progressive addition lenses on myopia progression in Japanese children: a prospective, randomized, double-masked, crossover trial. Invest Ophthalmol Vis Sci. 2008;49(7):2781–9.
215. Cheng D, Woo GC, Drobe B, Schmid KL. Effect of bifocal and prismatic bifocal spectacles on myopia progression in children: three-year results of a randomized clinical trial. JAMA Ophthalmol. 2014;132(3):258–64.
216. Lam CSY, Lee PK, Lam CSY, Tang WC, Lee PK, et al. Myopic control with multi-segment of myopic defocus (MSMD) spectacle lens: a randomized clinical trial. Birmingham, UK. 2017.
217. Sankaridurg P, Donovan L, Varnas S, et al. Spectacle lenses designed to reduce progression of myopia: 12-month results. Optom Vis Sci. 2010;87(9):631–41.

218. Kanda H, Oshika T, Hiraoka T, et al. Effect of spectacle lenses designed to reduce relative peripheral hyperopia on myopia progression in Japanese children: a 2-year multicenter randomized controlled trial. Jpn J Ophthalmol. 2018;62(5):537–43.
219. Walline JJ, Jones LA, Mutti DO, Zadnik K. A randomized trial of the effects of rigid contact lenses on myopia progression. Arch Ophthalmol. 2004;122(12):1760–6.
220. Katz J, Schein OD, Levy B, et al. A randomized trial of rigid gas permeable contact lenses to reduce progression of children's myopia. Am J Ophthalmol. 2003;136(1):82–90.
221. Cho P, Cheung SW, Edwards M. The longitudinal orthokeratology research in children (LORIC) in Hong Kong: a pilot study on refractive changes and myopic control. Curr Eye Res. 2005;30(1):71–80.
222. Kakita T, Hiraoka T, Oshika T. Influence of overnight orthokeratology on axial elongation in childhood myopia. Invest Ophthalmol Vis Sci. 2011;52(5):2170–4.
223. Cho P, Cheung SW. Retardation of myopia in Orthokeratology (ROMIO) study: a 2-year randomized clinical trial. Invest Ophthalmol Vis Sci. 2012;53(11):7077–85.
224. Hiraoka T, Kakita T, Okamoto F, Takahashi H, Oshika T. Long-term effect of overnight orthokeratology on axial length elongation in childhood myopia: a 5-year follow-up study. Invest Ophthalmol Vis Sci. 2012;53(7):3913–9.
225. Charm J, Cho P. High myopia-partial reduction ortho-k: a 2-year randomized study. Optom Vis Sci. 2013;90(6):530–9.
226. Wen D, Huang J, Chen H, et al. Efficacy and acceptability of orthokeratology for slowing myopic progression in children: a systematic review and meta-analysis. J Ophthalmol. 2015;2015:360806.
227. Sun Y, Xu F, Zhang T, et al. Orthokeratology to control myopia progression: a meta-analysis. PLoS One. 2015;10(4):e0124535.
228. Lee YC, Wang JH, Chiu CJ. Effect of orthokeratology on myopia progression: twelve-year results of a retrospective cohort study. BMC Ophthalmol. 2017;17(1):243.
229. Yen MY, Liu JH, Kao SC, Shiao CH. Comparison of the effect of atropine and cyclopentolate on myopia. Ann Ophthalmol. 1989;21(5):180–182, 187.
230. Kinoshita N, Konno Y, Hamada N, Kanda Y, Shimmura-Tomita M, Kakehashi A. Additive effects of orthokeratology and atropine 0.01% ophthalmic solution in slowing axial elongation in children with myopia: first year results. Jpn J Ophthalmol. 2018;62(5):544–53.
231. Young AL, Leung AT, Cheng LL, Law RW, Wong AK, Lam DS. Orthokeratology lens-related corneal ulcers in children: a case series. Ophthalmology. 2004;111(3):590–5.
232. Rah MJ, Walline JJ, Jones-Jordan LA, et al. Vision specific quality of life of pediatric contact lens wearers. Optom Vis Sci. 2010;87(8):560–6.
233. Walline JJ, Gaume A, Jones LA, et al. Benefits of contact lens wear for children and teens. Eye Contact Lens. 2007;33(6 Pt 1):317–21.
234. Benavente-Perez A, Nour A, Troilo D. Axial eye growth and refractive error development can be modified by exposing the peripheral retina to relative myopic or hyperopic defocus. Invest Ophthalmol Vis Sci. 2014;55(10):6765–73.
235. Li SM, Kang MT, Wu SS, et al. Studies using concentric ring bifocal and peripheral add multifocal contact lenses to slow myopia progression in school-aged children: a meta-analysis. Ophthalmic Physiol Opt. 2017;37(1):51–9.
236. Shih YF, Chen CH, Chou AC, Ho TC, Lin LL, Hung PT. Effects of different concentrations of atropine on controlling myopia in myopic children. J Ocul Pharmacol Ther. 1999;15(1):85–90.
237. Chua WH, Balakrishnan V, Chan YH, et al. Atropine for the treatment of childhood myopia. Ophthalmology. 2006;113(12):2285–91.
238. Chia A, Chua WH, Cheung YB, et al. Atropine for the treatment of childhood myopia: safety and efficacy of 0.5%, 0.1%, and 0.01% doses (Atropine for the Treatment of Myopia 2). Ophthalmology. 2012;119(2):347–54.
239. Tong L, Huang XL, Koh AL, Zhang X, Tan DT, Chua WH. Atropine for the treatment of childhood myopia: effect on myopia progression after cessation of atropine. Ophthalmology. 2009;116(3):572–9.

240. Chia A, Chua WH, Wen L, Fong A, Goon YY, Tan D. Atropine for the treatment of childhood myopia: changes after stopping atropine 0.01%, 0.1% and 0.5%. Am J Ophthalmol. 2014;157(2):451–457 e451.
241. Ashby R, Ohlendorf A, Schaeffel F. The effect of ambient illuminance on the development of deprivation myopia in chicks. Invest Ophthalmol Vis Sci. 2009;50(11):5348–54.
242. Seidemann A, Schaeffel F. Effects of longitudinal chromatic aberration on accommodation and emmetropization. Vis Res. 2002;42(21):2409–17.
243. Flitcroft DI. The complex interactions of retinal, optical and environmental factors in myopia aetiology. Prog Retin Eye Res. 2012;31(6):622–60.
244. Hung LF, Arumugam B, She Z, Ostrin L, Smith EL. Narrow-band, long-wavelength lighting promotes hyperopia and retards vision-induced myopia in infant rhesus monkeys. Exp Eye Res. 2018;176:147–60.

2

Prevalence of Myopia: A Global Perspective

Saiko Matsumura, Cheng Ching-Yu, and Seang-Mei Saw

Key Points

- The prevalence of myopia in children is high in urban East Asian countries.
- The myopia and HM prevalence among young adults is much higher in East Asia than in Western countries.
- The burden of HM is huge because HM can cause PM changes and visual impairment.
- The prevalence of PM among adults has been relatively low, but it is likely to increase in future.
- It is important to develop public policies and preventive measures to retard the epidemic myopia.

S. Matsumura
Singapore Eye Research Institute, Singapore, Singapore
e-mail: matsumura.saiko@seri.com.sg

C. Ching-Yu
Singapore National Eye Centre, Singapore, Singapore

National University of Singapore, Singapore, Singapore

Duke-NUS Medical School, Singapore, Singapore
e-mail: chingyu.cheng@duke-nus.edu.sg

S.-M. Saw (✉)
Singapore Eye Research Institute, Singapore, Singapore

National University of Singapore, Singapore, Singapore

Saw Swee Hock School of Public Health, National University of Singapore, Singapore, Singapore
e-mail: ephssm@nus.edu.sg, saw.seang.mei@seri.com.sg

2.1 Introduction

Myopia has become a significant global public health and socioeconomic problem [1–4]. Developed countries, especially among East Asia, have been faced with high prevalence of myopia and high myopia (HM) and the same trend has been shown in other parts of the world with less extent [5, 6]. (The definition of myopia and HM is spherical equivalence (SE) of −0.50 diopters (D) or less and SE −5.00 D or −6.00 D, respectively.) The prevalence of myopia and HM in young adults in urban area of East Asian countries has risen to 80–90% and around 20%, respectively [7, 8]. According to a summary of 145 studies regarding the global prevalence of myopia and HM, there are approximately 1950 million (28.3% of the global population) and 277 million (4.0% of the global population) cases, and they are predicted to increase to 4758 million (49.8% of the global population) for myopia, and 938 million (9.8% of the global population) for HM by 2050 [9].

Most cases of myopia are considered as a benign condition because vision is corrected with spectacles, contact lenses, or refractive surgery. However, severe cases of myopia are associated with the risk of irreversible vision impairment and blindness due to pathological changes in retina, choroid, and sclera. One study has shown that 25% of HM will develop pathologic myopia (PM) and 50% of those with PM will have low vision as older adults. Thus, HM and PM are likely to increase drastically in the older generation. Based on the global prediction of HM on 2050, PM may increase to over 200 million in future [9]. Treatment strategies against PM have not been effective and costly [10]. Considering the burden of PM in the future, it is important to develop public policies and preventive and early interventional measures to retard the epidemic myopia. In this chapter, we summarize data on the prevalence of myopia and HM in different generations and the prevalence of PM from recent epidemiological studies.

2.2 Prevalence of Myopia in Children

In children, cycloplegic refraction is a common procedure to measure refractive error because children have a possibility to have an overestimation of myopic refraction, due to increased tone of the ciliary muscle and a constant accommodative effort during the examination, and makes the refraction overestimated approximately over −1 to −2 D [11, 12]. Many population-based studies on children have proved that the prevalence of myopia is higher in urbanized East Asian countries. In surveys of 12-year-old children, the prevalence of myopia is higher in Singapore (62.0%) [13], Hong Kong (53.1%) [14], and Guangzhou, China (49.7%) [15] than in the United States (20.0%) [16], Northern Ireland (17.7%) [17], Australia (11.9%) [18], urban India (9.7%) [19], Nepal (16.5%) [20], and Cambodia (6.0%) [21]. We summarized the prevalence of myopia among children in population studies using cycloplegic refraction between Asian countries (Table 2.1) and non-Asian countries (Table 2.2).

Table 2.1 Summary of prevalence of myopia and high myopia in children in population-based studies using cycloplegic refraction in Asian countries

Study (authors, year)	Location	Number	Race	Age (year)	Response rate (%)	Description of source	Prevalence (%)	95%CI
East Asian countries								
Hsu et al. (2016) [22]	Taipei, Taiwan	$N = 11{,}590$	Taiwanese	8	59.8	Citywide cohort study	M: 36.4% HM: –	NA
Lai et al. (2009) [23]	Kaohsiung, Taiwan	$N = 618$	Taiwanese	3–6	97.7	The screening nationwide programs for schools	M: 5.5% HM: –	(3.6–7.4%)
Lin et al. (2004) [7]	Taiwan	$N = 10{,}889$	Taiwanese	7–18	91.0	Cross-sectional surveys	M: 20.0% (7 years) M: 61.0% (12 years) M: 81.0% (15 years)	NA
Li (2017) [24]	Beijing, China	$N = 3676$	Chinese	15.25 ± 0.46	NA	School-based longitudinal study	M: 65.5% HM: 6.7% (≤ −6.0 D)	NA
Ma et al. (2016) [25]	Shanghai, China	$N = 8398$	Chinese	3–10	70.0	Random selection of 7 kindergartens and 7 primary schools	M: 20.1% HM: 0.33%	NA
Li et al. (2013) [26]	Rural area, China	$N = 1675$	Chinese	5–18	90.8	Random selection of geographically defined clusters	M: 5.0% HM: –	(4.8–5.4%)
Pi et al. (2012) [27]	Yongchuan, Suburban area, China	$N = 3070$	Chinese	6–15	NA	Random cluster sampling door-to-door surveys	M: 13.7% HM: –	NA
He (2007) [28]	Rural area, Guangdong, China	$N = 2454$	Chinese	13–17	NA	Stratified cluster sampling in 17 county schools	M: 42.4% HM: –	(35.8–49.0%)

(continued)

Table 2.1 (continued)

Study (authors, year)	Location	Number	Race	Age (year)	Response rate (%)	Description of source	Prevalence (%)	95%CI
He et al. (2004) [15]	Urban area, Guangzhou, China	$N = 4364$	Chinese	5–15	86.4	Random selection of geographically defined clusters	M: 38.1% HM: –	(36.3–39.8%)
Zhao et al. (2000) [29]	Shunyi, North east of Beijing, China	$N = 5884$	Chinese	5–15	95.9	Random selection of village-based clusters	M: 14.9% HM: –	NA
Fan et al. (2011) [30]	Hong Kong	$N = 601$ $N = 823$	Chinese	3–6	96.5 99.3	Random selection of kindergartens	M: 2.3% M: 6.3%	NA
Dirani et al. (2010) [31]	Singapore	$N = 2369$	Chinese	6M–6	72.3	Stratified random sampling, door-to-door surveys	M: 11.0% HM: 0.2%	(10.9–11.2%) (0.08–0.50%)
Saw et al. (2005) [13]	Singapore	$N = 1453$	Chinese	7–9	67.6	School-based cross-sectional study	M: 36.7% HM:	(34.2–39.2%)
Rest of Asian countries								
Murthy et al. (2002) [19]	New Delhi, India	$N = 6447$	Indian	5–15	92.0	Random selection of geographically defined clusters	M: 7.4%	(5.0%–9.7%)
Dandona et al. (2002) [32]	1 urban 3 rural areas, India	$N = 11786$	Indian	<15 >15	NA	Stratified random cluster sampling	M: 3.19% (<15) M: 19.45% (>15) HM: –	(2.24–4.13%) (17.88–21.02%)
Yekta et al. (2010) [33]	Shiraz, Iran	$N = 1854$	Iranian	7–15	87.9	Random cluster sampling	M: 4.4% HM:	(2.89–5.82%)
Jamali et al. (2009) [34]	Shahrood, Iran	$N = 815$	Iranian	6	NA	Random selection of primary schools	M: 1.7% HM: –	NA

Fotouhi et al. (2007) [35]	Rural area Dezful, Iran	$N = 5544$	Iranian	7–15	96.8	Random cluster sampling, selection of 460 schools	M: 3.4% HM: –	(2.5–4.4%)
Hashemi et al. (2004) [36]	Tehran, Iran	$N = 809$	Iranian	5–15	70.3	Stratified random cluster sampling, door-to-door surveys	M: 7.2% HM: –	(5.3–9.2%)
Sapkota et al. (2008) [20]	Rural area Kathmandu, Nepal	$N = 4282$	Aryan Mongol Tibetan	10–15	95.1	Stratified random selection of classes from secondary private schools	M: 19.0% HM: –	(17.8–20.2%)
Yingyong et al. (2010) [37]	Thailand	$N = 2360$	Thai	6–12	NA	Random selection of geographically defined clusters	M: 11.1% HM: –	NA

NA not applicable, *M* myopia, *HM* high myopia

Table 2.2 Summary of prevalence of myopia and high myopia in children in population-based studies using cycloplegic refraction in non-Asian countries

Study (authors, year)	Location	Number	Race	Age (year)	Response rate (%)	Description of source	Prevalence (%)	95%CI
Wen et al. (2013) [38]	LA, USA	$N = 1501$ $N = 1507$	NHW Asian	6M–6	NA	Population-based cohort study, door-to-door surveys	M: 1.2% (NHM) M: 3.98% (Asian) HM: –	(0.76–1.89%) (3.11–5.09%)
Giordano et al. (2009) [39]	Baltimore, USA	$N = 2298$	White A-A	6M–6	62	Population-based cohort study, door-to-door surveys	M: 0.7% (White) M: 5.5% (A-A) (Myopia <−1.0 D) HM: –	NA
Tideman (2018) [40]	The Netherlands	$N = 5711$	Euro non-Euro	6	68.4	Population-based birth cohort study	M: 2.4% HM: –	(2.13–5.10%)
Logan et al. (2011) [41]	England	$N = 327$ $N = 269$	Mix ethnicity	6–7 12–13	NA	Random selection of geographically defined clusters	M: 9.4% (6–7 years) M: 29.4% (12–13 years) HM: –	NA
O'Donoghue et al. (2010) [42]	Northern Ireland	$N = 661$ $N = 392$	Euro non-Euro	6–7 12–13	65.0	Random cluster sampling	M: 2.8% (6–7 years) M: 17.7% (12–13 years) HM: –	(1.3–4.3%) (13.2–22.2%)
Czepita et al. (2007) [43]	Poland	$N = 4422$	Euro	6–18	95.8	Random selection of elementary and secondary schools	M: 13.3% HM: –	NA
French et al. (2013) [44]	Sydney, Australia	$N = 2760$	Mix ethnicity	12	50.5	Random stratified cluster-sample of 55 schools	M: 18.9% (12 years) HM: 0.1% (12 years)	(7.5–30.4%)

Ip et al. (2008) [18]	Australia	$N = 2353$	Mix ethnicity	11–15	75.3	Random cluster-sample of 21 secondary schools	M: 11.9% HM: –	(6.6–17.2%)
Ojaimi et al. (2005) [45]	Australia	$N = 1765$	Mix ethnicity	5–8	79.0	Random stratified cluster-sample of schools	M: 1.43% HM: –	(0.94–2.18%)
Kumah et al. (2013) [46]	Ghana	$N = 2435$	African	12–15	99.2	Random selection of geographically defined clusters	M: 3.4% HM: –	(2.7–4.2%)
Naidoo et al. (2003) [47]	South Africa	$N = 4890$	African	5–15	87.3	Random selection of geographically defined clusters	M: 4.0% HM: –	(3.3–4.8%)

NA not applicable, *NHW* non-Hispanic White, *A-A* African-American, *Euro* European, *M* myopia, *HM* high myopia

2.2.1 Asian Countries

2.2.1.1 East Asian Countries and Singapore

Taiwanese school children have the highest prevalence of myopia among all school children worldwide. The prevalence of myopia among 8-year-old children is 36.4% in Taiwan [22], followed by 34.7% in Singapore [13], 30.8% in Shanghai [25] and 14.0% in Malaysia [48]. Lai et al. reported that the prevalence of myopia among 618 preschool Taiwanese children were also as high as 3.0%, 4.2%, 4.7%, and 12.2% in the age groups of 3, 4, 5, and 6 years, respectively [23]. A nationwide myopia survey in Taiwan showed that the prevalence of myopia among 7-year-olds increased from 5.8% in 1983 to 21% in 2000. At the age of 12, the prevalence of myopia was 36.7% in 1983 increasing to 61% in 2000, corresponding figures for 15-year-olds being 64.2% and 81%, respectively [7]. In China, Ma et al. reported that the prevalence of myopia in Shanghai was 20.1% among 3-year-old to 10-year-old children. They also showed that the prevalence increased dramatically from 5.2% in 6-year-old children and 14.3% in 7-year-old children to 52.2% in 10-year-old children [25]. In the urban city of Guangzhou, the prevalence of myopia was 7.7% in 7-year-old, 30.1% in 10-year-old, and 78.4% in 15-year-old children, with an overall prevalence of 38.1% among 4364 children aged 5–15 years [15]. In a rural area of Beijing, Zhao et al. reported that the prevalence of myopia among school children aged 5–7 and 14–15 years were 1.2% and 38.8%, respectively, with an overall prevalence of 14.9% among 5884 children aged 5–15 years [29]. In a suburban area, the prevalence of myopia among 3070 school children aged 6, 7, 10, and 14 years was 0.42%, 1.92%, 9.4%, and 28.8%, respectively [27]. In another rural area of northern China, the prevalence of myopia among 1675 school children aged 5–9, 10–14, and 15–18 years was 0.9%, 4.5%, and 8.2%, respectively, with an overall prevalence rate of 5.0% [49]. In Hong-Kong, 2 population-based surveys were conducted in children aged 3–6 years during 1996–1997 and 2006–2007, which revealed that prevalence of myopia increased 2.3–6.3% in a decade [30]. In Singapore, the school-based population study of the Singapore Cohort Study of Risk factors for Myopia (SCORM) showed that the prevalence of myopia was 29.0% in 7-year-olds, 34.7% in 8-year-olds, and 53.1% in 9-year-olds [50]. In younger ages from 6 months to 6 years, the Strabismus, Amblyopia, and Refractive Error in Singapore (STARS) Study reported that the prevalence of myopia was 11.0% in Chinese children [31].

2.2.1.2 Rest of Asian Countries

On the other hand, the prevalence of myopia is generally lower in other countries in Asia. In India, 6447 school children aged 5–15 years had 7.4% of the myopia prevalence in an urban population in New Delhi [19]. A population-based cross-sectional study was conducted among children in 1 urban and 3 rural areas. It reported that the prevalence of myopia among children ≤15 years of age and >15 years of age was 3.2% and 20.0%, respectively [32]. In Iran, the prevalence of myopia among 1854 school children aged 7, 10, and 14 years were 1.7%, 2.4%, and 7.6%, respectively, with an overall prevalence rate of 4.4% among 7-year-old to 15-year-old children in Shiraz [33]. In 4282 Nepalese secondary school children aged 10–15 years, the myopia prevalence was ranged from 10.9% in 10-year-olds to 27.3% in 15-year-olds [20]. In Thailand, the prevalence of myopia was 11.1% in 2360 children aged 6–12 years [37].

2.2.2 Non-Asian Countries

Nowadays, a rise of the myopia prevalence has also been shown in non-East-Asian countries that previously were only mildly or moderately affected, such as the UK, Australia, and the United States, although the prevalence is still lower than that in Asian countries. In the United States, the prevalence of myopia among 6–month-old to 6-year-old children was 1.20% and 3.98% in 1501 non-Hispanic White and 1507 Asian ethnicity children, respectively, as per the Multi-Ethnic Pediatric Eye Disease Study [38]. In the Baltimore Eye Study, the prevalence of myopia (SE <-1.00 D) was 1.2% in Whites, 6.6% in African-Americans among children aged 6 years, and an overall prevalence among 6-month-old to 71-month-old children was 0.7% and 5.5% in 1030 Whites and 1268 African-Americans, respectively [39]. Although few reports have been published on the prevalence of myopia in children in Europe, regional differences from country to country were shown even within the same geographical area. In England, the Aston Eye Study (AES) reported that the prevalence was 9.4% among children aged 6–7 years, and 29.4% among children aged 12–13 years, whereas the prevalence was 2.8% and 17.7% among children in the same age groups in Northern Ireland [17, 41]. In the Netherlands, the myopia prevalence rate was as low as 2.4% in 5711 children aged 6 years [40]. In Poland, the myopia prevalence was lower: 2.0% in 6-year-old, 8.4% in 8-year-old, and 14.7% in 12-year-old children [43]. In Australia, the Sydney Myopia Study (SMS) reported that myopia was present in 1.43% in 1765 children aged 7 years, with 0.79% in European children and 2.73% in other ethnicity children [45]. The Sydney Adolescent Vascular and Eye Study (SAVES) reported the myopia prevalence to be 18.9% among 12-year-old children, with 52.5% in East Asian, 8.6% in European Caucasian, and 12.0% in other ethnicity groups [44]. However, these ethnic differences may not be based solely on genetic differences. Studies on migrant populations suggest that the prevalence of myopia among Asian children living in non-Asian countries such as Australia is not as high as those living in East Asian countries [51]. Finally, in population-based studies, the lowest prevalence appears to be in Africa. The prevalence of myopia was 3.4% in 12-year-old to 15-year-old children in Ghana and 4.0% in 5-year-old to 15-year-old children in South Africa [46].

2.2.3 Urban and Rural Areas

Collectively, there are significant differences in the prevalence of myopia between urban areas and rural areas. In China, the prevalence of myopia was 38.1% in children aged 5–15 years in urban area, Guangzhou, whereas the prevalence of myopia was 5.0% in children aged 5–18 years in rural area. In an urban area,

Tehran, the prevalence of myopia was 7.2% in 809 children aged 5–15 years in the Tehran Eye Study, while a rural area, Dezful, had a lower prevalence of myopia which was 3.4% in children aged 7–15 years [35, 36]. A recent meta-analysis found a 2.6 times higher risk of developing myopia in children of urban residence compared with those who lived in rural areas [52]. These differences in the myopia prevalence among children may be caused by a rigorous education system which children especially living in urbanized are exposed to. Especially in Eastern Asian countries, academic success is important, and most children are enrolled in competitive, academically oriented schooling at a very early age [51]. It is influenced by enduring patterns of behavior and cultural attitudes that may result in the myopic environmental factors, such as higher levels of more intense near-work and lower levels of outdoor activity.

In summary, the prevalence of myopia in children is higher in East Asian countries (49.7–62.0% among 12-year-old children) compared with non-Asian countries and other Asian countries (6.0–20.0%). The prevalence of myopia has remained consistently high among Chinese children in urban settings, but the evidence does not support the idea that it is caused by purely genetic difference [53]. The association of an urbanized setting with high myopia rates is likely to be influenced by possible modifiable risk factors such as near-work and outdoor time.

2.3 Prevalence of Myopia and HM in Teenagers and Young Adults

2.3.1 East Asian Countries

The prevalence of myopia in young adults is more than 80% in urbanized East Asian countries (Table 2.3). A remarkable increase in the myopia and HM prevalence was seen in the past decades. In China, Chen et al. conducted a 15-year population-based survey using noncycloplegic autorefraction to investigate trends in the prevalence of myopia among 43,858 high school students in Fenghua city, eastern China, from 2001 to 2015. The overall prevalence of myopia and HM increased from 79.5% to 87.7% and 7.9% to 16.6%, respectively, during the 15-year period [54]. In Shandong, another city in eastern China, the prevalence of myopia and HM using cycloplegic autorefraction in school children aged 17 years was 84.6% and 13.9%, respectively [55]. A cross-sectional study among 5083 university students in Shanghai showed that 95.5% were myopic and 19.5% were high myopic (SE <−6.0 D) [56]. In Korea, the prevalence of myopia and HM (SE <−6.0 D) using cycloplegic autorefraction was higher in an urban population (96.5% and 21.6%) [8], compared to a rural population (83.3% and 6.8%) [26], among 19-year-old males in military conscripts. In Taiwan, the prevalence of myopia and HM (SE <−6.0 D) was 86.1% and 21.2%, respectively, in males aged 18–24 years in military conscripts [57]. In Singapore, the overall myopia and HM prevalence in 28,906 young males aged 16–25 years increased from 79.2% and 13.1% in 1996–1997 to 81.6% and 14.7% in 2009–2010, respectively [58].

Table 2.3 Summary of prevalence of myopia and high myopia in teenager and adolescent in East Asian countries

Study (authors, year)	Location	Number	Race gender	Age (year)	Refraction method	Response rate (%)	Description of source	Prevalence (%)	95% CI
Chen et al. (2018) [54]	Fenghua suburban, China	$N = 2932$	Chinese male/ female	18.31 ± 0.60	Noncycloplegic autorefraction	NA	Population-based national college entrance examination	M: 87.7% HM: 16.6% (≤−6.0 D)	NA
Wu et al. (2013) [55]	Shandong, China	$N = 6026$	Chinese male/ female	17	Cycloplegic autorefraction	94.7	Random cluster sampling in a cross-sectional school-based study design	M: 84.6% HM: 13.9%	(78.0–91.0%) (7.8–19.9%)
Sun et al. (2012) [56]	Shanghai, China	$N = 5083$	Chinese male/ female	20.2 ± 2.8	Noncycloplegic autorefraction	92.8	Specific population of Chinese University students	M: 95.5% HM: 19.5% (≤−6.0 D)	(94.9–96.1%) (18.4–20.6%)
Lee et al. (2013) [26]	Rural area, South Korea	$N = 02805$	Korean male	19	Cycloplegic autorefraction	100	Population-based male compulsory conscripts	M: 83.3% HM: 6.8% (≤−6.0 D)	(81.8–84.7%)
Jung et al. (2012) [8]	South Korea	$N = 23{,}616$	Korean male	19	Cycloplegic autorefraction	100	Population-based male compulsory conscripts	M: 96.5% HM: 21.6% (≤−6.0 D)	(96.3–96.8%) (20.5–22.8%)
Lee et al. (2013) [57]	Taiwan	$N = 5048$	Chinese male	18–24	Noncycloplegic autorefraction	98.1	Population-based Male compulsory conscripts	M: 86.1% HM: 21.2% (≤−6.0 D)	NA
Koh et al. (2014) [58]	Singapore	$N = 28{,}908$	Chinese Malay Indian male	19.8 ± 1.2	Noncycloplegic autorefraction	99.9	Population-based male compulsory conscripts	M: 81.6% HM: 14.7%	(81.1–82.0%) (14.3–15.1%)

NA not applicable, *M* myopia, *HM* high myopia

2.3.2 Rest of East Asian Countries

In contrast to the uniformly high prevalence in Eastern Asian countries, the prevalence of myopia and HM in young adult populations in other countries varies among different ethnicity and geography (Table 2.4). In Israel, a 13-year series of population-based prevalence survey was conducted on young adults aged 16–22 years during the years 1990–2002. The overall prevalence of myopia and HM (SE <−6.0 D) using noncycloplegic autorefraction increased from 20.3% and 1.7% in 1990 to 28.3% and 2.05% in 2002, respectively [59]. In the Tehran Eye Study, the prevalence of myopia using cycloplegic autorefraction was 29.3% among young adults aged 16–25 years [36]. In Australia, the prevalence of myopia was 20.4% in a population-based cohort using cycloplegic autorefraction in mostly White subjects aged 19–22 years [60]. In the Sydney Adolescent Vascular and Eye Study (SAVES), myopia was present in 30.8%, with 59.1% in East Asian, 17.7% in European Caucasian, and 34.9% in other ethnicity group; and HM (SE <−6.00 D) was present in 1.9% among 17-year-old young adults [44]. In Europe, the prevalence of myopia and HM (SE <−6.50 D) among 4681 Danish conscripts was 12.8% and 0.3%, respectively [61]. A population-based study in Norway reported that 35.0% were myopic among 1248 young adults aged 20–25 years [62]. In the United States, the myopic prevalence rate was 27.7% in young adults aged 18–24 years [63].

As shown above, the myopia prevalence among young adults in East Asia is much higher than in Western countries. This is most likely reflecting the higher myopia prevalence among school children in Eastern Asia and can be further accelerated by their education system. This age population usually spend much time in study and are expected to achieve high scores for competitive college entrance examination, especially in Asia. In one study conducted in China, the prevalence of myopia in postgraduates was higher than in undergraduates [56], suggesting that associated factors, such as higher school achievement and prolonged near-work and less outdoor time, might contribute to the increasing prevalence of myopia [51]. We summarized the myopia prevalence in East Asian countries (Table 2.3) and rest of East Asian countries (Table 2.4). When comparing the results, we must be cautious because some conscript-based studies investigated only men, and conducted eye examination without cycloplegic refraction, which may make the refraction overestimated approximately over −0.50 D in younger adults [64].

2.4 Prevalence of Myopia and HM in Adults

In adults, the prevalence rates of myopia vary widely with age reflecting the hyperopic shift by aging in older generations. According to the results from the Beaver Dam Eye Study, the prevalence of myopia was likely to decrease with age among individuals aged above 43 years [65]. Wong et al. showed that the highest prevalence of myopia was in the age group of 40 years and above 70 years among Chinese-Singaporean adults aged 40–81 years old [66]. It suggested that the prevalence in elderly adults older 70 years could be overestimated due to lens nuclear sclerosis

Table 2.4 Summary of prevalence of myopia and high myopia in teenager and adolescent in rest of East Asian countries

Study (authors, year)	Location	Number	Race gender	Age (year)	Refraction method	Response rate (%)	Description of source	Prevalence (%)	95%CI
Bar Dayan et al. (2005) [59]	Israel	$N = 919,929$	Male/ female	16–22	Noncycloplegic autorefraction		Retrospective study, based on 13 repeated prevalence surveys	M: 28.3% HM: 2.0% (M) HM: 2.3% (F) (≤−6.0 D)	NA
Hashemi (2004) [36]	Tehran, Iran	$N = 974$	Iranian male/ female	16–25	Cycloplegic autorefraction	70.3	Stratified random cluster sampling, door-to-door surveys	M: 29.3%	(26.0–32.7%)
McKnight et al. (2014) [60]	Australia	$N = 1315$	Mix ethnicity male/ female	19–22	Cycloplegic autorefraction	97.8	Population-based cross-sectional study	M: 20.4% HM: –	(21.4–25.9%)
French (2013) [44]	Australia	$N = 1157$	Mix ethnicity male/ female	17	Cycloplegic autorefraction	51.5	Random stratified cluster-sample of 55 schools	M: 30.8% HM: 1.9%	(22.5–39.0%)
Jacobsen et al. (2007) [61]	Denmark	$N = 4681$	Danish male	19.3 ± 1.6	Noncycloplegic autorefraction	NA	Population-based male compulsory conscripts	M: 12.8% HM: 0.3% (≤−6.5 D)	(11.8–13.8%) (0.2–0.5%)
Midelfart et al. (2002) [62]	Norway	$N = 1248$	Euro male/ female	20–25	Noncycloplegic autorefraction	NA	Population-based sample in a health study (HUNT)	M: 35.0% HM: –	NA
Sperduto et al. (1983) [63]	USA	$N = 9882$	Mix male/ female	18–24	Noncycloplegic autorefraction	69.9	Population-based sample in a National Health Nutrition Examination Survey	M: 27.7%	NA

NA not applicable, *Euro* European, *M* myopia, *HM* high myopia

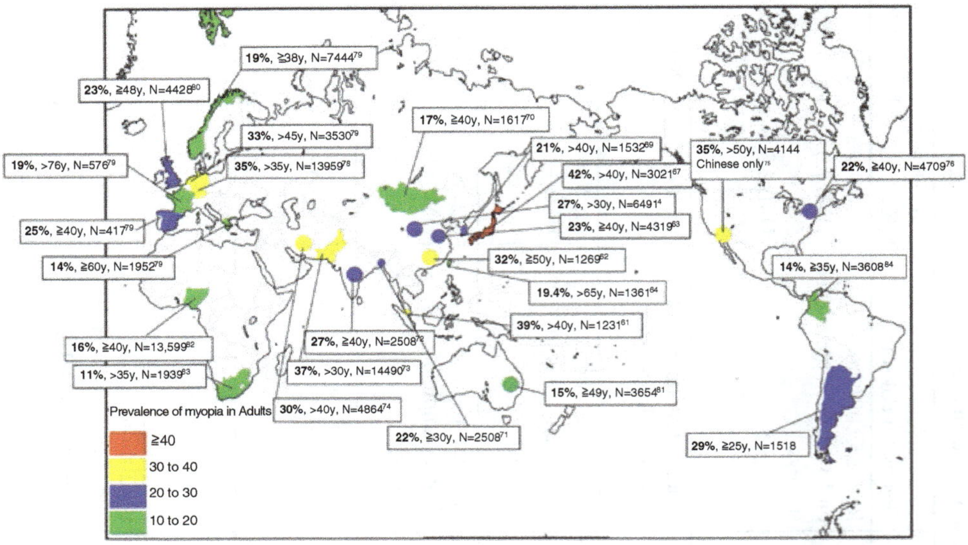

Fig. 2.1 Reported prevalence of myopia in adult population based on population studies

inducing refractive myopia. Population-based data indicate that Asian adult population is more susceptible to myopia compared with similarly aged western population. However, compared to the prevalence of myopia in children, the regional difference is not obvious in adults. We summarized the prevalence of myopia in adult population-based studies in the world (Fig. 2.1). It must be noted that there is lack of consensus in definitions of myopia and HM, and the definition varies among studies and that there is a difference of age population affecting by nuclear cataract, thus not directly comparable among different studies.

2.4.1 Asian Countries

2.4.1.1 East Asian Countries

In China, the prevalence of myopia and HM (SE <−6.0 D) was 32.3% and 5.0%, respectively, in 1269 adults aged 50 or more years in the Liwan Eye Study [67] conducted in an urban city of Guangzhou. In rural areas, 26.7% were myopic and 1.8% were high myopic in 6491 adults aged 30 or more years in the Handan Eye Study [4]. The Beijing Eye Study reported that the myopia and HM (SE <−6.0 D) prevalence was 22.9% and 2.6%, respectively, in 4319 adults aged 40 or more years in urban and rural Chinese populations [68]. However, these data may lead to substantial underestimation of the myopia prevalence because refraction data were obtained only from those with visual impairment. In Taiwan, the Shinpai Eye Study in adults aged over 65 years reported that the prevalence of myopia and HM (SD <−6.0 D) was 19.4% and 2.4%, respectively [69]. In Singapore, the prevalence of myopia in Singaporean-Chinese, Malay, and Indians was 38.7% [66], 26.2% [70], and 28.0% [71], and corresponding figures for HM being 9.1%, 3.9%, and 4.1%, respectively. In Japan, the prevalence of myopia and HM in urban areas is relatively high, 41.8% and 8.2%, respectively, in 3021 adults above 40 years in the Tajimi Study [72]. However, the myopia rates may be overestimated because of the use of noncycloplegic refraction for the younger population who may have excessive residual accommodation. A latest population-based study from a rural area showed that the prevalence of myopia and HM was 29.5% and 1.9%, respectively, among adults aged 40 years or older in the Kumejima Study [73]. In this study, the prevalence of myopia was nearly the same as those in urban areas of China, while the prevalence of HM was similar to that reported in rural areas of other Asian countries. In South Korea, the prevalence of myopia and HM was 20.5% and 1.0%, respectively, among adults above 40 years in the Namil Study [74]. Relatively low prevalence in the study was reflected by rural lesions, it was similar to that of rural Chinese population.

2.4.1.2 Rest of East Asian Countries

In other Asian developing countries, the prevalence of myopia is slightly lower: 17.2% among adults aged 40 or more years in Mongolia, and 22.1% among adults aged 30 or more years in Bangladesh [75, 76]. Further, the myopia rate in the Bangladesh study may be overestimated because of the use of noncycloplegic refraction for the younger group aged 30–39 years who may have excessive residual accommodation. In a rural area in India, the prevalence of myopia and HM was 27.0% and 3.7%, respectively, in 2508 Indian adults aged above 39 years [77]. Relatively high prevalence in rural Indian population may be caused by higher rates of nuclear cataract. The prevalence of myopia is slightly higher at 36.5% among adults aged 30 or more years in Pakistan, and at 30.2% among adults aged 40 or more years in Iran [78, 79]. The myopia rate in the Pakistan study may be overestimated because of the cohort effect of younger group aged 30–39 years.

2.4.2 Non-Asian Countries

In the USA, the latest report in the Chinese American study showed the relatively high prevalence of myopia and HM, 35.1% and 7.4%, respectively, in 4144 Chinese adults aged 50 years or older [80]. This result is similar to or slightly higher than same Chinese populations from other studies in urban Asian countries (38.7% in the Tanjong Pagar Study, Singapore and 32.3% in the Liwan Eye Study). The Barbados Eye Study reported the prevalence of myopia was 21.9% in 4709 African-Americans aged 40–84 years [81]. Another population-based study in Latino showed that the overall prevalence of myopia (SE <-1.00 D) and HM in the worse eye was 16.8% and 2.4%, respectively, among 5927 adults aged 40 years or older [82]. In Europe, although the myopia rate varies across the countries, two latest population-based studies proved that it was nearly the same as those in urban Asian countries. The Gutenburg Health Study in Germany reported that the prevalence of myopia and HM was 35.1% and 5.6%, respectively, in 13,959 adults aged 35–74 years. The high prevalence of myopia in the study can be explained by the fact that this cohort had younger participants than most other studies [83]. In the Netherlands, the prevalence of myopia was 32.5% in a total of 3530 adults aged above 46 years in the Rotterdam study [84]. This study may have overestimated the prevalence of myopia because the refraction method was subjective refraction. In UK, a population-based study showed that 23.0% were myopic among a total of 7444 adults aged above 48 years [85]. In other European countries, the prevalence of myopia is slightly lower: 19.4% among adults aged 38 or more years in Norway, 19.1% among adults aged 76 or more years in France, and 14.2% among adults aged 60 or more years in Greece [84]. In Australia, the prevalence of myopia was relatively lower, 15.0% in 3654 adults aged over 49 years in the Blue Mountain Eye Study in 1999 [86]. In the two population-based studies, the lowest prevalence appears to be in Africa. In Nigeria, the prevalence of myopia and HM was 16.1% and 2.1%, respectively, among 13,599 adults aged over 40 years as per the Nigeria National Blindness and Visual Impairment Study [87]. In South Africa, the prevalence of myopia was 11.4% in 1939 adults aged over 35 years [88]. In the same vein, the prevalence of myopia was relatively low 14.4% among adults aged 35–55 years in MIROR Study in Colombia [89].

2.4.3 Generational Gap

There is a difference in myopia and HM prevalence among age groups. In general, the generational differences of prevalence of myopia and HM are seen with the highest rates in young adults and the lowest rates in older adults. We have shown the higher prevalence rates of myopia (65.5–96.5%) and HM (14.7–21.6%) in East Asian young adults in the previous section [8, 57, 58]. By contrast, the lower prevalence rates of myopia (approximately 25–40%) and HM (2.4–8.2%) were reported among East Asian middle-aged and elderly adults [69, 72, 90]. Particularly, the burden of HM is important because HM is more likely to develop PM changes that tend to be visually disabling. Some studies supported the idea of two types of HM, one is related to educational parameters such as near-work and frequent among young adults, and the other is more likely related to the earlier onset of myopia by genetic factors in contrast to environmental factors and occurs in older adults [91, 92]. Jonas et al. compared highly myopic young individuals and highly myopic adult individuals and assessed the association of the prevalence of HM with parameters of education. It revealed that education-related parameters did not show a clear association with HM in older generation, while in contrast, HM in school children showed a strong association with education [91]. Thus, it has been assumed that the development of pathologic myopia (PM) in later life may be different depending on two forms of HM with different etiologies. One form of HM is caused by mutations of genes responsible to scleral modeling and leading to abnormal deformity and thin sclera [93], while the other form caused by insufficient outdoor time in younger adults may be driven by reduced release of retinal dopamine [1].

In summary, the higher prevalence rates of myopia were also seen in urban East Asian countries (approximately 25–40%) and in Western Europe or the United States (approximately 20–35%), compared to other developing Asian countries and some countries in Western populations such as Australia (approximately 15–20%). Similarly, urban Asian countries have higher prevalence rates of HM (5–9%), compared with other Asian countries (2–5%) or non-Asian countries (2–7%). However, the geographic difference of myopia prevalence in older populations is not pronounced compared to that in younger populations. From a viewpoint of ethnicity difference, Chinese have a substantially higher prevalence of myopia compared with other racial groups, and a similar pattern of even greater magnitude was seen in HM prevalence. The prevalence of myopia and HM in Chinese ethnicity in western countries is similar to other studies of Chinese in urban Asian countries [80].

2.5 The Prevalence of PM

Pathologic myopia (PM) has been reported as one of the most common causes of blindness worldwide. Studies reported that PM is the major cause of blindness or visual impairment (VI) in 7% in Western populations and in 12–27% in Asian populations [94–99]. According to a review to estimate blindness and VI with myopic macular degeneration (MMD), 10.0 million people had VI from MMD (0.13%), 3.3 million of whom were blind (0.04%) in 2015, and furthermore 55.7 million people will have VI from MMD (0.33%), 18.5 million of whom will be blind (0.19%) in 2050 [100].

Before we discuss the prevalence of PM in detail, it must be noted that the definition of PM has been inconsistent in previous studies. Avila et al. proposed a definition of myopic maculopathy that included posterior staphyloma, and it has been used most frequently in earlier studies [101]. However, this classification was not based on the actual progression pattern. In 2015, the META-analysis for Pathologic Myopia (META-PM) study group proposed a new classification system for PM for use in future studies [102]. In this classification, myopic macular degeneration (MMD) is categorized into 5 categories according to severity: no myopic retinal lesions (category 0); tessellated fundus only (category 1); diffuse chorioretinal atrophy (category 2); patchy chorioretinal atrophy (category 3); and macula atrophy (category 4). And three additional lesions of MMD that cause central vision loss were included as plus sign: lacquer cracks, myopic choroidal neovascularization (CNV), Fuchs spot. PM is defined if an eye has category 2 or above, or presence of plus sign, or the presence of posterior staphyloma. We summarized population-based studies on PM prevalence in adult populations (Fig. 2.2).

In China, the Beijing Eye Study showed a high PM prevalence, 3.1%, among 4319 Chinese subjects aged 40 years or older [103]. PM was defined with myopic chorioretinal atrophy or staphyloma or lacquer cracks or Fuch's spot. In the same definition, the Handan Eye Study showed that the prevalence of PM and HM was 0.9% and 2.1%, respectively, among 6603 Chinese subjects aged 30 years or older

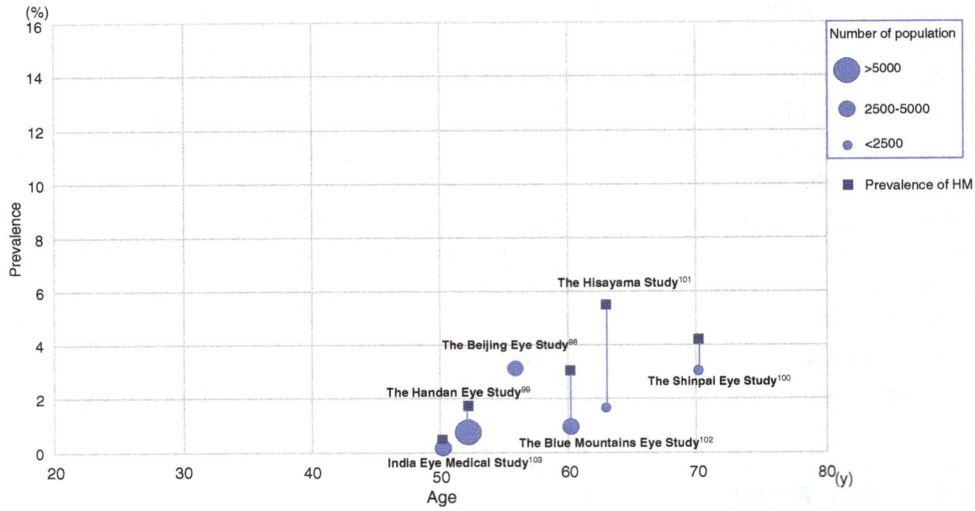

Fig. 2.2 Prevalence of pathologic myopia (PM) among adults in population-based studies

[104]. The much lower prevalence in this study than Beijing might be due to urban and rural differences. Among 1058 Taiwanese subjects aged 65 years or older in the Shinpai Eye study, the prevalence of PM and HM was 3% and 4.2%, respectively, with the definition by Avila et al. [105]. The high prevalence was influenced by its older population than other population-based studies. The Hisayama study reported the prevalence of PM and HM was 1.7% and 5.7%, respectively, among 1892 Japanese aged 40 years or older with the definition of PM as myopic chorioretinal atrophy, lacquer cracks, or Fuch's spot [106]. However, this study cannot exclude the possibility of sampling bias because the response rate was only 44.4%. In Western countries, the Blue Mountain Eye Study was performed in 3583 adults aged 49 years or older, who were mainly White urban population of Australia, using the same PM definition with two studies in China [107]. The prevalence of PM and HM was 1.2% and 2.7%, respectively. Using the new META-PM classification, the prevalence of PM and HM was 0.2% and 0.5%, respectively, among 4561 Indian subjects aged 30 years or older in rural central India [108]. However, the population in this study may not be adequately representative of the whole population of India because this study was conducted in rural tribal regions.

As shown above, the prevalence of PM among adult populations was relatively low in the world. Furthermore, the prevalence of PM among middle-aged and elderly adults is higher in urban East Asian populations (1.7–3.1%) than rural Asian populations (0.2–0.9%) and non-Asian populations (1.2%) [109]. It is consistent with the results of higher prevalence of HM in East Asian countries because the risk of PM increases with HM [109]. Both the prevalence and severity of PM become higher in adult population aged 40 years and with severe high myopia. Compared to the PM prevalence in adult populations, adolescents and children have significantly lower prevalence [27, 110]. It supports the idea that myopic macular changes are time-dependent changes as a result of mechanical stretching of the retina from axial elongation. However, a recent report revealed that myopia-related changes of the optic disc and macula were commonly found in highly myopic eyes in young adults [111].

Thus, the disease burden of PM due to high myopia is likely to increase in future, contributed by the aging effect where young adults who have high rates of high myopia will grow older.

2.6 Conclusion

In children, the prevalence of myopia is substantially higher in urban East Asian countries (49.7–62.0% among 12-year-old children) compared with other countries (6.0–20.0% among 12-year-old children). Similarly, in teenagers and young adults, the prevalence of myopia is higher in East Asian countries (65.5–96.5%) compared with other countries (12.8–35.0%). However, the geographic difference of myopia prevalence in older populations is less than that of younger populations. The prevalence rates of myopia in adults in urban East Asian countries are only slightly higher than in Western countries.

A relationship between myopia prevalence and community development is apparent, and most data have shown urban areas have a higher prevalence of myopia than rural areas. The association of an urbanized environment with myopia development in Asia could be mediated by factors such as intensive education and greater levels of near-work and less outdoor time. Overall, the prevalence of myopia in child population seems to be strongly related to the region where they grow up and the environmental factors such as urbanization, economy, and education.

Generational differences are seen with the highest rates in young adults (myopia 65.5–96.5% and HM 6.8–21.6%) and the lowest rates in older adults (myopia 25.0–40.0% and HM 2.4–8.2%). The disease progression pattern of HM and subsequent development of PM may be different between young adults and older adults due to generational differences, or changes in the lifestyle factors such as the education system and near-work and outdoor time exposure in rapidly developing urban Asian countries.

Current data show a relatively low prevalence of PM among middle-aged and elderly adults so far, and PM increases with age over 40 years and severity of myopia. Despite the relatively low prevalence in general population, PM is the major cause of blindness or visual impairment in both Asian populations and Western populations. According to a previous study, early grades of PM lesions are observed in young highly myopic adults in urban Asian population, and these structure changes are likely to worsen with age [111]. Considering the increasing prevalence of HM among young generations, we must be prepared for the expected increase of disease burden of PM in the near future.

References

1. Dolgin E. The myopia boom. Nature. 2015;519(7543):276–8.
2. Vitale S, Cotch MF, Sperduto RD. Prevalence of visual impairment in the United States. JAMA. 2006;295(18):2158–63.
3. Zheng YF, Pan CW, Chay J, Wong TY, Finkelstein E, Saw SM. The economic cost of myopia in adults aged over 40 years in Singapore. Invest Ophthalmol Vis Sci. 2013;54(12):7532–7.

4. Liang YB, Wong TY, Sun LP, Tao QS, Wang JJ, Yang XH, et al. Refractive errors in a rural Chinese adult population the Handan eye study. Ophthalmology. 2009;116(11):2119–27.
5. Morgan IG, Ohno-Matsui K, Saw S-M. Myopia. Lancet. 2012;379(9827):1739–48.
6. Morgan IG. What public policies should be developed to deal with the epidemic of myopia? Optom Vis Sci. 2016;93(9):1058–60.
7. Lin LL, Shih YF, Hsiao CK, Chen CJ. Prevalence of myopia in Taiwanese school children: 1983 to 2000. Ann Acad Med. 2004;33(1):27–33.
8. Jung SK, Lee JH, Kakizaki H, Jee D. Prevalence of myopia and its association with body stature and educational level in 19-year-old male conscripts in Seoul, South Korea. Invest Ophthalmol Vis Sci. 2012;53(9):5579–83.
9. Holden BA, Fricke TR, Wilson DA, Jong M, Naidoo KS, Sankaridurg P, et al. Global prevalence of myopia and high myopia and temporal trends from 2000 through 2050. Ophthalmology. 2016;123(5):1036–42.
10. Wong TY, Ferreira A, Hughes R, Carter G, Mitchell P. Epidemiology and disease burden of pathologic myopia and myopic choroidal neovascularization: an evidence-based systematic review. Am J Ophthalmol. 2014;157(1):9–25.e12.
11. Zhao J, Mao J, Luo R, Li F, Pokharel GP, Ellwein LB. Accuracy of noncycloplegic autorefraction in school-age children in China. Optom Vis Sci. 2004;81(1):49–55.
12. Fotedar R, Rochtchina E, Morgan I, Wang JJ, Mitchell P, Rose KA. Necessity of cycloplegia for assessing refractive error in 12-year-old children: a population-based study. Am J Ophthalmol. 2007;144(2):307–9.
13. Saw SM, Tong L, Chua WH, Chia KS, Koh D, Tan DT, et al. Incidence and progression of myopia in Singaporean school children. Invest Ophthalmol Vis Sci. 2005;46(1):51–7.
14. Fan DS, Lam DS, Lam RF, Lau JT, Chong KS, Cheung EY, et al. Prevalence, incidence, and progression of myopia of school children in Hong Kong. Invest Ophthalmol Vis Sci. 2004;45(4):1071–5.
15. He M, Zeng J, Liu Y, Xu J, Pokharel GP, Ellwein LB. Refractive error and visual impairment in urban children in Southern China. Invest Ophthalmol Vis Sci. 2004;45(3):793–9.
16. Zadnik K. The Glenn A. Fry Award Lecture (1995). Myopia development in childhood. Optom Vis Sci. 1997;74(8):603–8.
17. O'Donoghue L, Kapetanankis VV, McClelland JF, Logan NS, Owen CG, Saunders KJ, et al. Risk factors for childhood myopia: findings from the NICER study. Invest Ophthalmol Vis Sci. 2015;56(3):1524–30.
18. Ip JM, Huynh SC, Robaei D, Kifley A, Rose KA, Morgan IG, et al. Ethnic differences in refraction and ocular biometry in a population-based sample of 11-15-year-old Australian children. Eye. 2008;22(5):649–56.
19. Murthy GV, Gupta SK, Ellwein LB, Munoz SR, Pokharel GP, Sanga L, et al. Refractive error in children in an urban population in New Delhi. Invest Ophthalmol Vis Sci. 2002;43(3): 623–31.
20. Sapkota YD, Adhikari BN, Pokharel GP, Poudyal BK, Ellwein LB. The prevalence of visual impairment in school children of upper-middle socioeconomic status in Kathmandu. Ophthalmic Epidemiol. 2008;15(1):17–23.
21. Gao Z, Meng N, Muecke J, Chan WO, Piseth H, Kong A, et al. Refractive error in school children in an urban and rural setting in Cambodia. Ophthalmic Epidemiol. 2012;19(1):16–22.
22. Hsu CC, Huang N, Lin PY, Tsai DC, Tsai CY, Woung LC, et al. Prevalence and risk factors for myopia in second-grade primary school children in Taipei: a population-based study. J Chin Med Assoc. 2016;79(11):625–32.
23. Lai YH, Hsu HT, Wang HZ, Chang SJ, Wu WC. The visual status of children ages 3 to 6 years in the vision screening program in Taiwan. J AAPOS. 2009;13(1):58–62.
24. Li Y, Liu J, Qi P. The increasing prevalence of myopia in junior high school students in the haidian district of beijing, china: A 10-year population-based survey. BMC Ophthalmol. 2017;17:88.
25. Ma Y, Qu X, Zhu X, Xu X, Zhu J, Sankaridurg P, et al. Age-specific prevalence of visual impairment and refractive error in children aged 3-10 years in Shanghai, China. Invest Ophthalmol Vis Sci. 2016;57(14):6188–96.

26. Lee JH, Jee D, Kwon JW, Lee WK. Prevalence and risk factors for myopia in a rural Korean population. Invest Ophthalmol Vis Sci. 2013;54(8):5466–71.
27. Pi LH, Chen L, Liu Q, Ke N, Fang J, Zhang S, et al. Prevalence of eye diseases and causes of visual impairment in school-aged children in Western China. J Epidemiol. 2012;22(1):37–44.
28. He M, Huang W, Zheng Y, Huang L, Ellwein LB. Refractive error and visual impairment in school children in rural southern china. Ophthalmology. 2007;114:374–82.
29. Zhao J, Pan X, Sui R, Munoz SR, Sperduto RD, Ellwein LB. Refractive error study in children: results from Shunyi District, China. Am J Ophthalmol. 2000;129(4):427–35.
30. Fan DS, Lai C, Lau HH, Cheung EY, Lam DS. Change in vision disorders among Hong Kong preschoolers in 10 years. Clin Exp Ophthalmol. 2011;39(5):398–403.
31. Dirani M, Chan YH, Gazzard G, Hornbeak DM, Leo SW, Selvaraj P, et al. Prevalence of refractive error in Singaporean Chinese children: the strabismus, amblyopia, and refractive error in young Singaporean Children (STARS) study. Invest Ophthalmol Vis Sci. 2010;51(3):1348–55.
32. Dandona R, Dandona L, Srinivas M, Giridhar P, McCarty CA, Rao GN. Population-based assessment of refractive error in India: the Andhra Pradesh eye disease study. Clin Exp Ophthalmol. 2002;30(2):84–93.
33. Yekta A, Fotouhi A, Hashemi H, Dehghani C, Ostadimoghaddam H, Heravian J, et al. Prevalence of refractive errors among schoolchildren in Shiraz, Iran. Clin Exp Ophthalmol. 2010;38(3):242–8.
34. Jamali P, Fotouhi A, Hashemi H, Younesian M, Jafari A. Refractive errors and amblyopia in children entering school: Shahrood, iran. Optom Vis Sci. 2009;86:364–9.
35. Fotouhi A, Hashemi H, Khabazkhoob M, Mohammad K. The prevalence of refractive errors among schoolchildren in Dezful, Iran. Br J Ophthalmol. 2007;91(3):287–92.
36. Hashemi H, Fotouhi A, Mohammad K. The age- and gender-specific prevalences of refractive errors in Tehran: the Tehran Eye Study. Ophthalmic Epidemiol. 2004;11(3):213–25.
37. Yingyong P. Refractive errors survey in primary school children (6-12 year old) in 2 provinces: Bangkok and Nakhonpathom (one year result). J Med Assoc Thail. 2010;93(10):1205–10.
38. Wen G, Tarczy-Hornoch K, McKean-Cowdin R, Cotter SA, Borchert M, Lin J, et al. Prevalence of myopia, hyperopia, and astigmatism in non-Hispanic white and Asian children: multi-ethnic pediatric eye disease study. Ophthalmology. 2013;120(10):2109–16.
39. Giordano L, Friedman DS, Repka MX, Katz J, Ibironke J, Hawes P, et al. Prevalence of refractive error among preschool children in an urban population: the Baltimore Pediatric Eye Disease Study. Ophthalmology. 2009;116(4):739–46.
40. Tideman JWL, Polling JR, Hofman A, Jaddoe VW, Mackenbach JP, Klaver CC. Environmental factors explain socioeconomic prevalence differences in myopia in 6-year-old children. Br J Ophthalmol. 2018;102(2):243–7.
41. Logan NS, Shah P, Rudnicka AR, Gilmartin B, Owen CG. Childhood ethnic differences in ametropia and ocular biometry: the Aston Eye Study. Ophthalmic Physiol Opt. 2011;31(5):550–8.
42. O'Donoghue L, McClelland JF, Logan NS, Rudnicka AR, Owen CG, Saunders KJ. Refractive error and visual impairment in school children in northern ireland. Br J Ophthalmol. 2010;94:1155–9.
43. Czepita D, Zejmo M, Mojsa A. Prevalence of myopia and hyperopia in a population of polish school children. Ophthalmic Physiol Opt. 2007;27(1):60–5.
44. French AN, Morgan IG, Burlutsky G, Mitchell P, Rose KA. Prevalence and 5- to 6-year incidence and progression of myopia and hyperopia in Australian school children. Ophthalmology. 2013;120(7):1482–91.
45. Ojaimi E, Rose KA, Morgan IG, Smith W, Martin FJ, Kifley A, et al. Distribution of ocular biometric parameters and refraction in a population-based study of Australian children. Invest Ophthalmol Vis Sci. 2005;46(8):2748–54.
46. Kumah BD, Ebri A, Abdul-Kabir M, Ahmed AS, Koomson NY, Aikins S, et al. Refractive error and visual impairment in private school children in Ghana. Optom Vis Sci. 2013;90(12):1456–61.
47. Naidoo KS, Raghunandan A, Mashige KP, Govender P, Holden BA, Pokharel GP, Ellwein LB. Refractive error and visual impairment in african children in south africa. Invest Ophthalmol Vis Sci. 2003;44:3764–70.

48. Goh PP, Abqariyah Y, Pokharel GP, Ellwein LB. Refractive error and visual impairment in school-age children in Gombak District, Malaysia. Ophthalmology. 2005;112(4):678–85.
49. Li Z, Xu K, Wu S, Lv J, Jin D, Song Z, et al. Population-based survey of refractive error among school-aged children in rural northern China: the Heilongjiang eye study. Clin Exp Ophthalmol. 2014;42(4):379–84.
50. Saw SM, Carkeet A, Chia KS, Stone RA, Tan DT. Component dependent risk factors for ocular parameters in Singapore Chinese children. Ophthalmology. 2002;109(11):2065–71.
51. Rose KA, Morgan IG, Smith W, Burlutsky G, Mitchell P, Saw SM. Myopia, lifestyle, and schooling in students of Chinese ethnicity in Singapore and Sydney. Arch Ophthalmol. 2008;126(4):527–30.
52. Rudnicka AR, Kapetanakis VV, Wathern AK, Logan NS, Gilmartin B, Whincup PH, et al. Global variations and time trends in the prevalence of childhood myopia, a systematic review and quantitative meta-analysis: implications for aetiology and early prevention. Br J Ophthalmol. 2016;100(7):882–90.
53. Ding BY, Shih YF, Lin LLK, Hsiao CK, Wang IJ. Myopia among schoolchildren in East Asia and Singapore. Surv Ophthalmol. 2017;62(5):677–97.
54. Chen M, Wu A, Zhang L, Wang W, Chen X, Yu X, et al. The increasing prevalence of myopia and high myopia among high school students in Fenghua city, eastern China: a 15-year population-based survey. BMC Ophthalmol. 2018;18(1):159.
55. Wu JF, Bi HS, Wang SM, Hu YY, Wu H, Sun W, et al. Refractive error, visual acuity and causes of vision loss in children in Shandong, China. The Shandong Children Eye Study. PLoS One. 2013;8(12):e82763.
56. Sun J, Zhou J, Zhao P, Lian J, Zhu H, Zhou Y, et al. High prevalence of myopia and high myopia in 5060 Chinese university students in Shanghai. Invest Ophthalmol Vis Sci. 2012;53(12):7504–9.
57. Lee YY, Lo CT, Sheu SJ, Lin JL. What factors are associated with myopia in young adults? A survey study in Taiwan Military Conscripts. Invest Ophthalmol Vis Sci. 2013;54(2):1026–33.
58. Koh V, Yang A, Saw SM, Chan YH, Lin ST, Tan MM, et al. Differences in prevalence of refractive errors in young Asian males in Singapore between 1996-1997 and 2009-2010. Ophthalmic Epidemiol. 2014;21(4):247–55.
59. Bar Dayan Y, Levin A, Morad Y, Grotto I, Ben-David R, Goldberg A, et al. The changing prevalence of myopia in young adults: a 13-year series of population-based prevalence surveys. Invest Ophthalmol Vis Sci. 2005;46(8):2760–5.
60. McKnight CM, Sherwin JC, Yazar S, Forward H, Tan AX, Hewitt AW, et al. Myopia in young adults is inversely related to an objective marker of ocular sun exposure: the Western Australian Raine cohort study. Am J Ophthalmol. 2014;158(5):1079–85.
61. Jacobsen N, Jensen H, Goldschmidt E. Prevalence of myopia in Danish conscripts. Acta Ophthalmol Scand. 2007;85(2):165–70.
62. Midelfart A, Kinge B, Midelfart S, Lydersen S. Prevalence of refractive errors in young and middle-aged adults in Norway. Acta Ophthalmol Scand. 2002;80(5):501–5.
63. Sperduto RD, Seigel D, Roberts J, Rowland M. Prevalence of myopia in the United States. Arch Ophthalmol. 1983;101(3):405–7.
64. Mimouni M, Zoller L, Horowitz J, Wygnanski-Jaffe T, Morad Y, Mezer E. Cycloplegic autorefraction in young adults: is it mandatory? Graefes Arch Clin Exp Ophthalmol. 2016;254(2):395–8.
65. Wang Q, Klein BE, Klein R, Moss SE. Refractive status in the Beaver Dam Eye Study. Invest Ophthalmol Vis Sci. 1994;35(13):4344–7.
66. Wong TY, Foster PJ, Hee J, Ng TP, Tielsch JM, Chew SJ, et al. Prevalence and risk factors for refractive errors in adult Chinese in Singapore. Invest Ophthalmol Vis Sci. 2000;41(9):2486–94.
67. He M, Huang W, Li Y, Zheng Y, Yin Q, Foster PJ. Refractive error and biometry in older Chinese adults: the Liwan eye study. Invest Ophthalmol Vis Sci. 2009;50(11):5130–6.
68. Xu L, Li J, Cui T, Hu A, Fan G, Zhang R, et al. Refractive error in urban and rural adult Chinese in Beijing. Ophthalmology. 2005;112(10):1676–83.
69. Cheng CY, Hsu WM, Liu JH, Tsai SY, Chou P. Refractive errors in an elderly Chinese population in Taiwan: the Shihpai Eye Study. Invest Ophthalmol Vis Sci. 2003;44(11):4630–8.

70. Saw SM, Chan YH, Wong WL, Shankar A, Sandar M, Aung T, et al. Prevalence and risk factors for refractive errors in the Singapore Malay Eye Survey. Ophthalmology. 2008;115(10):1713–9.
71. Pan CW, Wong TY, Lavanya R, Wu RY, Zheng YF, Lin XY, et al. Prevalence and risk factors for refractive errors in Indians: the Singapore Indian Eye Study (SINDI). Invest Ophthalmol Vis Sci. 2011;52(6):3166–73.
72. Sawada A, Tomidokoro A, Araie M, Iwase A, Yamamoto T. Refractive errors in an elderly Japanese population: the Tajimi study. Ophthalmology. 2008;115(2):363–70.e3.
73. Nakamura Y, Nakamura Y, Higa A, Sawaguchi S, Tomidokoro A, Iwase A, et al. Refractive errors in an elderly rural Japanese population: the Kumejima study. PLoS One. 2018;13(11):e0207180.
74. Yoo YC, Kim JM, Park KH, Kim CY, Kim TW. Refractive errors in a rural Korean adult population: the Namil Study. Eye. 2013;27(12):1368–75.
75. Wickremasinghe S, Foster PJ, Uranchimeg D, Lee PS, Devereux JG, Alsbirk PH, et al. Ocular biometry and refraction in Mongolian adults. Invest Ophthalmol Vis Sci. 2004;45(3):776–83.
76. Bourne RR, Dineen BP, Ali SM, Noorul Huq DM, Johnson GJ. Prevalence of refractive error in Bangladeshi adults: results of the national blindness and low vision survey of Bangladesh. Ophthalmology. 2004;111(6):1150–60.
77. Raju P, Ramesh SV, Arvind H, George R, Baskaran M, Paul PG, et al. Prevalence of refractive errors in a rural South Indian population. Invest Ophthalmol Vis Sci. 2004;45(12):4268–72.
78. Shah SP, Jadoon MZ, Dineen B, Bourne RR, Johnson GJ, Gilbert CE, et al. Refractive errors in the adult pakistani population: the national blindness and visual impairment survey. Ophthalmic Epidemiol. 2008;15(3):183–90.
79. Hashemi H, Khabazkhoob M, Jafarzadehpur E, Yekta AA, Emamian MH, Shariati M, et al. High prevalence of myopia in an adult population, Shahroud, Iran. Optom Vis Sci. 2012;89(7):993–9.
80. Varma R, Torres M, McKean-Cowdin R, Rong F, Hsu C, Jiang X. Prevalence and risk factors for refractive error in adult Chinese Americans: The Chinese American Eye Study. Am J Ophthalmol. 2017;175:201–12.
81. Wu SY, Nemesure B, Leske MC. Refractive errors in a black adult population: the Barbados Eye Study. Invest Ophthalmol Vis Sci. 1999;40(10):2179–84.
82. Tarczy-Hornoch K, Ying-Lai M, Varma R. Myopic refractive error in adult Latinos: the Los Angeles Latino Eye Study. Invest Ophthalmol Vis Sci. 2006;47(5):1845–52.
83. Wolfram C, Hohn R, Kottler U, Wild P, Blettner M, Buhren J, et al. Prevalence of refractive errors in the European adult population: the Gutenberg Health Study (GHS). Br J Ophthalmol. 2014;98(7):857–61.
84. Williams KM, Verhoeven VJ, Cumberland P, Bertelsen G, Wolfram C, Buitendijk GH, et al. Prevalence of refractive error in Europe: the European Eye Epidemiology (E(3)) Consortium. Eur J Epidemiol. 2015;30(4):305–15.
85. Sherwin JC, Khawaja AP, Broadway D, Luben R, Hayat S, Dalzell N, et al. Uncorrected refractive error in older British adults: the EPIC-Norfolk Eye Study. Br J Ophthalmol. 2012;96(7):991–6.
86. Attebo K, Ivers RQ, Mitchell P. Refractive errors in an older population: the Blue Mountains Eye Study. Ophthalmology. 1999;106(6):1066–72.
87. Ezelum C, Razavi H, Sivasubramaniam S, Gilbert CE, Murthy GV, Entekume G, et al. Refractive error in Nigerian adults: prevalence, type, and spectacle coverage. Invest Ophthalmol Vis Sci. 2011;52(8):5449–56.
88. Mashige KP, Jaggernath J, Ramson P, Martin C, Chinanayi FS, Naidoo KS. Prevalence of refractive errors in the INK Area, Durban, South Africa. Optom Vis Sci. 2016;93(3):243–50.
89. Galvis V, Tello A, Otero J, Serrano AA, Gomez LM, Camacho PA, et al. Prevalence of refractive errors in Colombia: MIOPUR study. Br J Ophthalmol. 2018;102(10):1320–3.
90. Pan CW, Zheng YF, Anuar AR, Chew M, Gazzard G, Aung T, et al. Prevalence of refractive errors in a multiethnic Asian population: the Singapore epidemiology of eye disease study. Invest Ophthalmol Vis Sci. 2013;54(4):2590–8.

91. Jonas JB, Xu L, Wang YX, Bi HS, Wu JF, Jiang WJ, et al. Education-related parameters in high myopia: adults versus school children. PLoS One. 2016;11(5):e0154554.
92. Morgan I, Rose K. How genetic is school myopia? Prog Retin Eye Res. 2005;24(1):1–38.
93. Li YT, Xie MK, Wu J. Association between ocular axial length-related genes and high myopia in a Han Chinese Population. Ophthalmologica. 2016;235(1):57–60.
94. Ohno-Matsui K, Lai TY, Lai CC, Cheung CM. Updates of pathologic myopia. Prog Retin Eye Res. 2016;52:156–87.
95. Cedrone C, Culasso F, Cesareo M, Nucci C, Palma S, Mancino R, et al. Incidence of blindness and low vision in a sample population: the Priverno Eye Study, Italy. Ophthalmology. 2003;110(3):584–8.
96. Klaver CC, Wolfs RC, Vingerling JR, Hofman A, de Jong PT. Age-specific prevalence and causes of blindness and visual impairment in an older population: the Rotterdam Study. Arch Ophthalmol. 1998;116(5):653–8.
97. Iwase A, Araie M, Tomidokoro A, Yamamoto T, Shimizu H, Kitazawa Y. Prevalence and causes of low vision and blindness in a Japanese adult population: the Tajimi Study. Ophthalmology. 2006;113(8):1354–62.
98. Xu L, Wang Y, Li Y, Wang Y, Cui T, Li J, et al. Causes of blindness and visual impairment in urban and rural areas in Beijing: the Beijing Eye Study. Ophthalmology. 2006;113(7):1134.e1–11.
99. Yamada M, Hiratsuka Y, Roberts CB, Pezzullo ML, Yates K, Takano S, et al. Prevalence of visual impairment in the adult Japanese population by cause and severity and future projections. Ophthalmic Epidemiol. 2010;17(1):50–7.
100. Fricke TR, Jong M, Naidoo KS, Sankaridurg P, Naduvilath TJ, Ho SM, et al. Global prevalence of visual impairment associated with myopic macular degeneration and temporal trends from 2000 through 2050: systematic review, meta-analysis and modelling. Br J Ophthalmol. 2018;102(7):855–62.
101. Avila MP, Weiter JJ, Jalkh AE, Trempe CL, Pruett RC, Schepens CL. Natural history of choroidal neovascularization in degenerative myopia. Ophthalmology. 1984;91(12):1573–81.
102. Ohno-Matsui K, Kawasaki R, Jonas JB, Cheung CM, Saw SM, Verhoeven VJ, et al. International photographic classification and grading system for myopic maculopathy. Am J Ophthalmol. 2015;159(5):877–83.e7.
103. Liu HH, Xu L, Wang YX, Wang S, You QS, Jonas JB. Prevalence and progression of myopic retinopathy in Chinese adults: the Beijing Eye Study. Ophthalmology. 2010;117(9):1763–8.
104. Gao LQ, Liu W, Liang YB, Zhang F, Wang JJ, Peng Y, et al. Prevalence and characteristics of myopic retinopathy in a rural Chinese adult population: the Handan Eye Study. Arch Ophthalmol. 2011;129(9):1199–204.
105. Chen SJ, Cheng CY, Li AF, Peng KL, Chou P, Chiou SH, et al. Prevalence and associated risk factors of myopic maculopathy in elderly Chinese: the Shihpai eye study. Invest Ophthalmol Vis Sci. 2012;53(8):4868–73.
106. Asakuma T, Yasuda M, Ninomiya T, Noda Y, Arakawa S, Hashimoto S, et al. Prevalence and risk factors for myopic retinopathy in a Japanese population: the Hisayama Study. Ophthalmology. 2012;119(9):1760–5.
107. Vongphanit J, Mitchell P, Wang JJ. Prevalence and progression of myopic retinopathy in an older population. Ophthalmology. 2002;109(4):704–11.
108. Jonas JB, Nangia V, Gupta R, Bhojwani K, Nangia P, Panda-Jonas S. Prevalence of myopic retinopathy in rural Central India. Acta Ophthalmol. 2017;95(5):e399–404.
109. Wong YL, Saw SM. Epidemiology of pathologic myopia in Asia and worldwide. Asia-Pac J Ophthalmol. 2016;5(6):394–402.
110. Samarawickrama C, Mitchell P, Tong L, Gazzard G, Lim L, Wong TY, et al. Myopia-related optic disc and retinal changes in adolescent children from singapore. Ophthalmology. 2011;118(10):2050–7.
111. Koh V, Tan C, Tan PT, Tan M, Balla V, Nah G, et al. Myopic maculopathy and optic disc changes in highly myopic young asian eyes and impact on visual acuity. Am J Ophthalmol. 2016;164:69–79.

3

Myopia and High Myopia: Societal and Economic Cost

Sharon Yu Lin Chua and Paul J. Foster

Key Points

- The prevalence of myopia has increased rapidly throughout Asia. In urban areas, 80–90% of young adults are myopic and 10–20% have high myopia. By 2050, it is estimated that five billion people will be myopic. Of these, one billion people will be highly myopic. World Health Organization lists uncorrected or under-corrected myopia as a major cause of visual impairment.

- Myopia may impair many aspects of life including educational and occupational activities. The annual direct cost of myopia correction for Asian adults has been estimated at US $328 billion/annum. The cost of care is also likely to increase significantly and will be exacerbated by an even greater increase in the prevalence of high myopia.

- High myopes have greater risk of developing several vision-threatening conditions including myopic macular degeneration, retinal detachment, glaucoma, and cataract. Those affected individuals incur costs for specialist eye care, or specialist optical aids for patients with visual impairment. These costs are in the region of US $250 billion/annum.

S. Y. L. Chua · P. J. Foster (✉)
Integrative Epidemiology Cluster, NIHR Biomedical Research Centre, UCL Institute of Ophthalmology and Moorfields Eye Hospital NHS Foundation Trust, London, UK
e-mail: p.foster@ucl.ac.uk

- Myopes, especially high myopes, tend to have reduced quality of life due to adverse influences from psychological, cosmetic, practical and financial factors. Hence, affecting productivity, mobility, and activities of daily living.
- Treatments such as under-correction of myopia, gas permeable contact lenses, and bifocal or multifocal spectacles have all been proven to be ineffective for myopia control. The most effective methods are the use of orthokeratology contact lenses, soft bifocal contact lenses, and topical pharmaceutical agents, such as low-dose atropine or pirenzepine. These will have differing implications for personal finances and quality of life. Hence, the best modality should be selected by the eye care practitioner, parent or individual, based on the lifestyle of the individual.

3.1 Introduction

The prevalence of myopia is most pronounced in the industrialized nations of East Asia, where rates of 95% among young adults have been recorded [1]. In this context, the impact of myopia is profound and far reaching, and recent study by Naidoo et al. [2] suggests that myopia has a global economic impact, with the greatest burden throughout Asia. Its economic impact is very significant. This chapter seeks to examine the impact of myopia on individuals and the wider society, both from the monetary perspective and also in terms of emotional well-being and quality of life. Peer-reviewed data on this subject are comparatively sparse, and in some areas, it is necessary to make inferences on the basis of indirect evidence.

The impact of myopia illustrates an interesting dichotomy. The condition appears to be an exaggerated adaptive response which has a predilection for the most affluent and educated in society. Low myopia [up to around −3 D (diopters)] is arguably an ideal state for the older urban professional, in that the frustration of presbyopia is avoided, and hence maximum efficiency in an office-based career is maintained, and the ability to pursue leisure activities, such as reading, creative arts, and many household tasks, is enhanced. Myopes are among the best educated and thus highest earning members of any society. Furthermore, they confer on their children a range of advantages—they are typically well educated, and in turn benefit from higher career prospects and incomes. The offspring are also more likely to be myopes [3].

3.2 Economic Impact of Myopia

Myopia is the most common distance refractive error. The global prevalence of myopia is expected to increase from 27% of the world's population in 2010 to 52% by 2050 [4]—a 2.6-fold increase. A recent meta-analysis estimated a significant increase in the global prevalence of myopia and high myopia, affecting nearly five billion people and one billion people, respectively, by 2050 [4]. The projected increases in myopia and high myopia may be due to environmental factors, such as a combination of decreased time outdoors and increased near work activities, among other factors [5]. Uncorrected distance refractive error was estimated in 2013 to affect 108 million people globally, and myopia is the most common refractive error [6]. It is the leading cause of moderate and severe vision impairment (VI; 42%) and a major cause of blindness (3%) [2]. Uncorrected myopia as low as −1.50 D will result in moderate VI, and uncorrected myopia of −4.00 D is sufficient refractive error to be classified as blindness [7]. Depending on national legislation, people with moderate VI may not be allowed to drive. Moderate VI may also require the use of aids and/or accommodations/adaptions for some tasks in the learning environment.

If the increasing prevalence of myopia is not addressed, a similar increase in uncorrected refractive error can be expected. These projections are based on conservative assumptions and, given the published relationship between level of education and myopia, increased provision of education could markedly increase these trends. Furthermore, uncorrected distance refractive error has been estimated to result in a global loss of productivity of international dollar (I$) 269 billion [8] (US $202 billion) annually [9], which will also increase if there is a significant increase in uncorrected myopia. International dollar allows comparison of prices and currency values between countries after adjustment of currency exchange rate. An international dollar has the same purchasing power as the U.S. dollar has in the United States [10]. A recent meta-analysis estimated the global potential loss associated with VI in 2015 was US $244 billion/annum [95% confidence interval (CI) US $49 billion—US $697 billion] from uncorrected myopia and US $6 billion/annum (95% CI US $2 billion–US $17 billion) from myopic macular degeneration [2]. The cost of care is also likely to increase significantly, and will be exacerbated by an even greater increase in the prevalence of high myopia, from 2.8% (190 million people) to 9.7% (924 million people) by 2050 [4], representing a 4.9-fold increase in high myopia. In some populations of young adults in Asia, the prevalence of high myopia has already reached 38% [11]. The annual direct cost of optical correction of myopia for Singaporean adults has been estimated at US $755 million. Refractive correction comprising of optometry visits, spectacles, and/or contact lenses is the most significant cost domain and it accounts for 65.2% of the total costs [12]. In Singapore, the estimates in an adult (SG $587 or US $455 per patient per year) is significantly higher than a child aged 7–9 years (SG $222 or US $175 per patient per year) [13]. The higher cost could be because of the greater likelihood that adults may undergo laser-assisted in situ keratomileusis (LASIK), wear contact lens, or develop ocular complications due to high myopia. Furthermore, adults tend to have higher spending power compared to a child. It has been estimated that if such prevalence rates were extrapolated to all cities in Asia in which the prevalence of myopia is approximately equal to the rates in Singapore, the estimated direct cost would be US $328 billion/annum. It is estimated that US $8.1 billion/annum was spent on vision products including eyeglass frames, lenses, and contact lenses in the USA in 1990 [14]. In United States, a cross-sectional study demonstrated that 110 million Americans could achieve normal vision with refractive correction and the estimated cost was US $3.8 billion/annum [15]. Of this amount, the annual cost of providing distance vision correction for adults older than 65 years old was US $780 million. The types of refractive error included correction for myopia, hyperopia, and presbyopia. This represents approximately US $35 per person or US $13 per capita annually, based on the cost of a pair of spectacles and refractive examination. Possible reasons for the difference in direct costs of refractive correction are the treatment costs may be borne by the individual, who may be willing to pay for other factors such as aesthetics. Whereas in some countries (e.g., the United Kingdom), some segments of the population are entitled to free eye glasses subsidized by the government. As the prevalence of myopia increase in East Asia, the total cost of treating myopia will be high. There is likely to be an increase in the demand for optical services as the number of older people increases and if, as suggested, the number of younger people with myopia increases. It is estimated that partial sight and blindness in adults costs the UK economy around £22 billion per year [16].

The cost of spectacles varies, but there may some individuals who may not be able to afford a basic pair of spectacles, and hence refractive error may not be fully corrected. Health economic analyses in the United States and Australia have reported the economic burden of refractive correction associated with medical care expenditure, informal care days, and healthy utility is greater than age-related macular degeneration, primary open-angle glaucoma, and diabetic retinopathy, while it was secondary to the medical cost of age-related cataract [17, 18]. As the economic costs of myopia are high, more efforts and resources could be directed toward having new strategies to prevent and slow down myopia progression to high myopia and its associated visually disabling ocular complications.

3.3 Secondary Impact of Myopia from Other Eye Diseases and Sight Loss

High myopia increases the risk of other eye diseases such as cataract, glaucoma, retinal detachment, and myopic macular degeneration (MMD), which may lead to irreversible vision loss. MMD has been reported to cause 12.1% of VI (approximately 200,000 people) in Japan [19]. Visual impairment and blindness impact the individuals, their families, caregivers, and the community, which lead to a significant cost burden. In Australia, visual disorders were ranked seventh among diseases in terms of economic burden on the health system, which is ahead of coronary heart disease, diabetes, depression, and stroke [20]. Naidoo et al. estimated the potential global economic productivity loss resulting from VI and blindness as a result of uncorrected myopia and MMD in 2015 [2]. Their study suggests that the greatest burden of VI resulting from uncorrected refractive error is older people in rural areas of the least developed countries. The regional productivity loss owing to VI resulting from myopia may be reflected in Southeast Asia, South Asia, and East Asia as having a percentage gross domestic product (GDP) of 1.35%, 1.3%, and 1.27%, respectively. Differences in productivity loss arises from the interplay between country-specific variables, such as myopia and high myopia prevalence, demographics, Health Development Index (HDI), health expenditure, urbanization, labor force participation, employment, GDP, and population. There are other components that contribute to the overall burden of myopia, such as cost of eye examinations, refractive corrections, managing pathologic consequences of myopia such as MMD, and related opportunity costs. The value of any investment to prevent myopia, slow progression of myopia, improve spectacle correction rates, and improve outcomes in MMD depends on a comparison of lost productivity owing to VI resulting from myopia with the cost of prevention and management interventions. Fricke et al. estimated the global cost of facilities and personnel for establishing refractive care services US $20 billion over 5 years [9]. Direct medical costs occur mostly due to hospitalization, the use of direct medical services, and medical products. Hospitalization and use of medical services around diagnosis and treatment at the onset of VI and blindness were the two largest components related to direct medical costs. The mean annual expenses per patient to be US$ purchasing power parities (PPPs) 12,175–14,029 for moderate VI, US$ PPPs 13,154–16,321 for severe VI, and US$ PPPs 14,882–24,180 for blindness [21]. PPPs account for differences in price levels between countries, and convert local currencies into international dollars by taking into account the purchasing power of different national currencies and eliminates the difference in price levels between countries [22]. Direct nonmedical costs include assistive devices and aids, home modifications, and costs for healthcare services such as home-based nursing or nursing home placements. The cost for support services and assistive devices increased from US$ PPP 54 for a person with visual acuity (VA) 20/20 or better up to US$ PPP 609 for a person with VA 20/80 or worse. Indirect costs include productivity losses, changes in employment (employer and/or area of work), loss of income, premature mortality, and dead-weight losses [21]. Dead-weight losses, also known as excess burden, describe the costs to society created by market inefficiency. In the study by Köberlein et al., it is referred to as an excess financial burden on society caused by VI and blindness [21]. The annual estimates of productivity losses and absenteeism range from US$ PPP 4974 to 5724 million and a decrease in workforce participation range was estimated to be US$ PPP 7.4 billion [21].

Value of the Commercial Optical Good Sector

In the UK in 2017, the optical goods and services industry had total consumer spending estimated at £3.1 billion (2.0 billion US$ = @ 0.66 £:$). Growth was estimated at 2% for 2017, and forecasts projected further 3.2% growth in 2018. Market research suggests this was primarily driven by an aging population. In the UK, 70% of consumers are reported to wear some form of prescription eyewear. Just 11% of those with vision correction need wear contact lenses, with this sector characterized by a high rate of premium and daily wear lenses. Contact lenses account for 20% of the total spending on optical products, with the sale of contact lens solutions made up an additional 3% of the market, compared to 60% market share for spectacle frames and lenses. Only one in six (18%) people have purchased optical products online. Reports suggest that consumers perceive buying prescriptions eyewear online as harder—49% of people buying prescription eyewear saying it is more difficult than buying in-store, although 45% of consumers who said they have not bought optical products online before, would consider doing so in the future [23].

3.4 Quality of Life

Quality of life is a multidimensional construct with different domains. The identified domains related to ophthalmic quality of life include activity limitation, mobility, convenience, health concerns, visual symptoms, ocular-comfort symptoms, general symptoms, emotional well-being, and social and economic issues [24]. Impaired vision will lead to significant reduction in activities associated with participation in society and religion, mobility, daily living, and visually intensive tasks. This may impact education, employment, child development, mental health, and functional capacity in older people, increasing the risk of hip fractures and the need for community or family support or nursing home placement [25–27]. A cross-sectional study in Germany reported that mild VI affected emotional well-being [28]. Depression was considered to cause further functional decline in visually impaired patients by reducing motivation, initiative, and resiliency [29–31]. Visual impairment and blindness associated with myopic macular degeneration will increase significantly, hence affecting the quality of life and causing socioeconomic impact [32]. A cross-sectional study reported the functional status in daily life and quality of life of pathologic myopia patients were reduced compared with control subjects [33]. The influence of pathologic myopia on a patient's daily life was primarily the result of three major factors: handicap, disability, and support. Wong et al. reported that those with VI, measured in terms of presenting vision (i.e., wearing their habitual correction), had statistically significantly lower scores for total quality of life (−3.8; 95% CI −7.1 to −0.5; $P = 0.03$), psychosocial functioning (−4.2; 95% CI −8.1 to −0.3; $P = 0.03$), and school functioning (−5.5; 95% CI −10.2 to −0.9; $P = 0.02$) [34]. Another study indicates that correction of refractive errors by the provision of spectacles in low socioeconomic areas in China would markedly improve educational outcomes since the major medium of instruction is the blackboard [35].

Patients with cataract may experience vision-related problems, such as decreased visual acuity, loss of contrast sensitivity, problems under glare conditions, and altered color recognition [36]. Studies in Japan and Canada reported a loss of well-being as disability adjusted life years (DALYs) and an associated cost of US$ PPP 51.8 billion/annum and US$ PPP 15.11 billion/annum, respectively [37, 38]. The global burden of diseases study 2010 estimated the burden of disease related to vision disorders has increased by 47% from 12,858,000 disability adjusted life years (DALYs) in 1990 to 18,837,000 DALYs in 2010 [39]. The Melbourne Visual Impairment Project (VIP) cohort showed the association between VI and mortality to increase linearly from 4.5% in people with a VA of 20/20 or better to 22.2% in blind people with VA of 20/200 or worse [40].

3.5 Impact of Myopia Treatments on Quality of Life

Current treatment options for control of myopia progression include optical correction such as bifocal spectacle lenses, progressive addition spectacle lenses, under-correction, orthokeratology, multifocal contact lenses, increased exposure to outdoor activities, and the use of atropine eye drops. Surgical techniques, such as LASIK, have become increasingly popular and over a million surgical procedures are performed annually in the United States [41]. Choice of refractive correction leads to various quality-of-life implications. Often, the type of refractive correction depends on prescription, lifestyle including occupational and recreational needs, economic issues, and personality. If refractive error may be corrected through the provision of corrective spectacles, visual acuity, and therefore functional vision could be improved. Patient reported outcomes (PROs) have been used to assess the outcomes of interventions on people's lives. A PRO is described as a report that comes directly from a patient regarding the impact of the condition and outcome of an intervention [42]. The Quality of Life Impact of Refractive Correction (QIRC) is useful to detect differences in quality of life impact from various refractive corrections (spectacles, contact lenses, and refractive surgery). Pesudovs et al. reported that QIRC score was highest in refractive surgery patients (mean QIRC score of 50.2 ± 6.3), followed by contact lens wearers (mean QIRC score 46.7 ± 5.5), and spectacle wears (mean QIRC score 44.1 ± 5.9) [43]. Orthokeratology (OrthoK) contact lenses (CL) are worn while sleeping to reshape the cornea and are used to correct refractive error and slow the progression of myopia [44]. Quality of life using the National Eye Institute Refractive Error Quality of Life (NEI RQL)-42 questionnaire was evaluated in a group of subjects with low to moderate myopia who had undergone four types of refractive correction, namely, LASIK, OrthoK, soft contact lens (SCL), and spectacles [45]. Results showed decrease in quality of life for most of the subscales in the treatment groups compared to emmetropic subjects. The average decrease in quality of life compared with emmetropes were −7.1% ($P = 0.021$) for LASIK, −13.0% ($P = 0.001$) for OrthoK, −15.8% ($P = 0.001$) for spectacles, and −17.3% ($P = 0.001$) for SCL. The subscales which were affected in LASIK and OrthoK patients compared to emmetropes were as follows: clarity of vision, expectations, glare, and worry. This suggests that both types of treatment affected the quality of life due to high-order aberrations [46]. LASIK and OrthoK are commonly associated with experiencing haloes and glare because of the dramatic changes in the corneal shape [47]. Spectacle wearers had the worse scores in expectations, dependence on correction, worry, and appearance as compared to the other three treatment modalities [45]. The primary motivation for undergoing LASIK was a desire to improve uncorrected visual acuity, without a need to wear glasses and improved ease to pursue sports or recreational activities [48]. Although LASIK patients may have excellent vision during day time, they may experience disturbances in night vision such as halo and glare disability [49]. An estimated 12–57% of patients experience night vision symptoms and 30% have difficulty with night driving after undergoing photorefractive keratectomy (PRK) and LASIK [50, 51]. In addition, these patients may experience poor vision in low light setting due to contrast sensitivity decreasing initially after LASIK [52].

OrthoK allows patients to enjoy good vision without needing to wear vision correction during their waking hours. This benefits patients who have an active lifestyle as they are more mobile without the need for refractive correction. OrthoK provides excellent vision and improves vision related quality of life [45, 53]. Side effects of OrthoK include halos secondary to spherical aberration, which may reduce visual acuity and contrast sensitivity or discomfort from the lenses [54]. Although the most serious complication with CL wear is infection, these occurrences are relatively rare [55, 56]. Most common complaints are related to intolerance or limited wearing time due to fluctuations of vision, dryness and discomfort [57]. Atropine has been used to control myopia progression [58]. As atropine causes pupil dilation and temporary paralysis of accommodation, patients may experience glare, discomfort, blurred vision, or allergic/hypersensitivity reactions. Complications of LASIK include corneal ectasia [59], dry eyes [60], and night vision disturbances [49].

Cataract surgery is a highly effective, cost-effective health-care intervention [61], and results in almost immediate visual rehabilitation. In addition to visual rehabilitation from media opacities, it offers once in a lifetime opportunity for refractive manipulation that benefits the majority of people with a refractive error. Previous studies have utilized Visual Functioning Index-14 (VF-14) or similar vision-functioning tools and reported the impact of cataract surgery can be translated beyond visual acuity. Evidence has shown several fold improvements in other critical daily tasks such as read critical daily living tasks such as reading newspapers or books; driving; watching TV; cooking; negotiating steps; sewing, knitting, crocheting, or doing handicrafts; noticing traffic, information or shop signs; and recognizing people [62]. In addition, there are improvements in several psychosocial aspects such as social interaction; mental and emotional well-being; psychological distress; adaptation; and coping.

3.6 Summary

Myopia is a major global public health concern due to its high and increasing prevalence in Asian countries, where it is a common cause of vision dysfunction. Uncorrected myopia is a leading cause of visual impairment. People with high myopia have increased risk of developing myopic pathologies which may lead to blindness. The economic burden of uncorrected distance refractive error, largely caused by myopia, is estimated to be US $202 billion annually. Direct cost of refractive correction comprises of cost from spectacles, contact lenses, and refractive surgeries. Other medical costs include those associated with treatment of ocular complications from high myopia, such as retinal detachment, myopic macular degeneration, glaucoma and cataract, and its associated visual impairment and blindness. This global cost will continue to increase as the number of people with myopia rises. Patients with higher myopic refractive error tend to have adverse effect on the quality of life and lead to lower health, economic, and social outcomes. Effective methods to control or correct myopia include the use of optical devices, pharmacological drops, surgical, or outdoor exposure. Each treatment method will have various quality of life implications; thus, it is important to ensure prescription, lifestyle including occupational and recreational needs, and economic issues are discussed. Although a broader societal perspective is useful for informing policy, the patient's perspective is essential for designing service models to improve the social interaction and mental and emotional well-being of these individuals. In conclusion, the impact that myopia and its associated visual impairment have on individuals is substantial. Myopia preferentially affects the more highly educated and potentially most productive sectors of the population, the individual and societal costs involved. Developing appropriate public health policies to prevent and reduce myopia progression will benefit the individual and the wider society.

References

1. Lin LL, Shih YF, Hsiao CK, Chen CJ. Prevalence of myopia in Taiwanese schoolchildren: 1983 to 2000. Ann Acad Med Singap. 2004;33(1):27–33.
2. Naidoo KS, Fricke TR, Frick KD, et al. Potential lost productivity resulting from the global burden of myopia: systematic review, meta-analysis, and modeling. Ophthalmology. 2018;126(3):338–46.
3. Mutti DO, Mitchell GL, Moeschberger ML, et al. Parental myopia, near work, school achievement, and children's refractive error. Invest Ophthalmol Vis Sci. 2002;43(12):3633–40.
4. Holden BA, Fricke TR, Wilson DA, et al. Global prevalence of myopia and high myopia and temporal trends from 2000 through 2050. Ophthalmology. 2016;123(5):1036–42.
5. Morgan IG, Ohno-Matsui K, Saw S-M. Myopia. Lancet. 2012;379(9827):1739–48.
6. Bourne RRA, Stevens GA, White RA, et al. Causes of vision loss worldwide, 1990–2010: a systematic analysis. Lancet Glob Health. 2013;1(6):e339–e49.
7. Rabbetts RB. Bennett & Rabbetts' clinical visual optics. New York: Elsevier/Butterworth Heinemann; 2007.
8. Smith TS, Frick KD, Holden BA, et al. Potential lost productivity resulting from the global burden of uncorrected refractive error. Bull World Health Organ. 2009;87(6):431–7.
9. Fricke T, Holden B, Wilson D. Global cost of correcting vision impairment from uncorrected refractive error. Bull World Health Organ. 2012;90:728–38.
10. World Health Organization. Purchasing power parity. 2005. https://www.who.int/choice/costs/ppp/en/. Accessed 20 June 2019.
11. Wang TJ, Chiang TH, Wang TH, et al. Changes of the ocular refraction among freshmen in National Taiwan University between 1988 and 2005. Eye. 2009;23(5):1168–9.
12. Zheng YF, Pan CW, Chay J, et al. The economic cost of myopia in adults aged over 40 years in Singapore. Invest Ophthalmol Vis Sci. 2013;54(12):7532–7.
13. Lim MC, Gazzard G, Sim EL, et al. Direct costs of myopia in Singapore. Eye. 2009;23(5):1086–9.
14. Letsch SW, Lazenby HC, Levit KR, Cowan CA. National health expenditures, 1991. Health Care Financ Rev. 1992;14(2):1–30.
15. Vitale S, Cotch MF, Sperduto R, Ellwein L. Costs of refractive correction of distance vision impairment in the United States, 1999-2002. Ophthalmology. 2006;113(12):2163–70.
16. England N. Improving eye health and reducing sight loss: a call to action. 2014. https://www.england.nhs.uk/2014/06/eye-cta/. Accessed 6 Feb 2019.
17. Frick KD, Gower EW, Kempen JH, Wolff JL. Economic impact of visual impairment and blindness in the United States. Arch Ophthalmol. 2007;125(4):544–50.
18. Keeffe JE, Chou SL, Lamoureux EL. The cost of care for people with impaired vision in Australia. Arch Ophthalmol. 2009;127(10):1377–81.
19. Yamada M, Hiratsuka Y, Roberts CB, et al. Prevalence of visual impairment in the adult Japanese population by cause and severity and future projections. Ophthalmic Epidemiol. 2010;17(1):50–7.
20. Taylor HR, Pezzullo ML, Keeffe JE. The economic impact and cost of visual impairment in Australia. Br J Ophthalmol. 2006;90(3):272–5.
21. Koberlein J, Beifus K, Schaffert C, Finger RP. The economic burden of visual impairment and blindness: a systematic review. BMJ Open. 2013;3(11):e003471.

22. Organisation for Economic Co-operation and Development. OECD health statistics. 2018. http://www.oecd.org/els/health-systems/health-data.htm. Accessed 6 Feb 2019.
23. Mintel. Optical goods retailing: UK. 2018. http://reports.mintel.com/display/858753/. Accessed 6 Feb 2019.
24. Khadka J, Fenwick E, Lamoureux E, Pesudovs K. Methods to develop the eye-tem bank to measure ophthalmic quality of life. Optom Vis Sci. 2016;93(12):1485–94.
25. Cieza A, Kocur I, Mariotti S, McCoy M. The future of eye care in a changing world. Bull World Health Organ. 2017;95:667.
26. Klein BE, Klein R, Lee KE, Cruickshanks KJ. Performance-based and self-assessed measures of visual function as related to history of falls, hip fractures, and measured gait time. The Beaver Dam Eye Study. Ophthalmology. 1998;105(1):160–4.
27. Mitchell P, Hayes P, Wang JJ. Visual impairment in nursing home residents: the Blue Mountains Eye Study. Med J Aust. 1997;166(2):73–6.
28. Finger RP, Fenwick E, Marella M, et al. The impact of vision impairment on vision-specific quality of life in Germany. Invest Ophthalmol Vis Sci. 2011;52(6):3613–9.
29. Rovner BW, Casten RJ, Tasman WS. Effect of depression on vision function in age-related macular degeneration. Arch Ophthalmol. 2002;120(8):1041–4.
30. Horowitz A, Reinhardt JP, Boerner K, Travis LA. The influence of health, social support quality and rehabilitation on depression among disabled elders. Aging Ment Health. 2003;7(5):342–50.
31. Tolman J, Hill RD, Kleinschmidt JJ, Gregg CH. Psychosocial adaptation to visual impairment and its relationship to depressive affect in older adults with age-related macular degeneration. Gerontologist. 2005;45(6):747–53.
32. Fricke TR, Jong M, Naidoo KS, et al. Global prevalence of visual impairment associated with myopic macular degeneration and temporal trends from 2000 through 2050: systematic review, meta-analysis and modelling. Br J Ophthalmol. 2018;102(7):855–62.
33. Takashima T, Yokoyama T, Futagami S, et al. The quality of life in patients with pathologic myopia. Jpn J Ophthalmol. 2001;45(1):84–92.
34. Wong HB, Machin D, Tan SB, et al. Visual impairment and its impact on health-related quality of life in adolescents. Am J Ophthalmol. 2009;147(3):505–11.e1.
35. Ma X, Zhou Z, Yi H, et al. Effect of providing free glasses on children's educational outcomes in China: cluster randomized controlled trial. BMJ. 2014;349:g5740.
36. Crabtree HL, Hildreth AJ, O'Connell JE, et al. Measuring visual symptoms in British cataract patients: the cataract symptom scale. Br J Ophthalmol. 1999;83(5):519–23.
37. Cruess AF, Gordon KD, Bellan L, et al. The cost of vision loss in Canada. 2. Results. Can J Ophthalmol. 2011;46(4):315–8.
38. Roberts CB, Hiratsuka Y, Yamada M, et al. Economic cost of visual impairment in Japan. Arch Ophthalmol. 2010;128(6):766–71.
39. Murray CJ, Vos T, Lozano R, et al. Disability-adjusted life years (DALYs) for 291 diseases and injuries in 21 regions, 1990-2010: a systematic analysis for the Global Burden of Disease Study 2010. Lancet. 2012;380(9859):2197–223.
40. McCarty CA, Nanjan MB, Taylor HR. Vision impairment predicts 5 year mortality. Br J Ophthalmol. 2001;85(3):322–6.
41. Hammond MD, Madigan WP, Bower KS. Refractive surgery in the United States Army, 2000-2003. Ophthalmology. 2005;112(2):184–90.
42. Denniston AK, Kyte D, Calvert M, Burr JM. An introduction to patient-reported outcome measures in ophthalmic research. Eye. 2014;28(6):637–45.
43. Pesudovs K, Garamendi E. Elliott DB. A quality of life comparison of people wearing spectacles or contact lenses or having undergone refractive surgery. J Refract Surg. 2006;22(1):19–27.
44. Lipson MJ, Brooks MM, Koffler BH. The role of orthokeratology in myopia control: a review. Eye Contact Lens. 2018;44(4):224–30.
45. Queiros A, Villa-Collar C, Gutierrez AR, et al. Quality of life of myopic subjects with different methods of visual correction using the NEI RQL-42 questionnaire. Eye Contact Lens. 2012;38(2):116–21.

46. Queiros A, Villa-Collar C, Gonzalez-Meijome JM, et al. Effect of pupil size on corneal aberrations before and after standard laser in situ keratomileusis, custom laser in situ keratomileusis, and corneal refractive therapy. Am J Ophthalmol. 2010;150(1):97–109.e1.
47. al-Kaff AS. Patient satisfaction after photorefractive keratectomy. J Refract Surg. 1997;13(5 Suppl):S459–60.
48. McGhee CN, Craig JP, Sachdev N, et al. Functional, psychological, and satisfaction outcomes of laser in situ keratomileusis for high myopia. J Cataract Refract Surg. 2000;26(4):497–509.
49. Villa C, Gutierrez R, Jimenez JR, Gonzalez-Meijome JM. Night vision disturbances after successful LASIK surgery. Br J Ophthalmol. 2007;91(8):1031–7.
50. Bailey MD, Mitchell GL, Dhaliwal DK, et al. Patient satisfaction and visual symptoms after laser in situ keratomileusis. Ophthalmology. 2003;110(7):1371–8.
51. Schein OD, Vitale S, Cassard SD, Steinberg EP. Patient outcomes of refractive surgery. The refractive status and vision profile. J Cataract Refract Surg. 2001;27(5):665–73.
52. Chan JWW, Edwards MH, Woo GC, Woo VCP. Contrast sensitivity after laser in situ keratomileusis: one-year follow-up. J Cataract Refract Surg. 2002;28(10):1774–9.
53. Hiraoka T, Okamoto C, Ishii Y, et al. Patient satisfaction and clinical outcomes after overnight orthokeratology. Optom Vis Sci. 2009;86(7):875–82.
54. Johnson KL, Carney LG, Mountford JA, et al. Visual performance after overnight orthokeratology. Cont Lens Anterior Eye. 2007;30(1):29–36.
55. Morgan PB, Efron N, Hill EA, et al. Incidence of keratitis of varying severity among contact lens wearers. Br J Ophthalmol. 2005;89(4):430.
56. Schein OD. Microbial keratitis associated with overnight orthokeratology: what we need to know. Cornea. 2005;24(7):767–9.
57. Pritchard N, Fonn D. Dehydration, lens movement and dryness ratings of hydrogel contact lenses. Ophthalmic Physiol Opt. 1995;15(4):281–6.
58. Pineles SL, Kraker RT, VanderVeen DK, et al. Atropine for the prevention of myopia progression in children: a report by the American Academy of Ophthalmology. Ophthalmology. 2017;124(12):1857–66.
59. Randleman JB, Russell B, Ward MA, et al. Risk factors and prognosis for corneal ectasia after LASIK. Ophthalmology. 2003;110(2):267–75.
60. De Paiva CS, Chen Z, Koch DD, et al. The incidence and risk factors for developing dry eye after myopic LASIK. Am J Ophthalmol. 2006;141(3):438–45.
61. Lansingh VC, Carter MJ, Martens M. Global cost-effectiveness of cataract surgery. Ophthalmology. 2007;114(9):1670–8.
62. Lamoureux EL, Fenwick E, Pesudovs K, Tan D. The impact of cataract surgery on quality of life. Curr Opin Ophthalmol. 2011;22(1):19–27.

4

Mechanisms and Pathogenesis of Myopia

Ranjay Chakraborty, Scott A. Read, and Stephen J. Vincent

Key Points

- Visual environment (or the quality of the retinal image) modulates the refractive development of the eye.
- Ocular response to form-deprivation and lens induced defocus is evident across a wide range of animal species, including humans.
- The visual system appears to be more sensitive to myopic than hyperopic defocus.
- Evidence suggests that greater time spent outdoors is protective against development and progression of myopia in children.

4.1 Emmetropization and Normal Ocular Growth in Human Eyes

When incident parallel rays of light from distant objects are brought to a focus upon the retina without accommodation, it is known as emmetropia. During postnatal eye growth, the precise matching of the axial length (the distance from the anterior corneal surface to the retina along the visual axis) and the optical power of the eye brings the eye to emmetropia [1, 2]. This active regulatory process that harmonizes the expansion of the eye with the optical power of the cornea and the crystalline lens

R. Chakraborty (✉)
Flinders University, Adelaide, SA, Australia
e-mail: ranjay.chakraborty@flinders.edu.au

S. A. Read · S. J. Vincent
Queensland University of Technology, Brisbane, QLD, Australia

is known as emmetropization [1]. Any disruption to these highly coordinated ocular changes results in the development of refractive errors, wherein distant images are focused either behind (hyperopia) or in front (myopia) of the retina [1].

Human eyes exhibit a distinctive pattern of eye growth during the early period of visual development. The distribution of refractive errors at birth appears to be normally distributed [3, 4]. Apart from some exceptions [5], the majority of newborn infants are moderately hyperopic (~+2.00 to +4.00 D) and this refractive error reduces significantly during the first 18 months of life [3, 6–8] (Fig. 4.1). By about 2–5 years of age, the distribution becomes leptokurtic with a peak around emmetropia to low hyperopia of about +0.50 to +1.00 D [5, 6, 8, 11, 12]. Although studies have reported small reductions in hyperopic refraction until the middle to late teen years [13, 14], emmetropization is believed to be largely completed by 5–6 years of age [5, 6, 8, 14].

Based on the visually guided ocular growth observed in a variety of animal models [15–17] (see Sect. 4.3), the growth of the human eye is also believed to be modulated by an active visual feedback from the hyperopic refractive error in neonatal eyes [18]. Studies have found a strong correlation between the rapid reduction in hyperopia and the changes in axial length during early ocular development [18, 19]. Human eyes are ~17 mm long after birth and grow to about 20 mm after the first year [11, 18–20]. This rapid expansion of the eye is largely attributed to the

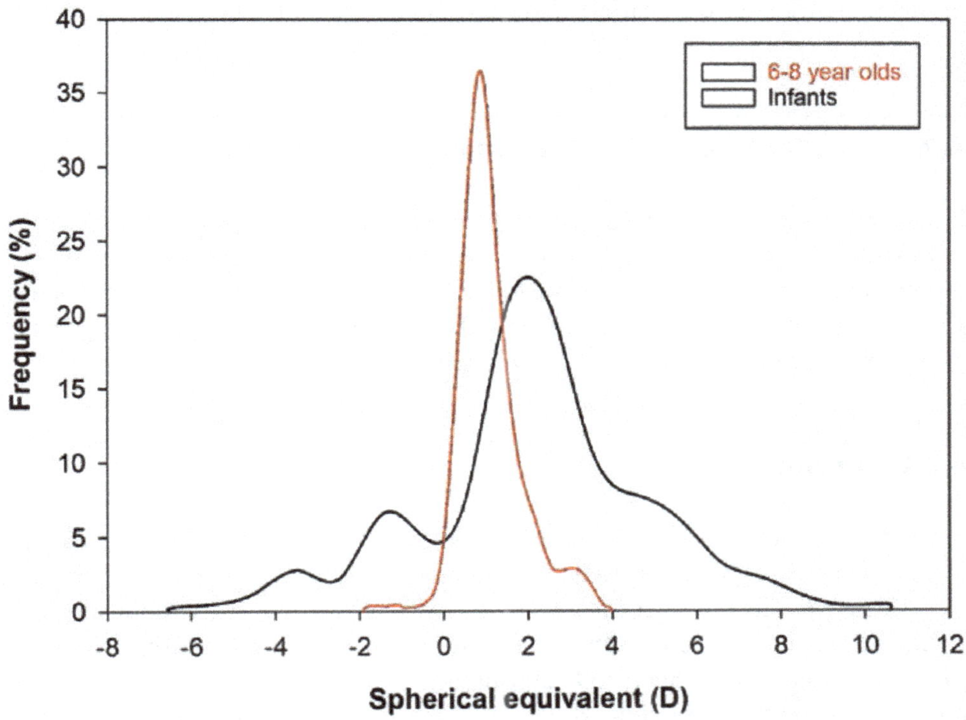

Fig. 4.1 Comparison of refractive error distribution among newborns [3] and 6–8-year-old children [9]. The distribution of refractive errors narrows between infancy to early childhood during the process of emmetropization. Adapted from FitzGerald and Duckman [10]

expansion of the vitreous chamber [18, 21]. From 2–3 years of age, axial elongation slows to approximately 0.4 mm/year until preschool age [11]. Consistent with changes in ocular refraction, the growth of the eye stabilizes further at 5–6 years, and only increases by 1–1.5 mm through the teenage years [11, 20, 21]. Together, these studies suggest that axial length is the most influential factor for emmetropization in human eyes.

In addition to changes in axial length, there is also a significant reduction in the refractive power of the cornea and the crystalline lens that contributes to the overall reduction in hyperopia in the first year of life [11, 18, 22]. Mutti et al. [18] reported a reduction of 1.07 and 3.62 D in corneal and crystalline lens powers, respectively, associated with flattening of the corneal and lens radii in newborn infants, between the ages of 3 and 9 months. Studies have also found higher degrees of corneal astigmatism in newborn infants [23–28], which reduces during the first 4 years of life and is associated with corneal flattening [24, 27, 29, 30]. Overall, these studies suggest that emmetropization in human eyes is largely attributed to the changes in axial length with minor contributions from corneal and crystalline lens powers.

Refractive errors occur as a result of either variations in (a) axial length with respect to the total refractive power of the eye (termed axial myopia or hyperopia) or (b) refractive power of the cornea and the crystalline lens with respect to the axial length of the eye (termed refractive myopia or hyperopia). This chapter focuses on the pathogenesis and potential underlying mechanisms of myopia, and the following section discusses the changes in different ocular parameters during myopic eye growth.

4.2 Ocular Biometric Changes in Human Myopia

As discussed earlier, the axial length of the eye is the primary biometric determinant of refractive error; however, the dimensions, curvature, and refractive index of each individual ocular structure contribute to the final refractive state. Ocular biometrics vary considerably throughout childhood, during the development and progression of myopia, and in response to clinical myopia control interventions.

4.2.1 Cornea

Several cross-sectional analyses have revealed a weak association between increasing corneal power (a steeper radius of curvature) and increasing levels of myopia [31–33], while others report no association [34], or the opposite relationship [35]. Longitudinal studies indicate that changes in corneal curvature during childhood [36–38] and early adulthood [39] are minimal and not associated with the magnitude of myopia progression. However, since the correlation between spherical equivalent refraction (SER) and the axial length to corneal radius ratio is typically stronger than that of axial length alone (by 15–20%) [40–43], corneal curvature does appear to make a modest contribution to the magnitude of myopia. Although corneal thickness does not vary systematically with refractive error [44–47], a reduction in corneal hysteresis (an estimate of corneal biomechanical strength or viscoelasticity) has been observed with increasing levels of myopia in children [48, 49] and adults [50–52]. However, the causal nature of this relationship remains unclear, or if such corneal metrics correlate with posterior scleral biomechanics.

4.2.2 Crystalline Lens and Anterior Chamber Depth

While the cornea flattens substantially during infancy and then remains relatively stable throughout childhood, the crystalline lens continues to thin, flatten, and reduce in optical power until approximately 10 years (a 0.25–0.50 D reduction per year), concurrent with lens fiber compaction [53–55]. These changes may be part of an emmetropization mechanism to compensate for continued axial elongation or a mechanical consequence of equatorial eye growth. Across a range of ethnicities, Mutti et al. [56] observed that within 1 year of myopia onset, compensatory crystalline lens thinning and flattening abruptly halted compared to children who remained emmetropic (Fig. 4.2), suggesting that childhood myopia is not purely axial in nature, but involves a decoupling of highly correlated anterior and posterior segment eye growth. In Singaporean children, Iribarren et al. [57] reported a transient acceleration in the reduction of lens power during myopia onset when the rate

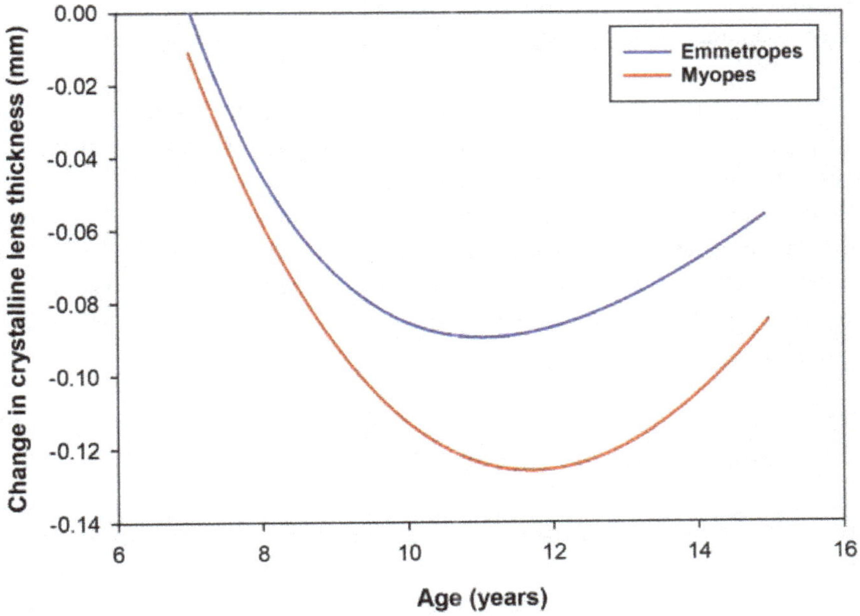

Fig. 4.2 The change in crystalline lens thickness as a function of age in myopes and emmetropes during childhood (after Mutti et al. [56]). Shortly after myopia onset (10–12 years), compensatory crystalline lens thinning abruptly halted compared to children who remained emmetropic suggesting that myopia development involves a decoupling of anterior and posterior segment eye growth

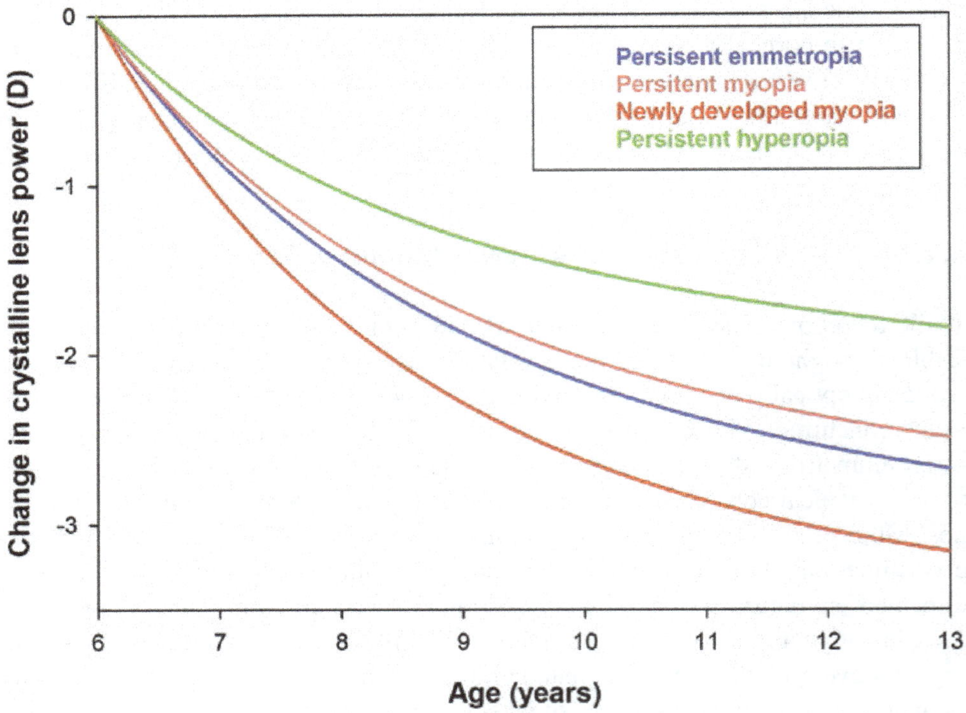

Fig. 4.3 The change in crystalline lens power during childhood (calculated from refraction and biometric measurements) in young Singaporean children for a range of refractive error groups (after Iribarren et al. [57]) The reduction in lens power increases during myopia onset (to a greater extent than other refractive error groups), but is not sustained throughout myopia progression

of axial growth was high, which was not sustained as myopia progressed (Fig. 4.3). Paradoxically, after 10 years of age, the lens continues to thicken and increase in curvature with the bedding down of additional fibers, but reduces in optical power, most likely due to a steepening of the gradient refractive index [58]. Changes in anterior chamber depth throughout childhood are inversely related to changes in lens thickness (as the lens thins, the anterior chamber deepens), and the anterior chamber is typically deeper in myopes compared to emmetropes and vice versa for the crystalline lens [53].

4.2.3 Vitreous Chamber and Axial Length

In contrast to the anterior segment, changes in the posterior segment (particularly, the vitreous chamber, choroid, and sclera) are more pronounced in myopic compared to non-myopic eyes (Fig. 4.4). Axial length, or more precisely, the vitreous chamber depth is the primary individual biometric contributor to refractive error in children, young adults, and the elderly [34, 59, 60], with the vitreous chamber depth accounting for over 50% of the observed variation in SER, followed by the cornea (~15%) and crystalline lens (~1%) [60]. Modeling of cross-sectional and

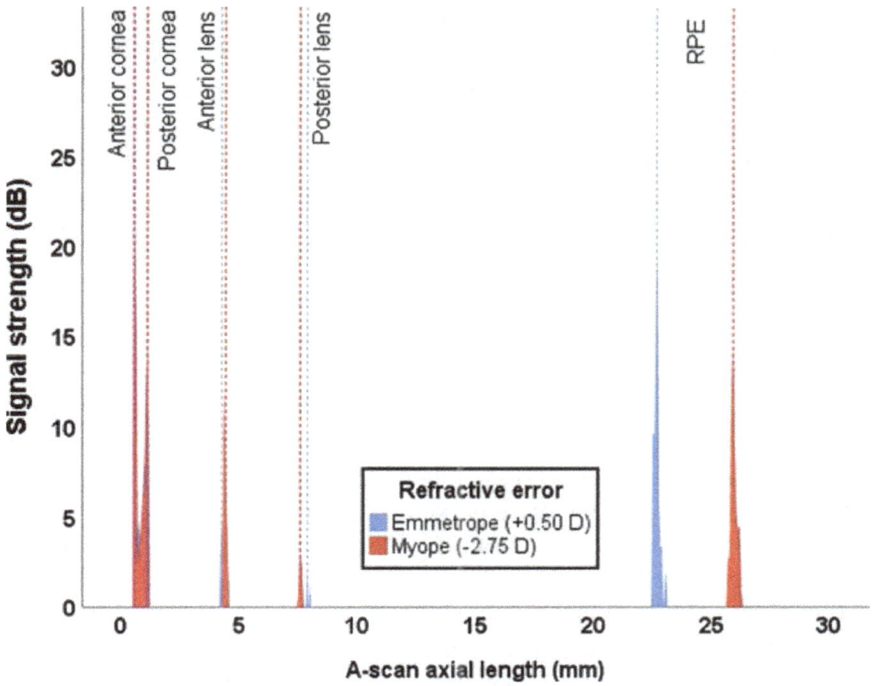

Fig. 4.4 Optical low coherence reflectometry A-Scan output from two 11-year-old males (one myope and one emmetrope). The predominant biometric differences are the deeper vitreous chamber (19.05 mm compared to 15.47 mm) and the longer axial length (25.87 mm compared to 22.69 mm) in the myopic eye. The anterior chamber depth is slightly shallower in the emmetropic eye (by 0.13 mm) while the crystalline lens is thicker (by 0.49 mm) in comparison to the myopic eye. The corneal thickness varies by only 0.04 mm

longitudinal data from emmetropic children indicates that axial length and vitreous chamber depth increase by approximately 0.16 mm per year from age 6–10 years, slowing to 0.05 mm per year from 11 to 14 years [61]. In myopic children aged between 6 and 11 years (corrected with single vision spectacles or contact lenses) average growth rates of approximately 0.30 mm per year have been reported [37, 62, 63], with greater vitreous chamber and axial elongation observed in younger females with myopic parents [37]. A range of myopia control interventions significantly slow the rate of eye growth and myopia progression during childhood, in some cases by up to 50% [64], and this reduction in axial elongation appears to be initially modulated by changes in the choroid underlying the retina.

4.2.4 Choroid

The choroid supplies the outer retina with oxygen and nutrients and regulates intraocular pressure and ocular temperature. The choroid is typically thinner in myopic compared to non-myopic eyes (most pronounced at the fovea [65, 66]) and thins with increasing myopia and axial length in both adults [67–74] and children [75–77]. Significant choroidal thinning is also observed in high myopia (<–6.00 D) or eyes with posterior staphyloma [78], and has been associated with the presence of lacquer cracks [79], choroidal neovascularization [80], and reduced visual acuity [81]. The choroid also appears to be a biomarker of ocular processes regulating eye growth given that the central macular choroid thins during the initial development and progression of myopia [82–84] and thickens in response to imposed peripheral myopic retinal image defocus [85, 86], topical anti-muscarinic agents [87, 88], and increased light exposure [89] (clinical interventions associated with a slowing of eye growth in children).

4.2.5 Sclera

Scleral thinning associated with axial myopia is primarily restricted to the posterior pole [90–92], due to scleral tissue redistribution [93]. Scleral thinning may alter the tissue strength surrounding the optic nerve head, rendering myopic eyes more susceptible to glaucomatous damage [94, 95]. Consequently, posterior reinforcement surgery using donor scleral tissue has been refined over the years to arrest further axial elongation and scleral thinning in highly myopic eyes [96, 97]. Although anterior scleral thickness is similar between myopic and non-myopic eyes [98–100], there is growing evidence that the anterior sclera thins slightly during accommodation, particularly in myopic eyes [101, 102], most likely due to biomechanical forces of the ciliary muscle. A greater thinning observed in myopic eyes may be a result of a thicker posterior ciliary muscle [103–105] or changes in biomechanical properties of the sclera reported in animal models of form-deprivation myopia [106, 107].

4.3 Visual Environment, Emmetropization, and Myopia: Evidence from Animal Models

Over the last four decades, numerous animal models have provided valuable insight into the mechanisms underlying emmetropization and refractive error development. Much of the knowledge on vision-dependent changes in ocular growth has emanated from animal experiments in which either the quality of image formed on the retina is degraded (known as form-deprivation [FD]), or the focal point of the image is altered with respect to the retinal plane (known as lens induced defocus). Both FD and lens induced defocus result in abnormal eye growth and development of refractive errors. This section summarizes the attributes of experimental ametropias derived from these two visual manipulations, their differences, and significance for understanding refractive error development in humans.

4.3.1 Form-Deprivation Myopia

FD is the most commonly used experimental paradigm to model axial myopia in animals. Depriving the retina of form or patterned vision through eyelid suture

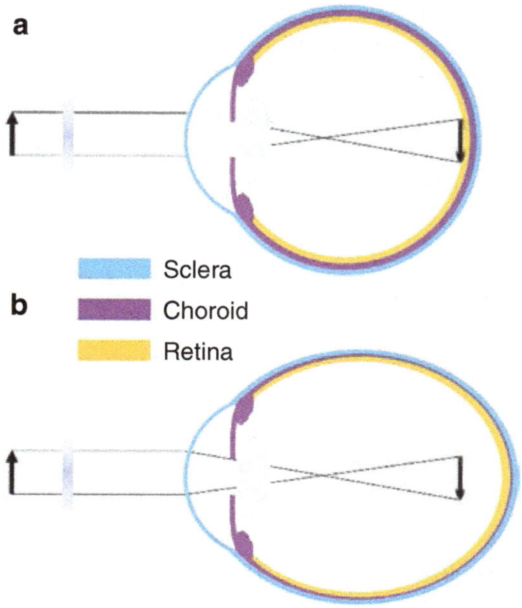

Fig. 4.5 Ocular compensation for form-deprivation (FD). (**a**) A diffuser causes nondirectional blur and a reduction in contrast of the retinal image. (**b**) The absence of visual feedback related to the effective refractive state of the eye causes a thinning of the posterior choroid and an increase in ocular growth, resulting in myopia

[108–110], or translucent diffusers [2, 15, 111–114] consistently produces axial myopia (Fig. 4.5). The use of noncontact translucent diffusers offers a more reliable representation of ocular changes with FD since they do not induce corneal changes (unlike eyelid fusion techniques). The ocular changes observed in response to FD clearly illustrate that degrading retinal image quality can produce robust myopic changes. Schaeffel et al. [115] proposed that FD is an open-loop condition, in which myopia develops as a result of uncoordinated ocular growth due to reduced retinal image contrast (or mid-range spatial frequency vision) [116] and the absence of visual feedback related to the effective refractive state of the eye [117].

The myopic response to FD varies among different animals. It is generally greatest in chickens (−9 D after 5 days of FD) [118], followed by tree shrews (−8 D after 12 days in young animals) [119] and guinea pigs (−6.6 D after 11 days) [113], and is less pronounced and much more variable in marmosets (−8 D after 4.5 weeks) [120] and rhesus monkeys (~−5 to −6 D after 17 weeks) [121, 122]. Variations observed between individual studies and animal models may be due to differences in experimental paradigms, the duration and extent of FD, inherent ocular anatomical variations, and/or differences in susceptibility to environmental myopia. Nevertheless, the myopic response to FD is conserved across a wide range of animal species (including fish, rabbit, mouse, and kestrel) [123]. In all species, axial myopia is predominantly caused by a significant elongation of the vitreous chamber, along with thinning of the choroid and the sclera [16, 17, 113, 124–132]. Few studies have also reported changes in corneal curvature and lens thickness with FD [131, 133–135]. Interestingly, ocular conditions that cause varying degrees of visual deprivation in humans such as ptosis [136], congenital cataract [137], corneal opacity [138], and vitreous hemorrhage [139] are associated with myopia, which may result from mechanisms similar to FD myopia observed in animals.

FD myopia is a graded phenomenon, where increasing degrees of image degradation are positively correlated with the magnitude of induced axial myopia [129, 140]. In addition, the effects of FD declines with age. Younger chicks [141, 142], macaques [143], tree shrews [119], and marmosets [144] show greater ocular changes in response to image degradation compared to older animals, potentially due to age-related reductions in sensory processing of blur stimuli or changes in scleral growth [144].

4.3.2 Lens Defocus Ametropias

Perhaps the strongest evidence of visual regulation of ocular growth comes from animal studies that show eyes can actively compensate for artificially induced myopic and hyperopic defocus by adjusting the axial length to the altered focal plane (i.e., emmetropization through the treatment lenses) (Fig. 4.6) [145]. Myopic defocus with plus lenses simulates artificial myopia that leads to a thickening of the choroid (moving the retina forward) and a reduction in the overall growth of the eye, thus, causing a hyperopic refractive error. Conversely, hyperopic defocus with minus lenses induces artificial hyperopia that leads to a thinning of the choroid

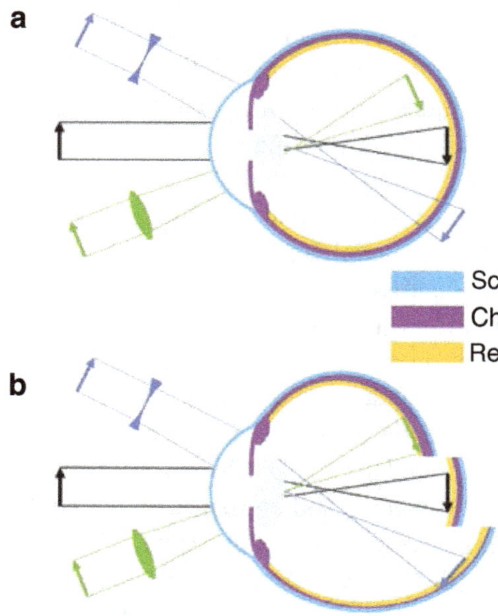

Fig. 4.6 (**a**) Schematic of imposed lens defocus. With no lens (black arrow), incident parallel rays of light from distant objects are focused on the retina. A plus lens (green, convex) causes the retinal image to focus in front of the retina known as myopic defocus, whereas a minus lens (blue, concave) focuses the image behind the retina known as hyperopic defocus. (**b**) A normal eye with no imposed lens defocus (black) exhibits normal ocular growth and choroidal thickness. Myopic defocus with plus lenses (green) causes a thickening of the choroid (moving the retina forward) and a reduction in the overall growth of the eye, causing a hyperopic refractive error. Hyperopic defocus with minus lenses (blue) leads to a thinning of the choroid (moving the retina backward) and an increase in ocular growth, resulting in myopia. Adapted from Wallman J and Winawer J, 2004 [1]

(moving the retina backward) and an increase in ocular growth, resulting in myopia to re-establish the optimal refractive state. This phenomenon was first documented in chicks [145], and has been extensively studied in chicks [16, 17, 146–148], tree shrews [149], rhesus monkeys [15, 150], marmosets [151], guinea pigs [152, 153], and mice [154] thereafter, indicating that the mechanisms regulating ocular growth can distinguish the sign of the imposed defocus in a wide range of animal species.

Chick eyes can compensate for a remarkable range of +15 to −10 D of imposed defocus [16, 147]. However, the operating range of defocus is much smaller for other animal species (monkey: −2 to +8 D [15], marmosets: −8 to <+4 D [151], tree shrew: −10 to +4 D [155], guinea pig: −7 to +4 D) [152, 156]. Compared to birds, the inability of primates to compensate for greater magnitudes of defocus may be due to bigger eye size [15, 150], the process of emmetropization [150], differences in the accommodative response to defocus stimuli, and/or the degree of independent accommodation between fellow eyes [15, 150, 157]. In all animals, the axial response to lens induced defocus is dependent upon the power of the treatment lens [147, 149–152, 158], and is predominantly attributed to the changes in vitreous chamber depth [16, 147, 159]. Similar to FD, the ocular response to lens induced defocus decreases with age [16]. Recent evidence suggests that the human visual system may also be able to detect the sign and magnitude of imposed defocus and make compensatory changes in axial length, similar to other animals. A number of studies have reported small bidirectional changes in axial length and choroidal thickness in response to 1–2 h of myopic and hyperopic defocus in children and young adults [160–165].

Studies have shown that the biological mechanisms underlying alterations in ocular growth to myopic and hyperopic defocus may be completely different (and not merely opposite to each other), and that the visual system is perhaps more sensitive to myopic defocus [166, 167]. In fact, the ocular response to lens induced defocus depends on the frequency and duration of lens wear, and not simply the "total duration" per day [166–169]. These findings argue for a nonlinear processing of myopic and hyperopic defocus signals across the retina [166, 167].

4.3.3 Comparing Form-Deprivation and Lens Defocus

Although FD and lens induced defocus use different visual stimuli to induce compensatory changes in ocular growth, there are features that are common to both visual manipulations. Removal of the visual manipulation triggers "recovery" from both FD and lens induced defocus [16, 17, 170]. During this recovery phase, the eyes quickly return to emmetropia by reversing the changes in choroidal thickness and axial eye growth (mainly by changing the vitreous chamber depth) [16, 17, 119, 150, 151, 170–173].

Further evidence from animal work suggests that the elimination of accommodation by cycloplegia, ciliary nerve section or damage to the Edinger-Westphal nucleus does not prevent the response to imposed FD [145, 174] or lens induced defocus [148, 175]. These results suggest that intact accommodation is not essential for visually guided growth [176] or there might be another accommodative pathway (not through ciliary and iris sphincter muscles) underlying optical defocus induced alterations in ocular growth [175].

Other studies argue that mechanisms underlying the response to FD and lens induced defocus may not be the same [177]. Some studies show different light paradigms selectively disrupt the response to FD or lens induced defocus [178–180]. For instance, high luminance levels inhibit myopia caused by FD in monkeys and chicks, but only slow the response to negative lenses [181, 182]. Furthermore, dopamine (a strong ocular growth inhibitor, see Sect. 4.4.1) may not signal eye growth in a similar manner for these two forms of experimental myopia [183]. While most studies indicate that dopamine agonists block increased axial elongation [177], one study reported that dopamine agonists inhibit FD, but not lens-induced myopia in guinea pigs [184]. More studies are needed to determine if these contradictory results are due to different regulatory mechanisms of eye growth or other parameters of the experimental paradigm.

4.4 Other Visual Cues for Emmetropization

Whilst the clarity of the retinal image dominates the nature of ocular growth, other visual cues may also influence the process of emmetropization. This section examines some of the important cues that could significantly affect retinal image quality, and hence ocular growth in human eyes.

4.4.1 Retinal Physiology

Work from animal models suggests that retinal defocus (or visual blur) initiates a signaling cascade that leads to a number of cellular and biochemical changes in the retina and the retinal pigment epithelium (RPE), which signal changes to the choroid, and eventually the sclera, leading to alterations in the overall growth and refractive state of the eye (Fig. 4.7) [16, 17, 185]. The retina is an integral part of this visual signaling as it is the first layer of photosensory neurons that detect

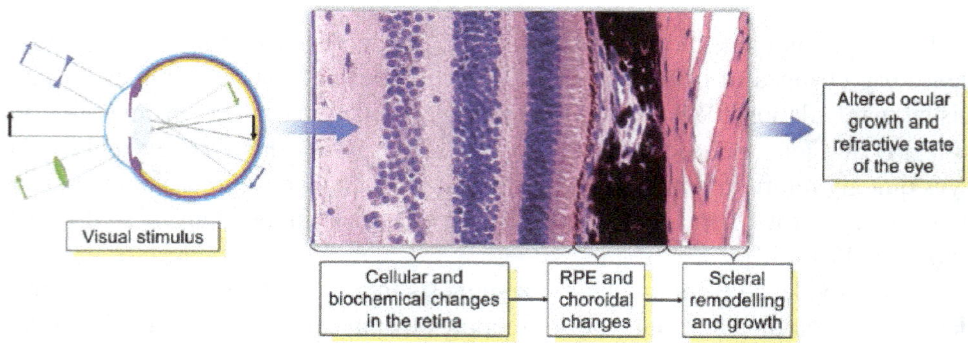

Fig. 4.7 A biochemical signal cascade beginning at the retina and ending at the sclera regulating ocular growth and the refractive state. Retinal defocus may initiate a signaling cascade that leads to a number of cellular and biochemical changes in the retina and the retinal pigment epithelium (RPE), the choroid, and eventually the sclera, leading to alterations in the overall growth and the refractive state of the eye

defocus [186]. Furthermore, ocular compensation for both FD and lens induced defocus are largely regulated at the retinal level. Severing the optic nerve in young chicks does not prevent the development of refractive errors in response to spectacle lenses [16, 187] or diffusers [130]. In both chicks [17, 188, 189] and primates [190], partial diffusers and hemifield spectacle lenses restricted to only half of the visual field cause corresponding myopic changes only in the visually deprived part of the globe. These studies demonstrate that the visual regulation of ocular growth in response to diffusers and lenses primarily occurs within the retina, with minimal input from the brain.

Retinal neurons also secrete a number of growth regulatory neurotransmitters (such as dopamine [191, 192], retinoic acid [153], nitric oxide [193, 194] and glucagon [195]) that can directly alter ocular growth in mammalian eyes. Dopamine, one of the most widely studied neurotransmitters with regard to myopia in animal models, has been implicated as a potent stop signal for myopic eye growth [183, 196]. In both chickens [191, 197] and primates [198], FD myopia is associated with lower levels of 3,4-dihydroxyphenylacetate (DOPAC, the primary metabolite of dopamine) and dopamine in the retina. Although the protective effects of outdoor light exposure on myopia development in children has been hypothesized to be mediated by greater dopamine synthesis in the eye (see Sect. 4.5), the exact mechanisms underlying the protective effects of dopamine on myopia are not fully known. Together, these studies suggest that alterations in normal retinal physiology and/or changes in retinal neurotransmitters may lead to the development of refractive errors, as shown in chickens [186, 199, 200] and mice [201–206]. Some features of retinal abnormalities and refractive errors are evident in humans as well; for instance, NYX [207] and GRM6 [208] retinal ON pathway mutations and retinal degenerations such as cone-rod dystrophy [209] and retinitis pigmentosa [210] are associated with myopia.

4.4.2 Aberrations

A long held belief is that myopia may develop due to the eye's emmetropization response to inherent ocular aberrations that degrade retinal image quality and trigger axial elongation [211]. Since there is minimal variation in longitudinal chromatic aberration between individuals or refractive error groups in humans [212], most investigations have focused on monochromatic higher order aberrations (HOAs) as a potential myopigenic stimulus. Evidence concerning the relationship between HOAs during distance viewing and refractive error from cross-sectional studies is conflicting [211, 213]. However, during or following near work tasks, adult myopic eyes tend to display a transient increase in corneal and total ocular HOAs (Figs. 4.8 and 4.9), suggesting a potential role for near work induced retinal image degradation in myopia development [214, 215]. Longitudinal studies of myopic children also indicate that eyes with greater positive spherical aberration demonstrate slower eye growth [63, 216].

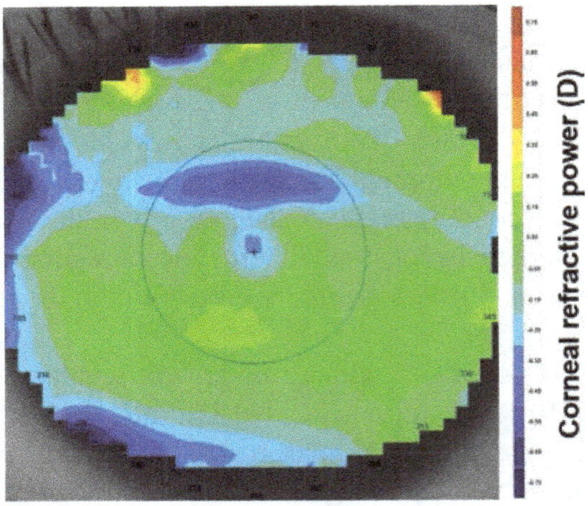

Fig. 4.8 Corneal refractive power difference map following a 10 min reading task at 25° downward gaze. The black circle denotes the pupil outline detected by the video keratoscope. A horizontal band of corneal flattening is observed in the superior aspect of the pupil corresponding to the position of the upper eyelid during downward gaze. This refractive change is equivalent to a 0.20 D hyperopic shift over the central 4 mm

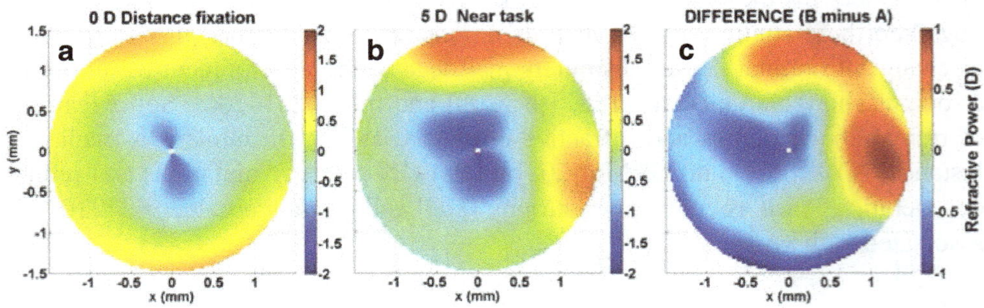

Fig. 4.9 Refractive power maps, a graphical representation of total ocular higher order aberrations, during (**a**) distance fixation (0 D accommodation demand), (**b**) a 5 D accommodation task, and (**c**) the difference (B minus A) over a 3 mm pupil diameter. A significant increase in negative spherical aberration of −0.10 μm is displayed

A number of myopia control interventions also alter the HOA and peripheral refraction profile. While relative peripheral refraction was initially thought to modulate central eye growth, recent longitudinal studies have found no association between peripheral refraction and myopia progression in children [217, 218]. Multifocal soft contact lenses and orthokeratology significantly increase the magnitude of positive spherical aberration [219, 220]. The anticholinergic agent atropine may also provide visual feedback that influences eye growth due to an increase in positive spherical aberration or horizontal coma associated with cycloplegia and pupil mydriasis, respectively [221]. Collectively, these findings suggest that changes in HOAs may influence eye growth and refractive development during childhood.

4.4.3 Accommodation

Given the association between near work and the development and progression of childhood myopia [222], numerous studies have compared various characteristics of accommodation between refractive error groups, typically the accuracy of the accommodation response, since a lag of accommodation (hyperopic retinal defocus) may stimulate axial elongation as observed in animal models. Using a range of experimental approaches, the accommodative response to a 3 D accommodative stimulus is ~0.25 to 1.00 D less in myopic adults compared to emmetropes [223–227]. The slowing of myopia progression during childhood with progressive addition or bifocal lenses, designed to improve accommodation accuracy and minimize a lag of accommodation, adds some weight to the role of accommodation in myopia development and progression [62, 228]. However, the exact underlying mechanism of myopia control with such lenses may be related to imposed peripheral retinal defocus or a reduction in the near vergence demand [229]. In a longitudinal study of young infants [230], a significant relationship was observed between the accommodative response and the reduction in neonatal refractive error in the first 2 years of life, supporting a potential role for accommodation-guided eye growth.

4.4.4 Circadian Rhythms

Like many of the human body's physiological processes, numerous ocular structures and functions exhibit cyclic variations over the course of the day. Visual inputs such as daily patterns of light exposure are considered critical factors in entraining the timing of these circadian rhythms. Findings from animal studies demonstrate that normal eye growth exhibits significant circadian variations, with the eye generally being longest during the day and shorter at night [231]. Choroidal thickness also exhibits a circadian rhythm in normal eyes, which is generally in antiphase to the rhythms in axial length [172]. Similar patterns of diurnal variation in axial length and choroidal thickness have also been documented in normal human eyes [232–234].

It has also been suggested that ocular circadian rhythms may play a role in eye growth regulation and the development of myopia, since altering the visual inputs that drive circadian rhythms (e.g., rearing animals in constant light [235] or constant darkness [236], or exposing the eye to bright light at night time [237]) can result in alterations in normal eye growth in animal models. Furthermore, when refractive errors (both hyperopic and myopic) are induced experimentally in animals, changes in the magnitude and phase of the normal circadian rhythms of axial length and choroidal thickness also occur, which also supports a potential role of circadian rhythms in the development of refractive errors [172, 238]. These findings from animal research were paralleled by studies in young adult humans, where changes in the normal diurnal rhythms of axial length and choroidal thickness occurred in response to short-term (12-h) exposure to monocular myopic [165], and hyperopic blur [163]. Although the exact role played by circadian rhythms in the regulation of human eye growth is not fully understood, human studies also indicate that myopes exhibit alterations in their systemic melatonin levels [239], and also exhibit altered sleep patterns [240] compared to non-myopic individuals.

4.5 Effects of Key Environmental Factors on Myopia

As discussed in Chaps. 1 and 2, myopia represents a "complex" disorder with both environmental and genetic origins [241, 242]. This section discusses some of the important environmental factors, and their influence on myopia.

4.5.1 Near Work and Education

Since the age when myopia normally develops and progresses coincides with the school years, myopia has long been suggested to be connected with increased levels of education. Indeed, numerous studies conducted across a range of different populations have consistently found that higher levels of education are associated with a higher prevalence of myopia [243–245]. The exact mechanism linking increased education with myopia, however, is less clear. Although it is possible that optical [214, 224] or biomechanical [246, 247] ocular changes associated with near work could potentially promote myopic eye growth in those with higher levels of education (and hence near work demands), population studies examining the link between near work activities and myopia have been conflicting, with some studies suggesting an association between near work and myopia [222, 248], and others indicating no significant effects [249]. The relatively inconsistent findings linking near work with myopia development suggests a potential role for other factors in the association between education and myopia, such as a lack of outdoor light exposure, discussed further below.

4.5.2 Urbanization

Aspects of the living environment may also be involved in the development and progression of myopia, since population-based studies consistently report a higher prevalence of myopia in children living in urban regions, compared to children living in rural regions [250, 251]. These associations between the urban environment and myopia could at least partially be explained by socioeconomic and educational differences between urban and rural regions, which could in turn result in differences in near work and outdoor activities. However, a number of recent studies indicate that a higher population density is significantly associated with increased myopia prevalence in children, independent of near work and outdoor activities [252, 253]. This suggests other aspects of the urban environment may potentially impact upon eye growth. Studies have also reported associations between housing type and myopia, with children living in smaller homes reported to have a significantly higher prevalence of myopia [253, 254]. Although further research is required to establish the causative nature and mechanisms underlying these associations, it has been hypothesized that a constricted living space may result in an increased exposure to hyperopic blur, thus promoting myopia.

4.5.3 Light Exposure

A number of recent studies report that the time children spend engaged in outdoor activities is negatively associated with their risk of myopia [241, 249, 255–259]. Both cross-sectional and longitudinal studies indicate that greater time spent outdoors is associated with a significantly lower myopia prevalence and reduced risk of myopia onset in childhood. Although some studies report significant associations between myopia progression and outdoor activity [257, 259], this is not a consistent finding across all longitudinal studies [260]. A recent meta-analysis of studies examining the relationship between outdoor time and myopia indicated that there was a 2% reduction in the odds of having myopia for each additional hour per week spent outdoors [261].

These associations [241, 255, 256] have prompted recent interest in the potential influence of light exposure in the regulation of eye growth and myopia. Since outdoor activity typically involves exposure to high intensity light, it has been hypothesized that increased exposure to bright light may be the important factor underlying these protective effects of outdoor activity [256]. Other factors, such as the typical pattern of retinal focus experienced in outdoor environments (which is likely to involve less near focusing and potentially less exposure to hyperopic blur), may also play a role [262].

Light Intensity and Myopia Animal studies indicate that the intensity of daily light exposure can influence refractive development. In normal growing young chickens, rearing animals under a normal daily light-dark cycle, but with daily bright ambient lighting (~10,000 lux) resulted in significantly less myopic refractive errors than when animals were reared under dim ambient lighting during the day (50 lux) [263]. Bright light exposure also inhibits the development of FD myopia in a range of different animal species [114, 181, 264], with the strength of inhibitory effects correlating significantly with the log of the intensity of ambient light exposure [264]. The effects of increased light intensity upon lens induced myopia (through imposing hyperopic defocus) in animals however are less consistent, with either a slowing of lens compensation (with no change in refractive endpoint) [182], or no significant effects on lens compensation reported [265].

Recent observational longitudinal studies in humans utilizing wearable light sensors to assess ambient light exposure have enabled the relationship between light exposure and axial eye growth in childhood to be examined [266, 267]. Similar to findings in animals, both of these recent studies have reported that slower axial eye growth is associated with greater daily ambient light exposure (with a 1-log unit increase in light exposure being associated with ~0.1 mm/year slower axial eye growth), with this relationship reaching statistical significance in the study with the larger sample size ($n = 102$) [266], and bordering on significance ($p = 0.07$, $n = 60$) in the other study [267]. A recent randomized, controlled trial in Taiwan examined the effect of increasing outdoor time during the school day (an extra 40 min of outdoor time during school recess) upon myopia development and axial eye growth over 12 months [268]. In this study, light exposure was also monitored using wearable light sensors, and a significant association between greater light exposure and slower myopia progression was also documented. Collectively, these studies suggest that increased light exposure is associated with slower axial eye growth in the human eye.

Increased light exposure may also underlie some of the differences in myopia prevalence found in different geographic locations. A recent study compared the habitual ambient light exposure (captured with wearable light sensors) of children living in Singapore (a country with some of the highest reported levels of childhood myopia prevalence [269]) with children living in Australia (where myopia prevalence is generally reported to be relatively low [270]) and found substantially lower levels of outdoor light exposure in the children living in Singapore (Fig. 4.10) [271].

Duration of Light Exposure and Myopia Animal studies examining the effects of increased light exposure upon myopia development have generally used experimental paradigms where elevated light levels were applied continuously for the full day. Lan et al. [272] examined the influence of different daily durations of bright light exposure upon inhibition of myopia in chickens. They found bright light applied for

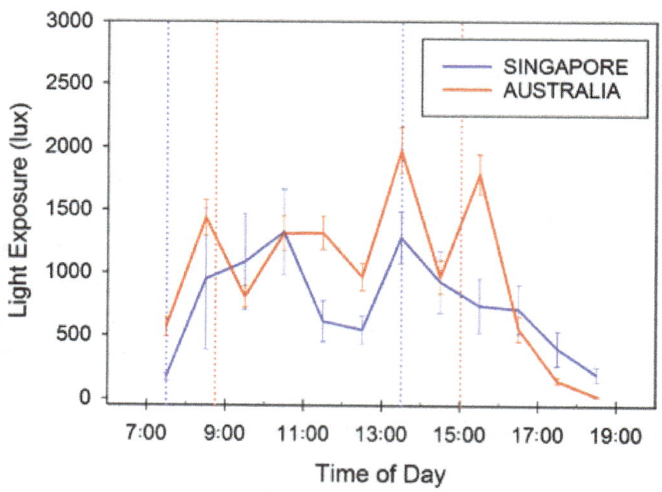

Fig. 4.10 Average hourly light exposure of Australian (red lines) and Singaporean (blue lines) children assessed during school weekdays using wearable light sensors. Note the substantially greater light exposure for the Australian children at a number of periods throughout the day [271]. This lower daily exposure to bright outdoor light may be one factor underlying the higher myopia prevalence typically observed in Singaporean children. Dashed lines indicate the average school start and finish times in Australia (red) and Singapore (blue). Error bars represent the standard error of the mean

only 1 or 2 h per day did not inhibit myopia, but 5 h of exposure did significantly protect against the development of FD myopia. Extending exposure duration further to 10 h per day did not appear to offer further protective benefit.

In a large longitudinal study, Jones et al. [249] reported that children who engaged in outdoor activities for 14 h per week or more, exhibited the lowest odds of developing myopia. A number of recent randomized controlled trials have reported that interventions that increase children's outdoor time (by 40–80 min a day) significantly reduce the onset of myopia in childhood [268, 273, 274]. In the "Role of outdoor activity in myopia study" [266], children who were habitually exposed to low ambient light levels (on average less than 60 min exposure to outdoor light per day) had significantly faster axial eye growth compared to children habitually exposed to moderate and high light levels. These findings from human studies suggest that children who are exposed to less than 60 min a day of bright outdoor light are at an increased risk of more rapid eye growth and myopia development, and that approximately 2 h or more of outdoor exposure each day is required to provide protection against myopia development in the human eye.

Spectral Composition of Light and Myopia Since the spectral characteristics of outdoor light are significantly different to typical indoor light, it has been suggested that the spectral composition of outdoor light may be an additional factor that underlies the protective effects of outdoor activity upon myopia development. Although some studies in humans suggest exposure to short-wavelength light may protect against myopia [275], there has only been limited work in humans examining the possible impact of the spectral composition of light on myopia.

Animal studies do suggest that the spectral content of light can influence the growth of the eye, since altered eye growth is observed in animals reared under narrow band spectral lighting conditions. However, the effects of the spectral content of light shows substantial interspecies differences [276–279]. In chickens and guineas pigs, raising animals in short-wavelength light appears to slow eye growth and reduce myopia development, whereas long-wavelength light appears to increase eye growth and lead to myopia development [276, 279]. Conversely long-wavelength light appears to slow eye growth and reduce myopia development in tree shrews and rhesus monkeys [277, 278]. Further research is required to understand the mechanisms underlying these effects (and interspecies differences) and to establish the impact of the spectral composition of light upon human myopia.

4.6 Conclusion

In conclusion, over the last 40 years, remarkable progress has been made in understanding the possible mechanisms and pathogenesis of myopia, with a large contribution to this knowledge coming from an extensive body of work in animal models. Importantly, laboratory research in animals have shown that the visual environment (i.e., quality and/or focus of the retinal image) influences ocular growth and refractive development, which has been a key to our current understanding of the process of emmetropization in humans. Similarities in features of defocus induced ocular changes in humans and experimental models of myopia, such as the eye's ability to detect the sign of retinal defocus and make compensatory changes in axial length, suggest that mechanisms of visually guided eye growth and refractive error development in animal models may be present in human eyes as well. Alongside animal research, a large body of clinical and epidemiological research has identified a number of other visual cues (e.g., aberrations, accommodation, and circadian rhythms) and environmental factors (e.g., light exposure, near work, and education) that could affect normal ocular growth and lead to the development of refractive errors. Experimental models continue to provide valuable information on cellular and biochemical mechanisms of eye growth, enabling the identification of potential new therapeutic targets for early diagnosis and treatment of myopia.

References

1. Wallman J, Winawer J. Homeostasis of eye growth and the question of myopia. Neuron. 2004;43:447–68.
2. Smith EL. Spectacle lenses and emmetropization: the role of optical defocus in regulating ocular development. Optom Vis Sci. 1998;75:388–98.
3. Cook RC, Glasscock R. Refractive and ocular findings in the newborn. Am J Ophthalmol. 1951;34:1407–13.
4. Banks MS. Infant refraction and accommodation. Int Ophthalmol Clin. 1980;20:205–32.
5. Mohindra I, Held R. Refraction in humans from birth to five years. In: Third International Conference on Myopia Copenhagen, August 24–27, 1980. New York: Springer; 1981. p. 19–27.
6. Ingram R, Barr A. Changes in refraction between the ages of 1 and 3 1/2 years. Br J Ophthalmol. 1979;63:339–42.
7. Wood I, Hodi S, Morgan L. Longitudinal change of refractive error in infants during the first year of life. Eye. 1995;9:551–7.
8. Gwiazda J, Thorn F, Bauer J, Held R. Emmetropization and the progression of manifest refraction in children followed from infancy to puberty. Clin Vis Sci. 1993;8:337–44.
9. Kempf GA, Collins SD, Jarman BL. Refractive errors in the eyes of children as determined by retinoscopie examination with a cycloplegic. Results of eye examinations of 1,860 white school children in Washington, DC. Public Health Bulletin. 1928;182:56.
10. Fitzgerald DE, Duckman R. Refractive error. In: Visual development, diagnosis, and treatment of the pediatric patient. Philadelphia: Lippincott Williams & Wilkins; 2006. p. 69–88.
11. Gordon RA, Donzis PB. Refractive development of the human eye. Arch Ophthalmol. 1985;103:785–9.
12. Saunders KJ. Early refractive development in humans. Surv Ophthalmol. 1995;40:207–16.
13. Hirsch MJ. Predictability of refraction at age 14 on the basis of testing at age 6—interim report from the Ojai Longitudinal Study of Refraction. Optom Vis Sci. 1964;41:567–73.
14. Zadnik K, Mutti DO, Friedman NE, Adams AJ. Initial cross-sectional results from the Orinda Longitudinal Study of Myopia. Optom Vis Sci. 1993;70:750–8.
15. Smith EL, Hung LF. The role of optical defocus in regulating refractive development in infant monkeys. Vis Res. 1999;39:1415–35.
16. Wildsoet C, Wallman J. Choroidal and scleral mechanisms of compensation for spectacle lenses in chicks. Vis Res. 1995;35:1175–94.

17. Wallman J, Wildsoet C, Xu A, et al. Moving the retina: choroidal modulation of refractive state. Vis Res. 1995;35:37–50.
18. Mutti DO, Mitchell GL, Jones LA, et al. Axial growth and changes in lenticular and corneal power during emmetropization in infants. Invest Ophthalmol Vis Sci. 2005;46:3074–80.
19. Pennie FC, Wood IC, Olsen C, White S, Charman WN. A longitudinal study of the biometric and refractive changes in full-term infants during the first year of life. Vis Res. 2001;41:2799–810.
20. Larsen JS. The sagittal growth of the eye: IV. Ultrasonic measurement of the axial length of the eye from birth to puberty. Acta Ophthalmol. 1971;49:873–86.
21. Larsen JS. The sagittal growth of the eye. 3. Ultrasonic measurement of the posterior segment (axial length of the vitreous) from birth to puberty. Acta Ophthalmol. 1971;49:441–53.
22. Sorsby A, Leary G, Richards MJ. Correlation ametropia and component ametropia. Vis Res. 1962;2:309–13.
23. Isenberg SJ, Del Signore M, Chen A, Wei J, Christenson PD. Corneal topography of neonates and infants. Arch Ophthalmol. 2004;122:1767–71.
24. Ehrlich DL, Braddick OJ, Atkinson J, et al. Infant emmetropization: longitudinal changes in refraction components from nine to twenty months of age. Optom Vis Sci. 1997;74:822–43.
25. Varughese S, Varghese RM, Gupta N, Ojha R, Sreenivas V, Puliyel JM. Refractive error at birth and its relation to gestational age. Curr Eye Res. 2005;30:423–8.
26. Friling R, Weinberger D, Kremer I, Avisar R, Sirota L, Snir M. Keratometry measurements in preterm and full term newborn infants. Br J Ophthalmol. 2004;88:8–10.
27. Rowland HC, Sayles N. Photokeratometric and photorefractive measurements of astigmatism in infants and young children. Vis Res. 1985;25:73–81.
28. Gwiazda J, Scheiman M, Mohindra I, Held R. Astigmatism in children: changes in axis and amount from birth to six years. Invest Ophthalmol Vis Sci. 1984;25:88–92.
29. Atkinson J, Braddick O, French J. Infant astigmatism: its disappearance with age. Vis Res. 1980;20:891–3.
30. Dobson V, Fulton A, Sebris SL. Cycloplegic refractions of infants and young children: the axis of astigmatism. Invest Ophthalmol Vis Sci. 1984;25:83–7.
31. Li SM, Iribarren R, Kang MT, et al. Corneal power, anterior segment length and lens power in 14-year-old Chinese children: the Anyang Childhood Eye Study. Sci Rep. 2016;6:20243.
32. Carney LG, Mainstone JC, Henderson BA. Corneal topography and myopia. A cross-sectional study. Invest Ophthalmol Vis Sci. 1997;38:311–20.
33. AlMahmoud T, Priest D, Munger R, Jackson WB. Correlation between refractive error, corneal power, and thickness in a large population with a wide range of ametropia. Invest Ophthalmol Vis Sci. 2011;52:1235–42.
34. Xie R, Zhou XT, Lu F, et al. Correlation between myopia and major biometric parameters of the eye: a retrospective clinical study. Optom Vis Sci. 2009;86:E503–8.
35. Zhang YY, Jiang WJ, Teng ZE, et al. Corneal curvature radius and associated factors in Chinese children: the Shandong Children Eye Study. PLoS One. 2015;10:e0117481.
36. Breslin KM, O'Donoghue L, Saunders KJ. A prospective study of spherical refractive error and ocular components among Northern Irish schoolchildren (the NICER study). Invest Ophthalmol Vis Sci. 2013;54:4843–50.
37. Saw SM, Chua WH, Gazzard G, Koh D, Tan DT, Stone RA. Eye growth changes in myopic children in Singapore. Br J Ophthalmol. 2005;89:1489–94.
38. Scheiman M, Gwiazda J, Zhang Q, et al. Longitudinal changes in corneal curvature and its relationship to axial length in the Correction of Myopia Evaluation Trial (COMET) cohort. J Opt. 2016;9:13–21.
39. Lin LL, Shih YF, Lee YC, Hung PT, Hou PK. Changes in ocular refraction and its components among medical studentsDOUBLEHYPHENa 5-year longitudinal study. Optom Vis Sci. 1996;73:495–8.
40. Ojaimi E, Rose KA, Morgan IG, et al. Distribution of ocular biometric parameters and refraction in a population-based study of Australian children. Invest Ophthalmol Vis Sci. 2005;46:2748–54.

41. He X, Zou H, Lu L, et al. Axial length/corneal radius ratio: association with refractive state and role on myopia detection combined with visual acuity in Chinese schoolchildren. PLoS One. 2015;10:e0111766.
42. Gonzalez Blanco F, Sanz Fernandez JC, Munoz Sanz MA. Axial length, corneal radius, and age of myopia onset. Optom Vis Sci. 2008;85:89–96.
43. Foo VH, Verkicharla PK, Ikram MK, et al. Axial length/corneal radius of curvature ratio and myopia in 3-year-old children. Transl Vis Sci Technol. 2016;5:5.
44. Ortiz S, Mena L, Rio-San Cristobal A, Martin R. Relationships between central and peripheral corneal thickness in different degrees of myopia. J Opt. 2014;7:44–50.
45. Pedersen L, Hjortdal J, Ehlers N. Central corneal thickness in high myopia. Acta Ophthalmol Scand. 2005;83:539–42.
46. Tong L, Saw SM, Siak JK, Gazzard G, Tan D. Corneal thickness determination and correlates in Singaporean schoolchildren. Invest Ophthalmol Vis Sci. 2004;45:4004–9.
47. Fam HB, How AC, Baskaran M, Lim KL, Chan YH, Aung T. Central corneal thickness and its relationship to myopia in Chinese adults. Br J Ophthalmol. 2006;90:1451–3.
48. Huang Y, Huang C, Li L, et al. Corneal biomechanics, refractive error, and axial length in Chinese primary school children. Invest Ophthalmol Vis Sci. 2011;52:4923–8.
49. Chang PY, Chang SW, Wang JY. Assessment of corneal biomechanical properties and intraocular pressure with the Ocular Response Analyzer in childhood myopia. Br J Ophthalmol. 2010;94:877–81.
50. Jiang Z, Shen M, Mao G, et al. Association between corneal biomechanical properties and myopia in Chinese subjects. Eye. 2011;25:1083–9.
51. Wang W, He M, He H, Zhang C, Jin H, Zhong X. Corneal biomechanical metrics of healthy Chinese adults using Corvis ST. Cont Lens Anterior Eye. 2017;40:97–103.
52. Shen M, Fan F, Xue A, Wang J, Zhou X, Lu F. Biomechanical properties of the cornea in high myopia. Vis Res. 2008;48:2167–71.
53. Shih YF, Chiang TH, Lin LL. Lens thickness changes among school children in Taiwan. Invest Ophthalmol Vis Sci. 2009;50:2637–44.
54. Wong HB, Machin D, Tan SB, Wong TY, Saw SM. Ocular component growth curves among Singaporean children with different refractive error status. Invest Ophthalmol Vis Sci. 2010;51:1341–7.
55. Jones LA, Mitchell GL, Mutti DO, Hayes JR, Moeschberger ML, Zadnik K. Comparison of ocular component growth curves among refractive error groups in children. Invest Ophthalmol Vis Sci. 2005;46:2317–27.
56. Mutti DO, Mitchell GL, Sinnott LT, et al. Corneal and crystalline lens dimensions before and after myopia onset. Optom Vis Sci. 2012;89:251–62.
57. Iribarren R, Morgan IG, Chan YH, Lin X, Saw SM. Changes in lens power in Singapore Chinese children during refractive development. Invest Ophthalmol Vis Sci. 2012;53:5124–30.
58. Dubbelman M, Van der Heijde GL. The shape of the aging human lens: curvature, equivalent refractive index and the lens paradox. Vis Res. 2001;41:1867–77.
59. Li SM, Li SY, Kang MT, et al. Distribution of ocular biometry in 7- and 14-year-old Chinese children. Optom Vis Sci. 2015;92:566–72.
60. Richter GM, Wang M, Jiang X, et al. Ocular determinants of refractive error and its age- and sex-related variations in the Chinese American Eye Study. JAMA Ophthalmol. 2017;135:724–32.
61. Zadnik K, Mutti DO, Mitchell GL, Jones LA, Burr D, Moeschberger ML. Normal eye growth in emmetropic schoolchildren. Optom Vis Sci. 2004;81:819–28.
62. Gwiazda J, Hyman L, Hussein M, et al. A randomized clinical trial of progressive addition lenses versus single vision lenses on the progression of myopia in children. Invest Ophthalmol Vis Sci. 2003;44:1492–500.
63. Lau JK, Vincent SJ, Collins MJ, Cheung SW, Cho P. Ocular higher-order aberrations and axial eye growth in young Hong Kong children. Sci Rep. 2018;8:6726.
64. Huang J, Wen D, Wang Q, et al. Efficacy comparison of 16 interventions for myopia control in children: a network meta-analysis. Ophthalmology. 2016;123:697–708.

65. Read SA, Collins MJ, Vincent SJ, Alonso-Caneiro D. Choroidal thickness in myopic and non-myopic children assessed with enhanced depth imaging optical coherence tomography. Invest Ophthalmol Vis Sci. 2013;54:7578–86.
66. Xiong S, He X, Deng J, et al. Choroidal thickness in 3001 Chinese children aged 6 to 19 years using swept-source OCT. Sci Rep. 2017;7:45059.
67. Chen FK, Yeoh J, Rahman W, Patel PJ, Tufail A, Da Cruz L. Topographic variation and interocular symmetry of macular choroidal thickness using enhanced depth imaging optical coherence tomography. Invest Ophthalmol Vis Sci. 2012;53:975–85.
68. Esmaeelpour M, Povazay B, Hermann B, et al. Three-dimensional 1060-nm OCT: choroidal thickness maps in normal subjects and improved posterior segment visualization in cataract patients. Invest Ophthalmol Vis Sci. 2010;51:5260–6.
69. Gupta P, Jing T, Marziliano P, et al. Distribution and determinants of choroidal thickness and volume using automated segmentation software in a population-based study. Am J Ophthalmol. 2015;159:293–301.e293.
70. Li XQ, Munkholm A, Larsen M, Munch IC. Choroidal thickness in relation to birth parameters in 11- to 12-year-old children: the Copenhagen Child Cohort 2000 Eye Study. Invest Ophthalmol Vis Sci. 2014;56:617–24.
71. Ouyang Y, Heussen FM, Mokwa N, et al. Spatial distribution of posterior pole choroidal thickness by spectral domain optical coherence tomography. Invest Ophthalmol Vis Sci. 2011;52:7019–26.
72. Tan CS, Cheong KX. Macular choroidal thicknesses in healthy adultsDOUBLEHYPHENrelationship with ocular and demographic factors. Invest Ophthalmol Vis Sci. 2014;55:6452–8.
73. Wei WB, Xu L, Jonas JB, et al. Subfoveal choroidal thickness: the Beijing Eye Study. Ophthalmology. 2013;120:175–80.
74. Sanchez-Cano A, Orduna E, Segura F, et al. Choroidal thickness and volume in healthy young white adults and the relationships between them and axial length, ammetropy and sex. Am J Ophthalmol. 2014;158:574–83.
75. He X, Jin P, Zou H, et al. Choroidal thickness in healthy Chinese children aged 6 to 12: The Shanghai Children Eye Study. Retina. 2017;37:368–75.
76. Jin P, Zou H, Zhu J, et al. Choroidal and retinal thickness in children with different refractive status measured by swept-source optical coherence tomography. Am J Ophthalmol. 2016;168:164–76.
77. Zhang JM, Wu JF, Chen JH, et al. Macular choroidal thickness in children: the Shandong Children Eye Study. Invest Ophthalmol Vis Sci. 2015;56:7646–52.
78. Zhou LX, Shao L, Xu L, Wei WB, Wang YX, You QS. The relationship between scleral staphyloma and choroidal thinning in highly myopic eyes: the Beijing Eye Study. Sci Rep. 2017;7:9825.
79. Wang NK, Lai CC, Chou CL, et al. Choroidal thickness and biometric markers for the screening of lacquer cracks in patients with high myopia. PLoS One. 2013;8:e53660.
80. Ikuno Y, Jo Y, Hamasaki T, Tano Y. Ocular risk factors for choroidal neovascularization in pathologic myopia. Invest Ophthalmol Vis Sci. 2010;51:3721–5.
81. Nishida Y, Fujiwara T, Imamura Y, Lima LH, Kurosaka D, Spaide RF. Choroidal thickness and visual acuity in highly myopic eyes. Retina. 2012;32:1229–36.
82. Read SA, Alonso-Caneiro D, Vincent SJ, Collins MJ. Longitudinal changes in choroidal thickness and eye growth in childhood. Invest Ophthalmol Vis Sci. 2015;56:3103–12.
83. Fontaine M, Gaucher D, Sauer A, Speeg-Schatz C. Choroidal thickness and ametropia in children: a longitudinal study. Eur J Ophthalmol. 2017;27:730–4.
84. Jin P, Zou H, Xu X, et al. Longitudinal changes in choroidal and retinal thicknesses in children with myopic shift. Retina. 2019;39:1091–9.
85. Chen Z, Xue F, Zhou J, Qu X, Zhou X. Effects of orthokeratology on choroidal thickness and axial length. Optom Vis Sci. 2016;93:1064–71.
86. Li Z, Cui D, Hu Y, Ao S, Zeng J, Yang X. Choroidal thickness and axial length changes in myopic children treated with orthokeratology. Cont Lens Anterior Eye. 2017;40:417–23.

87. Sander BP, Collins MJ, Read SA. The effect of topical adrenergic and anticholinergic agents on the choroidal thickness of young healthy adults. Exp Eye Res. 2014;128:181–9.
88. Zhang Z, Zhou Y, Xie Z, et al. The effect of topical atropine on the choroidal thickness of healthy children. Sci Rep. 2016;6:34936.
89. Read SA. Ocular and environmental factors associated with eye growth in childhood. Optom Vis Sci. 2016;93:1031–41.
90. Elsheikh A, Geraghty B, Alhasso D, Knappett J, Campanelli M, Rama P. Regional variation in the biomechanical properties of the human sclera. Exp Eye Res. 2010;90:624–33.
91. Norman RE, Flanagan JG, Rausch SM, et al. Dimensions of the human sclera: thickness measurement and regional changes with axial length. Exp Eye Res. 2010;90:277–84.
92. Vurgese S, Panda-Jonas S, Jonas JB. Scleral thickness in human eyes. PLoS One. 2012;7:e29692.
93. McBrien NA, Gentle A. Role of the sclera in the development and pathological complications of myopia. Prog Retin Eye Res. 2003;22:307–38.
94. Downs JC, Ensor ME, Bellezza AJ, Thompson HW, Hart RT, Burgoyne CF. Posterior scleral thickness in perfusion-fixed normal and early-glaucoma monkey eyes. Invest Ophthalmol Vis Sci. 2001;42:3202–8.
95. Nemeth J. The posterior coats of the eye in glaucoma. An echobiometric study. Graefes Arch Clin Exp Ophthalmol. 1990;228:33–5.
96. Xue A, Bao F, Zheng L, Wang Q, Cheng L, Qu J. Posterior scleral reinforcement on progressive high myopic young patients. Optom Vis Sci. 2014;91:412–8.
97. Xue A, Zheng L, Tan G, et al. Genipin-crosslinked donor sclera for posterior scleral contraction/reinforcement to fight progressive myopia. Invest Ophthalmol Vis Sci. 2018;59:3564–73.
98. Read SA, Alonso-Caneiro D, Vincent SJ, et al. Anterior eye tissue morphology: scleral and conjunctival thickness in children and young adults. Sci Rep. 2016;6:33796.
99. Buckhurst HD, Gilmartin B, Cubbidge RP, Logan NS. Measurement of scleral thickness in humans using anterior segment optical coherent tomography. PLoS One. 2015;10:e0132902.
100. Pekel G, Yagci R, Acer S, Ongun GT, Cetin EN, Simavli H. Comparison of corneal layers and anterior sclera in emmetropic and myopic eyes. Cornea. 2015;34:786–90.
101. Consejo A, Radhakrishnan H, Iskander DR. Scleral changes with accommodation. Ophthalmic Physiol Opt. 2017;37:263–74.
102. Woodman-Pieterse EC, Read SA, Collins MJ, Alonso-Caneiro D. Anterior scleral thickness changes with accommodation in myopes and emmetropes. Exp Eye Res. 2018;177:96–103.
103. Bailey MD, Sinnott LT, Mutti DO. Ciliary body thickness and refractive error in children. Invest Ophthalmol Vis Sci. 2008;49:4353–60.
104. Kuchem MK, Sinnott LT, Kao CY, Bailey MD. Ciliary muscle thickness in anisometropia. Optom Vis Sci. 2013;90:1312–20.
105. Muftuoglu O, Hosal BM, Zilelioglu G. Ciliary body thickness in unilateral high axial myopia. Eye. 2009;23:1176–81.
106. Phillips JR, Khalaj M, McBrien NA. Induced myopia associated with increased scleral creep in chick and tree shrew eyes. Invest Ophthalmol Vis Sci. 2000;41:2028–34.
107. Siegwart JT Jr, Norton TT. Regulation of the mechanical properties of tree shrew sclera by the visual environment. Vis Res. 1999;39:387–407.
108. Sherman SM, Norton TT, Casagrande VA. Myopia in the lid-sutured tree shrew (Tupaia glis). Brain Res. 1977;124:154–7.
109. Wallman J, Turkel J, Trachtman J. Extreme myopia produced by modest change in early visual experience. Science. 1978;201:1249–51.
110. Wilson J, Sherman S. Differential effects of early monocular deprivation on binocular and monocular segments of cat striate cortex. J Neurophysiol. 1977;40:891–903.
111. Hodos W, Kuenzel WJ. Retinal-image degradation produces ocular enlargement in chicks. Invest Ophthalmol Vis Sci. 1984;25:652–9.
112. Wallman J, Ledoux C, Friedman MB. Simple devices for restricting the visual fields of birds. Behav Res Methods Instrum. 1978;10:401–3.

113. Howlett MH, McFadden SA. Form-deprivation myopia in the guinea pig (Cavia porcellus). Vis Res. 2006;46:267–83.
114. Ashby R, Ohlendorf A, Schaeffel F. The effect of ambient illuminance on the development of deprivation myopia in chicks. Invest Ophthalmol Vis Sci. 2009;50:5348–54.
115. Schaeffel F, Howland HC. Properties of the feedback loops controlling eye growth and refractive state in the chicken. Vis Res. 1991;31:717–34.
116. Schmid KL, Wildsoe CF. Contrast and spatial-frequency requirements for emmetropization in chicks. Vis Res. 1997;37:2011–21.
117. Wiesel TN, Raviola E. Myopia and eye enlargement after neonatal lid fusion in monkeys. Nature. 1977;266(5597):66–8.
118. Wildsoet CF, Schmid KL. Optical correction of form deprivation myopia inhibits refractive recovery in chick eyes with intact or sectioned optic nerves. Vis Res. 2000;40:3273–82.
119. Siegwart JT Jr, Norton TT. The susceptible period for deprivation-induced myopia in tree shrew. Vis Res. 1998;38:3505–15.
120. Troilo D, Nickla DL. The response to visual form deprivation differs with age in marmosets. Invest Ophthalmol Vis Sci. 2005;46:1873–81.
121. Smith EL, Hung L-F, C-s K, Qiao Y. Effects of brief periods of unrestricted vision on the development of form-deprivation myopia in monkeys. Invest Ophthalmol Vis Sci. 2002;43:291–9.
122. Smith EL, Li-Fang H, Harwerth RS. Effects of optically induced blur on the refractive status of young monkeys. Vis Res. 1994;34:293–301.
123. Schaeffel F, Feldkaemper M. Animal models in myopia research. Clin Exp Optom. 2015;98:507–17.
124. McBrien NA, Lawlor P, Gentle A. Scleral remodeling during the development of and recovery from axial myopia in the tree shrew. Invest Ophthalmol Vis Sci. 2000;41:3713–9.
125. Troilo D, Nickla DL, Wildsoet CF. Choroidal thickness changes during altered eye growth and refractive state in a primate. Invest Ophthalmol Vis Sci. 2000;41:1249–58.
126. Gottlieb MD, Joshi HB, Nickla DL. Scleral changes in chicks with form-deprivation myopia. Curr Eye Res. 1990;9:1157–65.
127. Hung LF, Wallman J, Smith EL. Vision-dependent changes in the choroidal thickness of macaque monkeys. Invest Ophthalmol Vis Sci. 2000;41:1259–69.
128. Funata M, Tokoro T. Scleral change in experimentally myopic monkeys. Graefes Arch Clin Exp Ophthalmol. 1990;228:174–9.
129. Smith EL 3rd, Hung LF. Form-deprivation myopia in monkeys is a graded phenomenon. Vis Res. 2000;40:371–81.
130. Troilo D, Gottlieb MD, Wallman J. Visual deprivation causes myopia in chicks with optic nerve section. Curr Eye Res. 1987;6:993–9.
131. Norton TT, Rada JA. Reduced extracellular matrix in mammalian sclera with induced myopia. Vis Res. 1995;35:1271–81.
132. Gottlieb MD, Fugate-Wentzek LA, Wallman J. Different visual deprivations produce different ametropias and different eye shapes. Invest Ophthalmol Vis Sci. 1987;28:1225–35.
133. Troilo D, Li T, Glasser A, Howland HC. Differences in eye growth and the response to visual deprivation in different strains of chicken. Vis Res. 1995;35:1211–6.
134. McKanna JA, Casagrande VA. Reduced lens development in lid-suture myopia. Exp Eye Res. 1978;26:715–23.
135. Napper GA, Brennan NA, Barrington M, Squires MA, Vessey GA, Vingrys AJ. The duration of normal visual exposure necessary to prevent form deprivation myopia in chicks. Vis Res. 1995;35:1337–44.
136. O'Leary D, Millodot M. Eyelid closure causes myopia in humans. Experientia. 1979;35:1478–9.
137. von Noorden GK, Lewis RA. Ocular axial length in unilateral congenital cataracts and blepharoptosis. Invest Ophthalmol Vis Sci. 1987;28:750–2.
138. Gee SS, Tabbara KF. Increase in ocular axial length in patients with corneal opacification. Ophthalmology. 1988;95:1276–8.
139. Miller-Meeks MJ, Bennett SR, Keech RV, Blodi CF. Myopia induced by vitreous hemorrhage. Am J Ophthalmol. 1990;109:199–203.

140. Bartmann M, Schaeffel F. A simple mechanism for emmetropization without cues from accommodation or colour. Vis Res. 1994;34:873–6.
141. Papastergiou GI, Schmid GF, Laties AM, Pendrak K, Lin T, Stone RA. Induction of axial eye elongation and myopic refractive shift in one-year-old chickens. Vis Res. 1998;38:1883–8.
142. Wildsoet C, Anchong R, Manasse J, Troilo D. Susceptibility to experimental myopia declines with age in the chick. Optom Vis Sci. 1998;75:265.
143. Bradley D, Fernandes A, Boothe R. Form deprivation myopia in adolescent monkeys. Optom Vis Sci. 1999;76:428–32.
144. Troilo D, Nickla DL, Wildsoet CF. Form deprivation myopia in mature common marmosets (Callithrix jacchus). Invest Ophthalmol Vis Sci. 2000;41:2043–9.
145. Schaeffel F, Glasser A, Howland HC. Accommodation, refractive error and eye growth in chickens. Vis Res. 1988;28:639–57.
146. Irving EL, Callender MG, Sivak JG. Inducing myopia, hyperopia, and astigmatism in chicks. Optom Vis Sci. 1991;68:364–8.
147. Irving EL, Sivak JG, Callender MG. Refractive plasticity of the developing chick eye. Ophthalmic Physiol Opt. 1992;12:448–56.
148. Schmid KL, Wildsoet CF. Effects on the compensatory responses to positive and negative lenses of intermittent lens wear and ciliary nerve section in chicks. Vis Res. 1996;36:1023–36.
149. Siegwart J, Norton T. Refractive and ocular changes in tree shrews raised with plus or minus lenses. Invest Ophthalmol Vis Sci. 1993;34:1208.
150. Hung LF, Crawford ML, Smith EL. Spectacle lenses alter eye growth and the refractive status of young monkeys. Nat Med. 1995;1:761–5.
151. Graham B, Judge SJ. The effects of spectacle wear in infancy on eye growth and refractive error in the marmoset (Callithrix jacchus). Vis Res. 1999;39:189–206.
152. Howlett MH, McFadden SA. Spectacle lens compensation in the pigmented guinea pig. Vis Res. 2009;49:219–27.
153. McFadden SA, Howlett MH, Mertz JR. Retinoic acid signals the direction of ocular elongation in the guinea pig eye. Vis Res. 2004;44:643–53.
154. Barathi VA, Boopathi VG, Yap EP, Beuerman RW. Two models of experimental myopia in the mouse. Vis Res. 2008;48:904–16.
155. Metlapally S, McBrien NA. The effect of positive lens defocus on ocular growth and emmetropization in the tree shrew. J Vis. 2008;8:1–12.
156. McFadden S, Wallman J. Guinea-pig eye growth compensates for spectacle lenses. Invest Ophthalmol Vis Sci. 1995;19106:S758.
157. Schaeffel F, Howland HC, Farkas L. Natural accommodation in the growing chicken. Vis Res. 1986;26:1977–93.
158. Whatham AR, Judge SJ. Compensatory changes in eye growth and refraction induced by daily wear of soft contact lenses in young marmosets. Vis Res. 2001;41:267–73.
159. Zhu X, Winawer JA, Wallman J. Potency of myopic defocus in spectacle lens compensation. Invest Ophthalmol Vis Sci. 2003;44:2818–27.
160. Chiang ST, Phillips JR, Backhouse S. Effect of retinal image defocus on the thickness of the human choroid. Ophthalmic Physiol Opt. 2015;35:405–13.
161. Read SA, Collins MJ, Sander BP. Human optical axial length and defocus. Invest Ophthalmol Vis Sci. 2010;51:6262–9.
162. Wang D, Chun RKM, Liu M, et al. Optical defocus rapidly changes choroidal thickness in school children. PLoS One. 2016;11:e0161535.
163. Chakraborty R, Read SA, Collins MJ. Hyperopic defocus and diurnal changes in human choroid and axial length. Optom Vis Sci. 2013;90:1187–98.
164. Chakraborty R, Read SA, Collins MJ. Monocular myopic defocus and daily changes in axial length and choroidal thickness of human eyes. Exp Eye Res. 2012;103:47–54.
165. Moderiano D, Do M, Hobbs S, et al. Influence of the time of day on axial length and choroidal thickness changes to hyperopic and myopic defocus in human eyes. Exp Eye Res. 2019;182:125–36.
166. Zhu X, Wallman J. Temporal properties of compensation for positive and negative spectacle lenses in chicks. Invest Ophthalmol Vis Sci. 2009;50:37–46.

167. Zhu X. Temporal integration of visual signals in lens compensation (a review). Exp Eye Res. 2013;114:69–76.
168. Winawer J, Wallman J. Temporal constraints on lens compensation in chicks. Vis Res. 2002;42:2651–68.
169. Zhu X, Park TW, Winawer J, Wallman J. In a matter of minutes, the eye can know which way to grow. Invest Ophthalmol Vis Sci. 2005;46:2238–41.
170. Wallman J, Adams JI. Developmental aspects of experimental myopia in chicks: susceptibility, recovery and relation to emmetropization. Vis Res. 1987;27:1139–63.
171. Norton TT. Experimental myopia in tree shrews. Ciba Found Symp. 1990;155:178–94.
172. Nickla DL, Wildsoet C, Wallman J. Visual influences on diurnal rhythms in ocular length and choroidal thickness in chick eyes. Exp Eye Res. 1998;66:163–81.
173. Troilo D, Wallman J. The regulation of eye growth and refractive state: an experimental study of emmetropization. Vis Res. 1991;31:1237–50.
174. Schaeffel F, Troilo D, Wallman J, Howland HC. Developing eyes that lack accommodation grow to compensate for imposed defocus. Vis Neurosci. 1990;4:177–83.
175. Schwahn HN, Schaeffel F. Chick eyes under cycloplegia compensate for spectacle lenses despite six-hydroxy dopamine treatment. Invest Ophthalmol Vis Sci. 1994;35:3516–24.
176. Chung KM. Critical review: effects of optical defocus on refractive development and ocular growth and relation to accommodation. Optom Vis Sci. 1993;70:228–33.
177. Morgan IG, Ashby RS, Nickla DL. Form deprivation and lens-induced myopia: are they different? Ophthalmic Physiol Opt. 2013;33:355–61.
178. C-S K, Marzani D, Wallman J. Differences in time course and visual requirements of ocular responses to lenses and diffusers. Invest Ophthalmol Vis Sci. 2001;42:575–83.
179. Bartmann M, Schaeffel F, Hagel G, Zrenner E. Constant light affects retinal dopamine levels and blocks deprivation myopia but not lens-induced refractive errors in chickens. Vis Neurosci. 1994;11:199–208.
180. Padmanabhan V, Shih J, Wildsoet CF. Constant light rearing disrupts compensation to imposed- but not induced-hyperopia and facilitates compensation to imposed myopia in chicks. Vis Res. 2007;47:1855–68.
181. Smith EL, Hung LF, Huang J. Protective effects of high ambient lighting on the development of form-deprivation myopia in rhesus monkeys. Invest Ophthalmol Vis Sci. 2012;53:421–8.
182. Ashby RS, Schaeffel F. The effect of bright light on lens compensation in chicks. Invest Ophthalmol Vis Sci. 2010;51:5247–53.
183. Feldkaemper M, Schaeffel F. An updated view on the role of dopamine in myopia. Exp Eye Res. 2013;114:106–19.
184. Dong F, Zhi Z, Pan M, et al. Inhibition of experimental myopia by a dopamine agonist: different effectiveness between form deprivation and hyperopic defocus in guinea pigs. Mol Vis. 2011;17:2824–34.
185. Harper AR, Summers JA. The dynamic sclera: extracellular matrix remodeling in normal ocular growth and myopia development. Exp Eye Res. 2015;133:100–11.
186. Crewther DP. The role of photoreceptors in the control of refractive state. Prog Retin Eye Res. 2000;19:421–57.
187. Wildsoet CF. Neural pathways subserving negative lens-induced emmetropization in chicks-insights from selective lesions of the optic nerve and ciliary nerve. Curr Eye Res. 2003;27:371–85.
188. Wallman J, Gottlieb MD, Rajaram V, Fugate-Wentzek LA. Local retinal regions control local eye growth and myopia. Science. 1987;237:73–7.
189. Diether S, Schaeffel F. Local changes in eye growth induced by imposed local refractive error despite active accommodation. Vis Res. 1997;37:659–68.
190. Smith EL, Huang J, Hung LF, Blasdel TL, Humbird TL, Bockhorst KH. Hemiretinal form deprivation: evidence for local control of eye growth and refractive development in infant monkeys. Invest Ophthalmol Vis Sci. 2009;50:5057–69.
191. Stone RA, Lin T, Laties AM, Iuvone PM. Retinal dopamine and form-deprivation myopia. Proc Natl Acad Sci U S A. 1989;86:704–6.

192. Iuvone PM, Tigges M, Stone RA, Lambert S, Laties AM. Effects of apomorphine, a dopamine receptor agonist, on ocular refraction and axial elongation in a primate model of myopia. Invest Ophthalmol Vis Sci. 1991;32:1674–7.
193. Nickla DL, Wilken E, Lytle G, Yom S, Mertz J. Inhibiting the transient choroidal thickening response using the nitric oxide synthase inhibitor l-NAME prevents the ameliorative effects of visual experience on ocular growth in two different visual paradigms. Exp Eye Res. 2006;83:456–64.
194. Nickla DL, Wildsoet CF. The effect of the nonspecific nitric oxide synthase inhibitor NG-nitro-L-arginine methyl ester on the choroidal compensatory response to myopic defocus in chickens. Optom Vis Sci. 2004;81:111–8.
195. Feldkaemper MP, Schaeffel F. Evidence for a potential role of glucagon during eye growth regulation in chicks. Vis Neurosci. 2002;19:755–66.
196. Zhou X, Pardue MT, Iuvone PM, Qu J. Dopamine signaling and myopia development: what are the key challenges. Prog Retin Eye Res. 2017;61:60–71.
197. Pendrak K, Nguyen T, Lin T, Capehart C, Zhu X, Stone RA. Retinal dopamine in the recovery from experimental myopia. Curr Eye Res. 1997;16:152–7.
198. Iuvone PM, Tigges M, Fernandes A, Tigges J. Dopamine synthesis and metabolism in rhesus monkey retina: development, aging, and the effects of monocular visual deprivation. Vis Neurosci. 1989;2:465–71.
199. Crewther DP, Crewther SG, Xie RZ. Changes in eye growth produced by drugs which affect retinal ON or OFF responses to light. J Ocul Pharmacol Ther. 1996;12:193–208.
200. Crewther DP, Crewther SG. Pharmacological modification of eye growth in normally reared and visually deprived chicks. Curr Eye Res. 1990;9:733–40.
201. Chakraborty R, Park H, Aung MH, et al. Comparison of refractive development and retinal dopamine in OFF pathway mutant and C57BL/6J wild-type mice. Mol Vis. 2014;20:1318–27.
202. Chakraborty R, Pardue MT. Molecular and biochemical aspects of the retina on refraction. Prog Mol Biol Transl Sci. 2015;134:249–67.
203. Chakraborty R, Park HN, Hanif AM, Sidhu CS, Iuvone PM, Pardue MT. ON pathway mutations increase susceptibility to form-deprivation myopia. Exp Eye Res. 2015;137:79–83.
204. Bergen MA, Chakraborty R, Landis EG, Sidhu C, He L, Iuvone PM, Pardue MT. Altered refractive development in mice with reduced levels of retinal dopamine. Invest Ophthalmol Vis Sci. 2016;57(10):4412–9.
205. Pardue MT, Faulkner AE, Fernandes A, et al. High susceptibility to experimental myopia in a mouse model with a retinal on pathway defect. Invest Ophthalmol Vis Sci. 2008;49:706–12.
206. Markand S, Baskin NL, Chakraborty R, et al. IRBP deficiency permits precocious ocular development and myopia. Mol Vis. 2016;22:1291–308.
207. Zhang Q, Xiao X, Li S, et al. Mutations in NYX of individuals with high myopia, but without night blindness. Mol Vis. 2007;13:330–6.
208. Xu X, Li S, Xiao X, Wang P, Guo X, Zhang Q. Sequence variations of GRM6 in patients with high myopia. Mol Vis. 2009;15:2094–100.
209. Pras E, Abu A, Rotenstreich Y, et al. Cone-rod dystrophy and a frameshift mutation in the PROM1 gene. Mol Vis. 2009;15:1709.
210. Sieving PA, Fishman GA. Refractive errors of retinitis pigmentosa patients. Br J Ophthalmol. 1978;62:163–7.
211. Charman WN. Aberrations and myopia. Ophthalmic Physiol Opt. 2005;25:285–301.
212. Wildsoet CF, Atchison DA, Collins MJ. Longitudinal chromatic aberration as a function of refractive error. Clin Exp Optom. 1993;76:119–22.
213. Little JA, McCullough SJ, Breslin KM, Saunders KJ. Higher order ocular aberrations and their relation to refractive error and ocular biometry in children. Invest Ophthalmol Vis Sci. 2014;55:4791–800.
214. Buehren T, Collins MJ, Carney LG. Near work induced wavefront aberrations in myopia. Vis Res. 2005;45:1297–312.
215. Vincent SJ, Collins MJ, Read SA, Carney LG, Yap MK. Corneal changes following near work in myopic anisometropia. Ophthalmic Physiol Opt. 2013;33:15–25.

216. Hiraoka T, Kotsuka J, Kakita T, Okamoto F, Oshika T. Relationship between higher-order wavefront aberrations and natural progression of myopia in schoolchildren. Sci Rep. 2017;7:7876.
217. Atchison DA, Li SM, Li H, et al. Relative peripheral hyperopia does not predict development and progression of myopia in children. Invest Ophthalmol Vis Sci. 2015;56:6162–70.
218. Lee TT, Cho P. Relative peripheral refraction in children: twelve-month changes in eyes with different ametropias. Ophthalmic Physiol Opt. 2013;33:283–93.
219. Cheng X, Xu J, Chehab K, Exford J, Brennan N. Soft contact lenses with positive spherical aberration for myopia control. Optom Vis Sci. 2016;93:353–66.
220. Hiraoka T, Okamoto C, Ishii Y, Kakita T, Oshika T. Contrast sensitivity function and ocular higher-order aberrations following overnight orthokeratology. Invest Ophthalmol Vis Sci. 2007;48:550–6.
221. Hiraoka T, Miyata K, Nakamura Y, et al. Influences of cycloplegia with topical atropine on ocular higher-order aberrations. Ophthalmology. 2013;120:8–13.
222. Huang HM, Chang DS, Wu PC. The association between near work activities and myopia in children-a systematic review and meta-analysis. PLoS One. 2015;10:e0140419.
223. Rosenfield M, Gilmartin B. Disparity-induced accommodation in late-onset myopia. Ophthalmic Physiol Opt. 1988;8:353–5.
224. Gwiazda J, Thorn F, Bauer J, Held R. Myopic children show insufficient accommodative response to blur. Invest Ophthalmol Vis Sci. 1993;34:690–4.
225. McBrien NA, Millodot M. The effect of refractive error on the accommodative response gradient. Ophthalmic Physiol Opt. 1986;6:145–9.
226. Gwiazda J, Bauer J, Thorn F, Held R. A dynamic relationship between myopia and blur-driven accommodation in school-aged children. Vis Res. 1995;35:1299–304.
227. Abbott ML, Schmid KL, Strang NC. Differences in the accommodation stimulus response curves of adult myopes and emmetropes. Ophthalmic Physiol Opt. 1998;18:13–20.
228. Cheng D, Schmid KL, Woo GC, Drobe B. Randomized trial of effect of bifocal and prismatic bifocal spectacles on myopic progression: two-year results. Arch Ophthalmol. 2010;128:12–9.
229. Berntsen DA, Barr CD, Mutti DO, Zadnik K. Peripheral defocus and myopia progression in myopic children randomly assigned to wear single vision and progressive addition lenses. Invest Ophthalmol Vis Sci. 2013;54:5761–70.
230. Mutti DO, Mitchell GL, Jones LA, et al. Accommodation, acuity, and their relationship to emmetropization in infants. Optom Vis Sci. 2009;86:666–76.
231. Weiss S, Schaeffel F. Diurnal growth rhythms in the chicken eye: relation to myopia development and retinal dopamine levels. J Comp Physiol A. 1993;172:263–70.
232. Chakraborty R, Read SA, Collins MJ. Diurnal variations in axial length, choroidal thickness, intraocular pressure, and ocular biometrics. Invest Ophthalmol Vis Sci. 2011;52:5121–9.
233. Brown JS, Flitcroft DI, Ying GS, et al. In vivo human choroidal thickness measurements: evidence for diurnal fluctuations. Invest Ophthalmol Vis Sci. 2009;50:5–12.
234. Stone RA, Quinn GE, Francis EL, et al. Diurnal axial length fluctuations in human eyes. Invest Ophthalmol Vis Sci. 2004;45:63–70.
235. Li T, Troilo D, Glasser A, Howland HC. Constant light produces severe corneal flattening and hyperopia in chickens. Vis Res. 1995;35:1203–9.
236. Guyton DL, Greene PR, Scholz RT. Dark-rearing interference with emmetropization in the rhesus monkey. Invest Ophthalmol Vis Sci. 1989;30:761–4.
237. Nickla DL, Totonelly K. Brief light exposure at night disrupts the circadian rhythms in eye growth and choroidal thickness in chicks. Exp Eye Res. 2016;146:189–95.
238. Nickla DL. The phase relationships between the diurnal rhythms in axial length and choroidal thickness and the association with ocular growth rate in chicks. J Comp Physiol A. 2006;192:399–407.
239. Kearney S, O'Donoghue L, Pourshahidi LK, Cobice D, Saunders KJ. Myopes have significantly higher serum melatonin concentrations than non-myopes. Ophthalmic Physiol Opt. 2017;37:557–67.

240. Jee D, Morgan IG, Kim EC. Inverse relationship between sleep duration and myopia. Acta Ophthalmol. 2016;94:e204–10.
241. Mutti DO, Mitchell GL, Moeschberger ML, Jones LA, Zadnik K. Parental myopia, near work, school achievement, and children's refractive error. Invest Ophthalmol Vis Sci. 2002;43:3633–40.
242. Morgan IG. The biological basis of myopic refractive error. Clin Exp Optom. 2003;86:276–88.
243. Au Eong KG, Tay TH, Lim MK. Education and myopia in 110,236 young Singaporean males. Singap Med J. 1993;34:489–92.
244. Williams KM, Bertelsen G, Cumberland P, et al. Increasing prevalence of myopia in Europe and the impact of education. Ophthalmology. 2015;122:1489–97.
245. Mirshahi A, Ponto KA, Hoehn R, et al. Myopia and level of education: results from the Gutenberg Health Study. Ophthalmology. 2014;121:2047–52.
246. Read SA, Collins MJ, Woodman EC, Cheong SH. Axial length changes during accommodation in myopes and emmetropes. Optom Vis Sci. 2010;87:656–62.
247. Woodman-Pieterse EC, Read SA, Collins MJ, Alonso-Caneiro D. Regional changes in choroidal thickness associated with accommodation. Invest Ophthalmol Vis Sci. 2015;56:6414–22.
248. Hepsen IF, Evereklioglu C, Bayramlar H. The effect of reading and near-work on the development of myopia in emmetropic boys: a prospective, controlled, three-year follow-up study. Vis Res. 2001;41:2511–20.
249. Jones LA, Sinnott LT, Mutti DO, Mitchell GL, Moeschberger ML, Zadnik K. Parental history of myopia, sports and outdoor activities, and future myopia. Invest Ophthalmol Vis Sci. 2007;48:3524–32.
250. He M, Zheng Y, Xiang F. Prevalence of myopia in urban and rural children in mainland China. Optom Vis Sci. 2009;86:40–4.
251. He M, Huang W, Zheng Y, Huang L, Ellwein LB. Refractive error and visual impairment in school children in rural southern China. Ophthalmology. 2007;114:374–82.
252. Zhang M, Li L, Chen L, et al. Population density and refractive error among Chinese children. Invest Ophthalmol Vis Sci. 2010;51:4969–76.
253. Ip JM, Rose KA, Morgan IG, Burlutsky G, Mitchell P. Myopia and the urban environment: findings in a sample of 12-year-old Australian school children. Invest Ophthalmol Vis Sci. 2008;49:3858–63.
254. Choi KY, Yu WY, Lam CHI, et al. Childhood exposure to constricted living space: a possible environmental threat for myopia development. Ophthalmic Physiol Opt. 2017;37:568–75.
255. Parssinen O, Lyyra AL. Myopia and myopic progression among schoolchildren: a three-year follow-up study. Invest Ophthalmol Vis Sci. 1993;34:2794–802.
256. Rose KA, Morgan IG, Ip J, et al. Outdoor activity reduces the prevalence of myopia in children. Ophthalmology. 2008;115:1279–85.
257. Guo Y, Liu LJ, Tang P, et al. Outdoor activity and myopia progression in 4-year follow-up of Chinese primary school children: The Beijing Children Eye Study. PLoS One. 2017;12:e0175921.
258. Guggenheim JA, Northstone K, McMahon G, et al. Time outdoors and physical activity as predictors of incident myopia in childhood: a prospective cohort study. Invest Ophthalmol Vis Sci. 2012;53:2856–65.
259. Parssinen O, Kauppinen M, Viljanen A. The progression of myopia from its onset at age 8-12 to adulthood and the influence of heredity and external factors on myopic progression. A 23-year follow-up study. Acta Ophthalmol. 2014;92:730–9.
260. Jones-Jordan LA, Sinnott LT, Cotter SA, et al. Time outdoors, visual activity, and myopia progression in juvenile-onset myopes. Invest Ophthalmol Vis Sci. 2012;53:7169–75.
261. Sherwin JC, Reacher MH, Keogh RH, Khawaja AP, Mackey DA, Foster PJ. The association between time spent outdoors and myopia in children and adolescents: a systematic review and meta-analysis. Ophthalmology. 2012;119:2141–51.
262. Flitcroft DI. The complex interactions of retinal, optical and environmental factors in myopia aetiology. Prog Retin Eye Res. 2012;31:622–60.
263. Cohen Y, Belkin M, Yehezkel O, Solomon AS, Polat U. Dependency between light intensity and refractive development under light-dark cycles. Exp Eye Res. 2011;92:40–6.

264. Karouta C, Ashby RS. Correlation between light levels and the development of deprivation myopia. Invest Ophthalmol Vis Sci. 2014;56:299–309.
265. Smith EL, Hung LF, Arumugam B, Huang J. Negative lens-induced myopia in infant monkeys: effects of high ambient lighting. Invest Ophthalmol Vis Sci. 2013;54:2959–69.
266. Read SA, Collins MJ, Vincent SJ. Light exposure and eye growth in childhood. Invest Ophthalmol Vis Sci. 2015;56:6779–87.
267. Ostrin LA, Sajjadi A, Benoit JS. Objectively measured light exposure during school and summer in children. Optom Vis Sci. 2018;95:332–42.
268. Wu PC, Chen CT, Lin KK, et al. Myopia prevention and outdoor light intensity in a school-based cluster randomized trial. Ophthalmology. 2018;125(8):1239–50.
269. Rudnicka AR, Kapetanakis VV, Wathern AK, et al. Global variations and time trends in the prevalence of childhood myopia, a systematic review and quantitative meta-analysis: implications for aetiology and early prevention. Br J Ophthalmol. 2016;100:882–90.
270. French AN, Morgan IG, Burlutsky G, Mitchell P, Rose KA. Prevalence and 5- to 6-year incidence and progression of myopia and hyperopia in Australian school children. Ophthalmology. 2013;120:1482–91.
271. Read SA, Vincent SJ, Tan CS, Ngo C, Collins MJ, Saw SM. Patterns of daily outdoor light exposure in Australian and Singaporean children. Transl Vis Sci Technol. 2018;7:8.
272. Lan W, Feldkaemper M, Schaeffel F. Intermittent episodes of bright light suppress myopia in the chicken more than continuous bright light. PLoS One. 2014;9:e110906.
273. He M, Xiang F, Zeng Y, et al. Effect of time spent outdoors at school on the development of myopia among children in China: a randomized clinical trial. JAMA. 2015;314:1142–8.
274. Wu PC, Tsai CL, Wu HL, Yang YH, Kuo HK. Outdoor activity during class recess reduces myopia onset and progression in school children. Ophthalmology. 2013;120:1080–5.
275. Torii H, Kurihara T, Seko Y, et al. Violet light exposure can be a preventive strategy against myopia progression. EBioMedicine. 2017;15:210–9.
276. Foulds WS, Barathi VA, Luu CD. Progressive myopia or hyperopia can be induced in chicks and reversed by manipulation of the chromaticity of ambient light. Invest Ophthalmol Vis Sci. 2013;54:8004–12.
277. Smith EL, Hung LF, Arumugam B, Holden BA, Neitz M, Neitz J. Effects of long-wavelength lighting on refractive development in infant rhesus monkeys. Invest Ophthalmol Vis Sci. 2015;56:6490–500.
278. Gawne TJ, Ward AH, Norton TT. Long-wavelength (red) light produces hyperopia in juvenile and adolescent tree shrews. Vis Res. 2017;140:55–65.
279. Jiang L, Zhang S, Schaeffel F, et al. Interactions of chromatic and lens-induced defocus during visual control of eye growth in guinea pigs (Cavia porcellus). Vis Res. 2014;94:24–32.

5

A Genetic Approach to Myopia

Milly S. Tedja, Annechien E. G. Haarman,
Magda A. Meester-Smoor, Virginie J. M. Verhoeven,
Caroline C. W. Klaver, and Stuart MacGregor

Key Points

- While the recent global rise of myopia prevalence is primarily attributable to environmental changes, within populations inherited factors play a large role in explaining why some individuals are affected by myopia while others are not.
- Early efforts to identify the specific genes underlying the heritability of refractive error used linkage and candidate gene designs to identify up to 50 loci and genes, although most remain unconfirmed.

M. S. Tedja · A. E. G. Haarman · M. A. Meester-Smoor
Department of Ophthalmology, Erasmus Medical Center, Rotterdam, The Netherlands

Department of Epidemiology, Erasmus Medical Center, Rotterdam, The Netherlands

V. J. M. Verhoeven
Department of Ophthalmology, Erasmus Medical Center, Rotterdam, The Netherlands

Department of Epidemiology, Erasmus Medical Center, Rotterdam, The Netherlands

Department of Clinical Genetics, Erasmus Medical Center, Rotterdam, The Netherlands

C. C. W. Klaver
Department of Ophthalmology, Erasmus Medical Center, Rotterdam, The Netherlands

Department of Epidemiology, Erasmus Medical Center, Rotterdam, The Netherlands

Department of Ophthalmology, Radboud University Medical Center, Nijmegen, The Netherlands

S. MacGregor (✉)
Statistical Genetics, QIMR Berghofer Medical Research Institute, Brisbane, QLD, Australia
e-mail: stuart.macgregor@qimrberghofer.edu.au

- As the sample size in genome-wide association studies (GWAS) has increased, the number of implicated loci has risen steadily, with 161 variants reported in the latest meta-analysis.
- Interrogation of loci uncovered by GWAS offers insight into the molecular basis of myopia—for example, pathway analysis implicates the light induced retina-to-sclera signaling pathway in myopia development.
- Although many loci have been uncovered by GWAS, statistical modelling shows there are many more genes to find—identifying these will further illuminate the molecular pathways leading to myopia and open up new avenues for intervention.

5.1 Introduction

This chapter addresses the scientific exploration of the genetic architecture of myopia. Myopia is the most common eye condition worldwide and its prevalence is increasing. Changes in environmental conditions where time spent outdoors has reduced relative to previous generations are the main hypothesized culprit. Despite these environmental trends, within populations, myopia is highly heritable; genes explain up to 80% of the variance in refractive error. Initial attempts to identify myopia genes relied on family studies using linkage analysis or candidate gene approaches with limited progress. For the last decade, genome-wide association study (GWAS) approaches have predominated, ultimately resulting in the identification of hundreds of genes for refractive error and myopia, providing new insights into its molecular machinery. Thanks to these studies, it was revealed that myopia is a complex trait, with many genetic variants of small effect influencing retinal signaling, eye growth and the normal process of emmetropization. However, the genetic architecture and its molecular mechanisms are still to be clarified and while genetic risk score prediction models are improving, this knowledge must be expanded to have impact on clinical practice.

Some sections of this report follow the framework described in a recent International Myopia Institute Genetics report by Tedja et al. [1]

5.2 Heritability

The tendency for myopia to run in families has long been noted, suggesting genetic factors play a role in determining risk [2]. While family studies show familial aggregation, twin studies are required to reliably separate the effects of genes and familial environment [3–6]. Benchmarking of the relative contribution of genetics and environment is done by computation of heritability, the proportion of the total trait variance (here, spherical equivalent) due to additive genetic factors. Since the contributions of genes and environment can vary across human populations, heritabilities are population and even time specific [7, 8]. The influence of environmental variance is well illustrated in the case of the heritability study in Alaskan Eskimos, where the rapid introduction of the American school system dramatically increased the contribution of the environment. As a result heritability estimates, computed based on families where the parents are less educated relative to their offspring, were very low at this time (10%) [7].

Across most human populations, environment is fairly constant and the estimates of spherical equivalent heritability are usually high (~80%) [9–11]. Although the aggregate contribution of genetic factors to variation in refractive error is high, initial studies were unable to determine the genetic architecture of myopia—that is, is myopia caused by rare mutations of large effect? Or is most variation driven by common variants, each with individually small effect on risk? With the advent of genotyping arrays, it became possible to estimate the aggregate effect of all common variants, with "array heritability" estimates of 35% from the ALSPAC study. Such estimates place a lower bound on the proportion of the heritability that is attributable to genetic variants which are common in the population. The remaining 45% (80%–35%) is likely attributable to rare genetic variants, to variants not covered by genotyping arrays or to non-additive genetic effects.

5.3 Syndromic Myopia

Syndromic myopia is generally monogenic and can occur within a wide spectrum of clinical presentations. This type of myopia is usually accompanied by other systemic or ocular disorders. Table 5.1 summarizes all syndromic and ocular conditions that present with myopia [12]. We are able to learn about myopia development by investigating these syndromes. For instance, several types of heritable syndromes result in extreme axial elongation, due to abnormalities in the development of connective tissue (i.e. Marfan syndrome, OMIM #154700; Stickler syndrome, OMIM #,108300 #604841, #614134, #614284 and Ehlers–Danlos syndrome, OMIM #225400, #601776). Similarly, inherited retinal dystrophies lead to myopia due to defects in photoreceptors, for instance, in X-linked retinitis pigmentosa (mutations in *RPGR*-gene) and congenital stationary night blindness [13].

Interestingly, several syndromic myopia genes were found in association to other ocular traits, such as CCT (*ADAMTS2*, *COL4A3*, *COL5A1*, *FBN1*) [14], and Fuchs's dystrophy (*TCF4*) [15]. However, the majority of the genes causing syndromic myopia have not been linked to common forms of myopia, except for *COL2A1* [16, 17] and *FBN1* [18, 19]. Nevertheless, a recent study found an overrepresentation for syndromic myopia genes in GWAS studies on refractive error and myopia [20], implying their important role in myopia development.

5.4 Linkage Studies

Linkage studies have been successfully applied for many Mendelian disorders, although the success has been much more limited in complex traits. The linkage approach searches for cosegregation of genetic markers with the trait of interest in

Table 5.1 Overview of syndromic forms of myopia

Syndrome	Gene and inheritance pattern	Ocular phenotype other than myopia
(A) Syndromes associated with myopia and associated ocular phenotype		
Acromelic frontonasal dysostosis	*ZSWIM6* (*AD*)	Telecanthus, ptosis (some patients), corneal dermoid cyst (rare), glaucoma (rare), segmental optic nerve hypoplasia (rare), persistent primary vitreous (rare)
Alagille syndrome	*JAG1* (*AD*)	Deep-set eyes, hypertelorism, upslanting palpebral fissures, posterior embryotoxon, anterior chamber anomalies, eccentric or ectopic pupils, chorioretinal atrophy, band keratopathy, cataracts, retinal pigment clumping, Axenfeld anomaly, microcornea, choroidal folds, strabismus, anomalous optic disc
Alport syndrome	*COL4A5* (*XLD*); *COL4A3* (*AR/AD*)	Anterior lenticonus, lens opacities, cataracts, pigmentary changes ("flecks") in the perimacular region, corneal endothelial vesicles, corneal erosions
Angelman syndrome	*UBE3A* (*IP*); *CH*	Strabismus (most frequently exotropia), ocular hypopigmentation, refractive errors (astigmatism, hyperopia, myopia)
Bardet–Biedl syndrome	*ARL6*; *BBS1*; *BBS2*; *BBS4*; *BBS5*; *BBS7*; *BBS9*; *BBS10*; *BBS12*; *CEP290*; *LZTFL1*; *MKKS*; *MKS1*; *SDCCAG8*; *TMEM67*; *TRIM32*; *TTC8*; *WDPCP* (*AR*)	Rod-cone dystrophy onset by end of 2nd decade, retinitis pigmentosa, retinal degeneration, strabismus, cataracts
Beals syndrome	*FBN2* (*AD*)	Ectopia lentis
Beaulieu–Boycott–Innes syndrome	*THOC6* (*AR*)	Deep-set eyes, short palpebral fissures, upslanting palpebral fissures
Bohring–Opitz syndrome	*ASXL1* (*AD*)	Prominent eyes, hypoplastic orbital ridges, hypertelorism, upslanting palpebral fissures, strabismus, retinal abnormalities, optic nerve abnormalities
Bone fragility and contractures; arterial rupture and deafness	*PLOD3* (*AR*)	Shallow orbits, cataracts
Branchiooculofacial syndrome	*TFAP2A* (*AD*)	Lacrimal sac fistula, orbital dermoid cyst, iris pigment epithelial cyst, combined hamartoma of the retina and retinal pigment epithelium, upslanting palpebral fissures, telecanthus, hypertelorism, ptosis, lacrimal duct obstruction, iris coloboma, retinal coloboma, microphthalmia, anophthalmia, cataract, strabismus

Table 5.1 (continued)

Syndrome	Gene and inheritance pattern	Ocular phenotype other than myopia
Cardiofaciocutaneous syndrome	*MAP2K2* (*AD*)	Ptosis, nystagmus, strabismus, downslanting palpebral fissures, hypertelorism, exophthalmos, epicanthal folds, optic nerve dysplasia, oculomotor apraxia, loss of visual acuity, absence of eyebrows, absence of eyelashes
Cohen syndrome	*VPS13B* (*AR*)	Downslanting palpebral fissures, almond-shaped eyes, chorioretinal dystrophy, decreased visual acuity, optic atrophy
Cornelia de Lange syndrome	*NIPBL* (*AD*); *HDAC8* (*XLD*)	Synophrys, long curly eyelashes, ptosis
Cowden syndrome	*PTEN* (*AD*)	Cataract, angioid streaks
Cranioectodermal dysplasia	*IFT122* (*AR*)	Telecanthus, hypotelorism, epicanthal folds, myopia (1 patient), nystagmus (1 patient), retinal dystrophy (1 patient)
Cutis laxa	*ATP6V0A2*; *ALDH18A1* (*AR*)	Downslanting palpebral fissures, strabismus
Danon disease	*LAMP2* (*XLD*)	Moderate central loss of visual acuity in males, normal to near-normal visual acuity in carrier females, fine lamellar white opacities on slit lamp exam in carrier females, near complete loss of peripheral retinal pigment in males, peppered pigmentary mottling of peripheral retinal pigment in carrier females, nonspecific changes on electroretinogram in carrier females
Deafness and myopia	*SLITRK6* (*AR*)	High myopia
Desanto–Shinawi syndrome	*WAC* (*AD*)	Hypertelorism, downslanting palpebral issues, synophrys, deep-set eyes, astigmatism, strabismus
Desbuquois dysplasia	*CANT1* (*AR*)	Prominent eyes, bulging eyes, congenital glaucoma
Donnai–Barrow syndrome	*LRP2* (*AR*)	Hypertelorism, high myopia, loss of vision, iris coloboma, iris hypoplasia, cataract, enlarged globes, downslanting palpebral fissures, underorbital skin creases, retinal detachment, retinal dystrophy, prominent eyes
DOORS	*TBC1D24* (*AR*)	Optic atrophy, blindness, high myopia, cataracts
Ehlers–Danlos syndrome	*COL5A1* (*AD*); *PLOD1* (*AR*); *CHST14* (*AR*); *ADAMTS2* (*AR*); *B3GALT6* (*AR*); *FKBP14* (*AR*)	Blue sclerae, ectopia lentis, epicanthal folds

(continued)

Table 5.1 (continued)

Syndrome	Gene and inheritance pattern	Ocular phenotype other than myopia
Emanuel syndrome	CH	Hooded eyelids, deep-set eyes, upslanting palpebral fissures, strabismus
Fibrochondrogenesis	*COL11A1* (*AR*)	–
Gyrate atrophy of choroid and retina with/without ornithinemia	*OAT* (*AR*)	Progressive chorioretinal degeneration, night blindness (onset in first decade, progressive loss of peripheral vision, blindness (onset in fourth or fifth decade), posterior subcapsular cataracts (onset in second or third decade)
Hamamy syndrome	*IRX5* (*AR*)	Severe hypertelorism, laterally sparse eyebrows, myopia (progressive severe)
Homocystinuria	*CBS* (*AR*)	Ectopia lentis, glaucoma
Joint laxity; short stature; myopia	*GZF1* (*AR*)	Exophthalmos, severe myopia, retinal detachment (some patients), iris coloboma (some patients), chorioretinal coloboma (some patients), glaucoma (1 patient)
Kaufman oculocerebrofacial syndrome	*UBE3B* (*AR*)	Blepharophimosis, ptosis, upward-slanting palpebral fissures, telecanthus, hypertelorism, astigmatism, strabismus, mild
Kenny–Caffey syndrome	*FAM111A* (*AD*)	Hyperopia (not myopia), microphthalmia, papilledema, corneal and retinal calcification, congenital cataracts (rare)
Kniest dysplasia	*COL2A1* (*AD*)	Retinal detachment, cataracts, prominent eyes
Knobloch syndrome	*COL18A1* (*AR*)	High myopia, vitreoretinal degeneration, retinal detachment (childhood), congenital cataract, syneresis, vitreous attachment at the disc, persistent foetal hyaloid vasculature, peripapillary atrophy, phthisis bulbi, band keratopathy, macular hypoplasia, irregular white dots at the vitreoretinal interface, visual loss, nystagmus
Lamb–Shaffer syndrome	*SOX5* (*AD*)	Downslanting palpebral fissures, epicanthal folds, strabismus
Lethal congenital contracture syndrome	*ERBB3* (*AR*)	High myopia, degenerative vitreoretinopathy
Leukodystrophy	*POLR1C*; *POLR3A*; *POLR3B*; *GJC2* (*AR*)	–
Linear skin defects with multiple congenital anomalies	*NDUFB11*; *COX7B* (*XLD*)	Lacrimal duct atresia, nystagmus, strabismus
Loeys–Dietz syndrome	*TGFBR1*; *TGFBR2* (*AD*)	Hypertelorism, exotropia, blue sclerae, proptosis

Table 5.1 (continued)

Syndrome	Gene and inheritance pattern	Ocular phenotype other than myopia
Macrocephaly/ megalencephaly syndrome	*TBC1D7* (*AR*)	Astigmatism
Marfan syndrome	*FBN1* (*AD*)	Enophthalmos, ectopia lentis increased axial globe length, corneal flatness, retinal detachment, iris hypoplasia, early glaucoma, early cataracts, downslanting palpebral fissures, trabeculodysgenesis, primary (some patients), strabismus (some patients), exotropia (some patients), esotropia (rare), hypertropia (rare)
Marshall syndrome	*COL11A1* (*AD*)	congenital cataracts, esotropia, retinal detachment, glaucoma, lens dislocation, vitreoretinal degeneration, hypertelorism, epicanthal folds
Microcephaly with/ without chorioretinopathy; lymphedema; and/or mental retardation	*KIF11* (*AD*)	Upslanting palpebral fissures, downslanting palpebral fissures (some patients), epicanthal folds (some patients), nystagmus, reduced visual acuity, hypermetropia, myopic astigmatism, hypermetropic astigmatism, corneal opacity, microcornea, microphthalmia, cataract, retrolenticular fibrotic mass, chorioretinopathy, retinal folds, falciform retinal folds, retinal detachment, temporal dragging of optic disc, retinal pigment changes (some patients), optic atrophy (uncommon)
Mohr–Tranebjaerg syndrome	*TIMM8A* (*XLR*)	Photophobia, cortical blindness, decreased visual acuity, constricted visual fields, abnormal electroretinogram
Mucolipidosis	*GNPTAG* (*AR*)	Fine corneal opacities
Muscular dystrophy	*TRAPPC11*; *POMT*; *POMT1*; *POMT2*; *POMGNT1*; *B3GALNT2*; *FKRP*; *DAG1*; *FKTN*(*AR*)	Cataracts, strabismus, alacrima (some patients)
Nephrotic syndrome	*LAMB2* (*AR*)	Nystagmus, strabismus, microcoria, aplasia/atrophy of the dilatator pupillae muscle, hypoplasia of the iris and ciliary body, lenticonus posterior, blindness, decreased or absent laminin beta-2 immunoreactivity in tissues of the anterior eye

(continued)

Table 5.1 (continued)

Syndrome	Gene and inheritance pattern	Ocular phenotype other than myopia
Noonan syndrome	*A2ML1*; *BRAF*; *CBL*; *HRAS*; *KRAS*; *MAP2K1*; *MAP2K2*; *NRAS*; *PTPN11*; *RAF1*; *RIT1*; *SOS1*; *SHOC2*; *SPRED1* (*AD*)	Ptosis, hypertelorism, downslanting palpebral fissures, epicanthal folds, blue-green irides
Oculocutaneous albinism	*TYR* (*AR*)	Absent pigment in iris and retina, translucent iris, pink irides (childhood), blue-gray irides (adult), choroidal vessels visible, foveal hypoplasia, decreased visual acuity, strabismus, nystagmus, photophobia, high refractive errors (hyperopia, myopia, with-the-rule astigmatism), albinotic optic disc, misrouting of the optic nerves at the chiasm, absent stereopsis due to anomalous decussation at the optic chiasm, positive angle kappa (appearance of exotropia but no shift on cover test), asymmetric visual evoked potentials
Oculodentodigital dysplasia	*GJA1* (*AR*)	Hypoplastic eyebrows, sparse eyelashes, telecanthus, short palpebral fissures, downslanting palpebral fissures, microphthalmia, microcornea, cataract, persistent pupillary membrane
Pallister–Killian syndrome	CH	Sparse eyebrows, sparse eyelashes, upslanting palpebral fissures, hypertelorism, ptosis, strabismus, epicanthal folds, cataracts, exophthalmos
Papillorenal syndrome	*PAX2* (*AD*)	Retinal coloboma, optic nerve anomalies (coloboma, gliosis, absent optic nerve head), optic disc anomalies (dysplasia, excavation, hyperplasia, morning glory optic disc, hypoplasia), orbital cysts, microphthalmia, abnormal retinal pigment epithelium, abnormal retinal vessels, chorioretinal degeneration, retinal detachment (rare). retinal staphyloma (rare), retinal edema (rare), macular degeneration (rare), papillomacular detachment (rare), hyperpigmentation of the macula (rare), cystic degeneration of the macula (rare), posterior lens luxation (rare), lens opacity (rare)

Table 5.1 (continued)

Syndrome	Gene and inheritance pattern	Ocular phenotype other than myopia
Peters-plus syndrome	*B3GLCT* (*AR*)	Hypertelorism, Peter's anomaly, anterior chamber cleavage disorder, nystagmus, ptosis, glaucoma, upslanting palpebral fissures, cataract, iris coloboma, retinal coloboma
Pitt–Hopkins syndrome	*TCF4* (*AD*)	Deep-set eyes, strabismus, astigmatism, upslanting palpebral fissures
Pontocerebellar hypoplasia	*CHMP1A* (*AR*)	Astigmatism, esotropia, strabismus, hyperopia, nystagmus (some patients), cortical visual impairment (some patients), poor visual tracking (some patients)
Poretti–Boltshauser syndrome	*LAMA1* (*AR*)	Strabismus, amblyopia, oculomotor apraxia, nystagmus, retinal atrophy, retinal dystrophy, retinal dysfunction, macular heterotopia
Prader–Willi syndrome	*NDN* (PC); *SNRPN* (IP); CH	Almond-shaped eyes, strabismus, upslanting palpebral fissures, hyperopia
Pseudoxanthoma elasticum	*ABCC6* (*AR*)	Peau d'orange retinal changes (yellow-mottled retinal hyperpigmentation), angioid streaks of the retina (85% of patients), macular degeneration, visual impairment (50–70% of patients), central vision loss, colloid bodies, retinal haemorrhage, choroidal neovascularization, optic head drusen (yellowish-white irregularities of optic disc), owl's eyes (paired hyperpigmented spots)
Renal hypomagnesemia	*CLDN16*; *CLDN19* (*AR*)	Strabismus, nystagmus, hyperopia, astigmatism
SADDAN	*FGFR3* (*AD*)	High myopia, exotropia
Schaaf–Yang syndrome	*MAGEL2* (*AD*)	Esotropia, strabismus, almond-shaped eyes, short palpebral fissures, bushy eyebrows
Schimke immunoosseous dysplasia	*SMARCAL1* (*AR*)	Corneal opacities, astigmatism
Schuurs–Hoeijmakers syndrome	*PACS1* (*AD*)	Full, arched eyebrows, long eyelashes, hypertelorism, downslanting palpebral fissures, ptosis, nystagmus, strabismus
Schwartz–Jampel syndrome	*HSPG2* (*AR*)	Narrow palpebral fissures, blepharophimosis, cataract, microcornea, long eyelashes in irregular rows, ptosis
Sengers syndrome	*AGK* (*AR*)	Cataracts (infantile), strabismus, glaucoma
Short stature; hearing loss; retinitis pigmentosa and distinctive facies	*EXOSC2* (*AR*)	Deep-set eyes, short palpebral fissures, upslanting palpebral fissures, retinitis pigmentosa (2 patients), corneal dystrophy (2 patients, young-adult onset), glaucoma (1 patient), nystagmus (1 patient), strabismus (1 patient)

(continued)

Table 5.1 (continued)

Syndrome	Gene and inheritance pattern	Ocular phenotype other than myopia
Short stature; optic nerve atrophy; and Pelger–Huet anomaly	*NBAS* (*AR*)	Thick and bush eyebrows, small orbits, bilateral exophthalmos, epicanthus, bilateral optic nerve atrophy, non-progressive decreased visual acuity, (in) complete achromatopsia, strabismus (some patients), hypertelorism (some patients), hypermetropia (rare), pigmented nevus (rare)
SHORT syndrome	*PIK3R1* (*AD*)	Deep-set eyes, Rieger anomaly, telecanthus, glaucoma, megalocornea, cataracts
Short-rib thoracic dysplasia with/without polydactyly	*WDR19* (*AR*)	Cataracts, attenuated arteries, macular anomalies
Shprintzen–Goldberg syndrome	*SKI* (*AD*)	Telecanthus, hypertelorism, proptosis, strabismus, downslanting palpebral fissures, ptosis, shallow orbits
Singleton–Merten syndrome	*IFIH1* (*AD*)	Glaucoma
Small vessel brain disease with/without ocular anomalies	*COL4A1* (*AD*)	Retinal arteriolar tortuosity, hypopigmentation of the fundus, episodic scotomas, episodic blurred vision, amblyopia (1 family), strabismus (1 family), high intraocular pressure (1 family). *Reported in some patients*: astigmatism, hyperopia, congenital cataracts, prominent or irregular Schwalbe line, iridocorneal synechiae, Axenfeld–Rieger anomalies, corneal opacities, microphthalmia, microcornea, iris hypoplasia, corectopia. *Rare*: decreased visual acuity, glaucoma, corneal neovascularization, polycoria, iridogoniodysgenesis, macular haemorrhage and Fuchs spots, peripapillary atrophy, choroidal atrophy
Smith–Magenis syndrome	*RAI1* (*AD*)	–
Spastic paraplegia and psychomotor retardation with or without seizures	*HACE1* (*AR*)	Strabismus, retinal dystrophy (some patients)
Split hand/foot malformation	CH	–
Stickler syndrome	*COL2A1* (*AD*); *COL11A1* (*AD*); *COL9A1* (*AR*); *COL9A2* (*AR*)	Retinal detachment, blindness, occasional cataracts, glaucoma, membranous (type I) vitreous phenotype

Table 5.1 (continued)

Syndrome	Gene and inheritance pattern	Ocular phenotype other than myopia
Syndromic mental retardation	*SETD5* (AD); *MBD5* (AD); *USP9X* (XLD); *NONO* (XLR); *RPL10* (XLR); *SMS* (XLR); *ELOVL4* (AR); *KDM5C* (XLR)	Synophrys, eyebrow abnormalities, upslanting and short palpebral fissures, epicanthal folds, mild hypertelorism, strabismus, cataracts, hypermetropia, astigmatism, poor vision
Syndromic microphthalmia	*OTX2*; *BMP4 (AD)*	Uni- or bilateral microphthalmia, uni- or bilateral anophthalmia, coloboma, microcornea, cataract, retinal dystrophy, optic nerve hypoplasia or agenesis
Temtamy syndrome	*C12orf57 (AR)*	Hypertelorism. "key-hole" iris, retina and choroid coloboma, dislocated lens (upward), downslanting palpebral fissures, arched eyebrows
White–Sutton syndrome	*POGZ (AD)*	Visual abnormalities, strabismus, astigmatism, hyperopia, optic atrophy, rod-cone dystrophy, cortical blindness
Zimmermann–Laband syndrome	*KCNH1 (AD)*	Thick eyebrows, synophrys, cataracts

AD autosomal dominant, *AR* autosomal recessive, *XLR* X linked recessive, *XLD* X linked dominant, *CH* chromosomal, *IP* imprinting defect

Table 5.1A Ocular conditions associated with myopia

Ocular condition	Gene and inheritance pattern
Achromatopsia	*CNGB3 (AR)*
Aland Island eye disease	*GPR143 (XLR)*
Anterior segment dysgenesis	*PITX3 (AD)*
Bietti crystalline corneoretinal dystrophy	*CYP4V2 (AD)*
Blue cone monochromacy	*OPN1LW*; *OPN1MW (XLR)*
Brittle cornea syndrome	*ZNF469*; *PRDM5 (AR)*
Cataract	*BFSP2*; *CRYBA2*; *EPHA2 (AD)*
Colobomatous macrophthalmia with microcornea	CH
Cone dystrophy	*KCNV2 (AD)*
Cone rod dystrophy	*C8orf37 (AR)*; *RAB28 (AR)*; *RPGR (XLR)*; *CACNA1F (XLR)*
Congenital microcoria	CH
Congenital stationary night blindness	*NYX (XLR)*; *CACNA1F (XLR)*; *GRM6 (AR)*; *SLC24A1 (AR)*; *LRIT3 (AR)*; *GNB3 (AR)*; *GPR179 (AR)*
Ectopia lentis et pupillae	*ADAMTSL4 (AR)*

(continued)

Ocular condition	Gene and inheritance pattern
High myopia with cataract and vitreoretinal degeneration	*P3H2* (*AR*)
Keratoconus	*VSX1* (*AD*)
Leber congenital amaurosis	*TULP1* (*AR*)
Microcornea, myopic chorioretinal atrophy, and telecanthus	*ADAMTS18* (*AR*)
Microspherophakia and/or megalocornea, with ectopia lentis and/or secondary glaucoma	*LTBP2* (*AR*)
Ocular albinism	*OCA2* (*AR*)
Primary open angle glaucoma	*MYOC*; *OPTN* (*AD*)
Retinal cone dystrophy	*KCNV2* (*AR*)
Retinal dystrophy	*C21orf2* (*AR*); *TUB* (*AR*)
Retinitis pigmentosa	*RP1* (*AD*); *RP2* (*XLR*); *RPGR* (*XLR*); *TTC8* (*AR*)
Sveinsson chorioretinal atrophy	*TEAD1* (*AD*)
Vitreoretinopathy	*ZNF408* (*AD*)
Wagner vitreoretinopathy	*VCAN* (*AD*)
Weill–Marchesani syndrome	*ADAMTS10* (*AR*); *FBN1*(*AD*); *LTBP2* (*AR*); *ADAMTS17* (*AR*)

AD autosomal dominant, *AR* autosomal recessive, *XLR* X linked recessive, *CH* chromosomal

pedigrees [21]. Families with genetic variants which show an autosomal dominant inheritance pattern were also most successful for myopia linkage studies. Up to now, 20 MYP loci [22–25] and several other loci [26–31] are identified for (high) myopia. Fine mapping led to candidate genes, such as the *IGF1* gene located in the MYP3 locus [32]. Linkage using a complex inheritance design found five additional loci [33–37].

Validation of candidate genes often resulted in no association, but other variants appeared associated with the non-Mendelian, common form of myopia. This hints towards a genetic overlap between Mendelian and common myopia [38]. As the GWAS era progressed, linkage studies fell by the wayside. Nevertheless, segregation analyses combined with linkage and next generation sequencing (i.e. whole exome sequencing) of regions in pedigrees with high myopia are, in theory, expected to facilitate the discovery of rare variants with large effects; an aspect which cannot be distilled from GWAS.

5.5 Candidate Gene Studies

In candidate gene studies the focus is on a gene with suspected biological, physiological or functional relevance to myopia, in particular high myopia. Although sometimes effective, candidate gene studies are limited by their reliance on this existing knowledge. Table 5.2 summarizes candidate gene studies on (high) myopia. Particularly

Table 5.2 Summary of candidate gene studies reporting positive association results with myopia

Gene symbol	Gene name	Hypothesized gene function	Associated phenotype	Ethnicity	Confirmation type (PMID)	Study (PMID)	Year
APLP2	Amyloid beta precursor like protein 2	Amacrine cell function modulation	Refractive error	Caucasian	n/a	Tkatchenko et al. [39] (26313004)	2015
BMP2K	Bone morphogenic protein-2-inducible protein kinase	Ocular development (embryogenesis) and retinal tissue remodelling	High myopia	Chinese	n/a	Liu et al. [40] (19927351)	2009
CHRM1	Cholinergic receptor muscarinic 1	Target of atropine	High myopia (−6.5 dpt)	Han Chinese	Expression study found no association with CHRM1 (19262686) and finding has been debated (20414262)	Lin et al. [41, 42] (19753311)	2010
CHRM1	Cholinergic receptor muscarinic 1	Target of atropine	High myopia (−6.5 dpt)	Han Chinese	Expression study found no association with CHRM1 (19262686) and finding has been debated (20414262)	Lin et al. [43, 44] (19753311)	2009
cMET (*alias HGFR*)	Tyrosine-protein kinase met	Hepatocyte growth factor and its receptor	Paediatric myopia (<−0.5 dpt)	Chinese	Replication independent high myopia cohort (24766640)	Khor et al. [45] (19500853)	2009
COL1A1	Collagen type I alpha 1 chain	Extracellular matrix	High myopia (<−9.25 dpt)	Japanese	Multiple systemic meta-analyses with contradicting results (27162737; 26131177; 27588274)	Inamori et al. [46] (17557158)	2007
COL2A1	Collagen type II alpha 1 chain	Extracellular matrix	High myopia (−5 dpt)	Caucasian	No replication independent high myopia cohort (21993774)	Metlapally et al. [47] (19387081)	2009
COL2A1	Collagen type II alpha 1 chain	Extracellular matrix	Paediatric myopia (<−0.75 dpt)	Caucasian	No replication independent high myopia cohort (21993774)	Mutti et al. [48] (17653045)	2007

(continued)

Table 5.2 (continued)

Gene symbol	Gene name	Hypothesized gene function	Associated phenotype	Ethnicity	Confirmation type (PMID)	Study (PMID)	Year
CRYBA4	Crystallin beta A4	Retinal and scleral remodelling	High myopia (<−8 dpt)	Chinese	No replication independent high myopia cohort (29263643)	Ho et al. [49] (22792142)	2012
HGF	Hepatocyte growth factor	Hepatocyte growth factor and its receptor	High myopia	Han Chinese	No replication independent high myopia cohort (19060265)	Han et al. [50] (16723436)	2006
HGF	Hepatocyte growth factor	Hepatocyte growth factor and its receptor	Refractive error	Caucasian	No replication independent high myopia cohort (19060265)	Veerappan et al. [51] (20005573)	2010
HGF	Hepatocyte growth factor	Hepatocyte growth factor and its receptor	High Myopia (−5 dpt)	Caucasian	No replication independent high myopia cohort (19060265)	Yanovitch et al. [52] (19471602)	2009
IGF1	Insulin-like growth factor 1	Hepatocyte growth factor and its receptor	High myopia (−5 dpt)	Caucasian	Systematic review and meta-analysis of studies in high myopics resulted in no association (28135889)	Metlapally et al. [53] (20435602)	2010
LAMA1	Laminin subunit alpha 1	Extracellular matrix	High myopia (<−6 dpt and axial length >26 mm)	Chinese	No replication independent high myopia cohort (29805427; 19668483)	Zhao et al. [54] (21541277)	2011
LUM	Lumican	Scleral and extracellular matrix remodelling	Extreme high myopia	Han Chinese	Meta-analysis of studies in high myopics resulted in no association (24927138)	Chen et al. [55] (19616852)	2009
LUM	Lumican	Scleral and extracellular matrix remodelling	High myopia	Han Chinese	Meta-analysis of studies in high myopics resulted in no association (24927138) and finding has been debated (20414262)	Lin et al. [41, 42] (19643966)	2010
LUM	Lumican	Scleral and extracellular matrix remodelling	High myopia (<−6.5 dpt)	Han Chinese	Meta-analysis of studies in high myopics resulted in no association (24927138)	Lin et al. [41, 42] (20010793)	2010

LUM	Lumican	Scleral and extracellular matrix remodelling	Extreme high myopia	Han Chinese	Meta-analysis of studies in high myopics resulted in no association (24927138)	Wang et al. [56] (16902402)	2006
MFN1	Mitofusin 1	Mitochondrial remodelling and apoptosis	Myopia	Caucasian	Expression study found association with myopia (27609161) and replication independent myopia cohort (26682159)	Andrew et al. [57] (18846214)	2008
MMP1	Matrix metallopeptidase 1	Extracellular matrix	Refractive error	Amish	No replication independent high myopia cohort (20435584; 23077567)	Wojciechowski et al. [58] (20484597)	2010
MMP1	Matrix metallopeptidase 1	Extracellular matrix	Refractive error	Caucasian	No replication independent high myopia cohort (20435584; 23077567)	Wojciechowski et al. [59] (23098370)	2013
MMP10	Matrix metallopeptidase 10	Extracellular matrix	Refractive error	Caucasian	No replication independent high myopia cohort (23077567)	Wojciechowski et al. [59] (23098370)	2013
MMP2	Matrix metallopeptidase 2	Extracellular matrix	Refractive error	Amish	Expression study found association with myopia (28402202; 29803830; 28900109; 24876280); no replication independent high myopia cohort (20435584; 23378725)	Wojciechowski et al. [58] (20484597)	2010
MMP2	Matrix metallopeptidase 2	Extracellular matrix	Refractive error	Caucasian	Expression study found association with myopia (28402202; 29803830; 28900109; 24876280); no replication independent high myopia cohort (20435584; 23378725)	Wojciechowski et al. [59] (23098370)	2013

(continued)

Table 5.2 (continued)

Gene symbol	Gene name	Hypothesized gene function	Associated phenotype	Ethnicity	Confirmation type (PMID)	Study (PMID)	Year
MMP3	Matrix metallopeptidase 3	Extracellular matrix	Refractive error	Caucasian	Expression study found no association with myopia (24876280); No replication independent high myopia cohort (20435584; 23077567; 16935611)	Hall et al. [60] (19279308)	2009
MMP9	Matrix metallopeptidase 9	Extracellular matrix	Refractive error	Caucasian	No replication independent high myopia cohort (23077567)	Hall et al. [60] (19279308)	2009
MYOC	Myocilin	Cytoskeletal function	High myopia	Chinese	No replication independent high myopia cohort (22809227; 24766640)	Tang et al. [61] (17438518)	2007
MYOC	Myocilin	Cytoskeletal function	High myopia	Caucasian	No replication independent high myopia cohort (22809227; 24766640)	Vatavuk et al. [62] (19260140)	2009
MYOC	Myocilin	Cytoskeletal function	High myopia	Caucasian	No replication independent high myopia cohort (22809227; 24766640)	Zayats et al. [63] (19180258)	2009
PAX6	Paired box 6	Ocular development (embryogenesis)	High myopia	Han Chinese	Systemic review and meta-analysis of studies in high and extreme myopics resulted in replication (24637479)	Han et al. [64] (19124844)	2009
PAX6	Paired box 6	Ocular development (embryogenesis)	High myopia (<−9 dpt)	Japanese	Systemic review and meta-analysis of studies in high and extreme myopics resulted in replication (24637479)	Kanemaki et al. [65] (26604670)	2015
PAX6	Paired box 6	Ocular development (embryogenesis)	High myopia (axial length >26 mm)	Japanese	Systemic review and meta-analysis of studies in high and extreme myopics resulted in replication (24637479)	Miyake et al. [66] (23213273)	2012

PAX6	Paired box 6	Ocular development (embryogenesis)	High myopia (<−6 dpt and axial length >26 mm)	Han Chinese	Systemic review and meta-analysis of studies in high and extreme myopics resulted in replication (24637479)	Ng et al. [67] (19907666)	2009
PAX6	Paired box 6	Ocular development (embryogenesis)	Extreme high myopia	Chinese	Systemic review and meta-analysis of studies in high and extreme myopics resulted in replication (24637479)	Tsai et al. [68] (17948041)	2008
PSARL	Presenilins-associated rhomboid-like protein	Mitochondrial remodelling and apoptosis	Myopia	Caucasian	n/a	Andrew et al. [57] (18846214)	2008
SOX2OT	Sex-determining region Y-box 2 overlapping transcript	Neurogenesis and vertebrate development (embryogenesis)	Myopia	Caucasian	n/a	Andrew et al. [57] (18846214)	2008
TGFβ1	Transforming growth factor beta 1	Extracellular matrix remodelling	High myopia (<−8 dpt)	Chinese	Replication GWAS-meta-analysis on refractive error (29808027)	Khor et al. [69] (20697017)	2010
TGFβ1	Transforming growth factor beta 1	Extracellular matrix remodelling	High myopia	Chinese	Replication GWAS-meta-analysis on refractive error (29808027)	Lin et al. [70] (16807529)	2006
TGFβ1	Transforming growth factor beta 1	Extracellular matrix remodelling	High myopia	Indian	Replication GWAS-meta-analysis on refractive error (29808027)	Rasool et al. [71] (23325483)	2013
TGFβ1	Transforming growth factor beta 1	Extracellular matrix remodelling	High myopia (<−8 dpt)	Chinese	Replication GWAS-meta-analysis on refractive error (29808027)	Zha et al. [72] (19365037)	2009

(continued)

Table 5.2 (continued)

Gene symbol	Gene name	Hypothesized gene function	Associated phenotype	Ethnicity	Confirmation type (PMID)	Study (PMID)	Year
TGFβ2	Transforming growth factor beta 2	Extracellular matrix remodelling	High myopia (<−6.5 dpt)	Han Chinese	Expression study found association with myopia (28900109; 29188062; 27214233; 24967344); expression study found no association with myopia (25112847)	Lin et al. [43, 44] (19710942)	2009
TGIF (*alias* *TGIF1*)	TGFB induced factor homeobox 1	Extracellular matrix remodelling	High myopia	Chinese	No replication independent high myopia cohort (19060265; 18172074; 17048038; 15223781)	Lam et al. [73] (12601022)	2003
TGIF1	TGFB induced factor homeobox 1	Extracellular matrix remodelling	High myopia	Indian	No replication independent high myopia cohort (19060265; 18172074; 17048038; 15223781)	Ahmed et al. [74] (24215395)	2014
UMODL1	Uromodulin like 1	Extracellular matrix	High myopia (<−9.25 dpt)	Japanese	No replication independent high myopia cohort (22857148)	Nishizaki et al. [75] (18535602)	2009

notable are genes encoding extracellular matrix-related proteins (*COL1A1*, *COL2A1* [16, 17] and *MMP1*, *MMP2*, *MMP3*, *MMP9*, *MMP10* [59, 60]). For candidates such as *PAX6* and *TGFB1*, the results were replicated in multiple independent extreme/high myopia studies and validated in a large GWAS meta-analysis in 2018, respectively [18, 76]. However in most other cases, the results were not independently validated: *LUM* and *IGF1* failed to confirm an association [77, 78]. Interestingly, in a few cases the candidates were subsequently implicated in GWAS of other ocular traits: *TGFβ2* and *LUM* for central corneal thickness (CCT), a glaucoma and keratoconus endophenotype [14], *PAX6* with optic disc area [79] and *HGF* [80].

5.6 Genome-Wide Association Studies

Generally, linkage studies are limited to identification of genetic variants with a large effect on myopia [81]. Given the limited number of genes identified by linkage, it became apparent in the 2000s that identifying large numbers of additional myopia genes was more practical with genome-wide association studies (GWASes), since it has dramatically higher statistical power. GWASes have greatly enhanced our knowl edge of the genetic architecture of (complex) diseases [82]. Most of the variants found via GWAS reside in non-exonic regions and their effect sizes are typically small [82 83]. For GWAS, 200 k–500 k genetic markers are usually genotyped and a further >10 million "imputed", taking advantage of the correlation structure of the genome. This approach is most effective for common variants (allele frequencies >0.01 in the popula tion, although with larger reference panels, rarer alleles can also be detected).

Initially, GWASes for myopia were performed as a dichotomous outcome (i.e. case-control, Table 5.3). Since myopia constitutes a dichotomization of the quantita tive trait spherical equivalent, considering the quantitative trait should be more informative for gene mapping. The first GWASes for spherical equivalent were conducted in 2010 [96, 97], with ~4000 individuals required to identify the first loci. The first loci to reach the genome-wide significance threshold ($P < 5 \times 10^{-8}$, the threshold reflecting the large number of statistical tests conducted genome-wide) were markers near the *RASGFR1* gene on 15q25.1 ($P = 2.70 \times 10^{-9}$) and markers near *GJD2* on 15q14 ($P = 2.21 \times 10^{-14}$). A subsequent analysis combining five cohorts ($N = 7000$) identified another locus at the *RBFOX1* gene on chromosome 16 ($P = 3.9 \times 10^{-9}$) [98

These early efforts made it clear that individual groups would have difficulty in mapping many genes for spherical equivalent, motivating the formation of the Consortium for Refractive Error and Myopia (CREAM) in 2010, which included researchers and cohorts from the USA, Europe, Asia and Australia. They replicated SNPs in the 15q14 loci [99], which was further affirmed by other studies on both spherical equivalent and axial length alongside with the replication of the 15q25 locus [100, 101].

In 2013, two major GWAS meta-analyses on refractive error traits (spherical equivalent and age of spectacle wear) identified 37 novel loci (Table 5.4), with robust replication of *GJD2*, *RFBOX1* and *RASGFR1* in both meta-analyses. The first was the collaborative work of CREAM based on a GWAS meta-analysis on spherical equivalent, comprising 35 individual cohorts ($N_{European} = 37{,}382$; $N_{SoutheastAsian} = 12{,}332$) [108]. 23andMe, a direct-to-consumer genetic testing com pany, performed the second major GWAS, replicating 8 of the novel loci found by CREAM and identifying another 11 novel loci based on a GWAS survival analysis

Table 5.3 Summary of case-control design GWASs and their highest associations with myopia

Authors (year)	Study description	Associations	Ethnicity	PMID
Nakanishi et al. (2009) [84]	Genome-wide association study (GWAS) 830 cases (pathologic myopia; AL >26 mm) 1911 controls	Strongest association with 11q24.1, 44kb upstream of the *BLID* gene and in the second intron of *LOC399959*	Japanese	19779542
Li et al. (2011) [85]	GWAS 287 cases (high myopia; SE ≤ -6D) 673 controls	Strongest suggestive association ($P = 1.51 \times 10^{-5}$) with 5p15.2 for an intronic SNP within the *CTNND2* gene, but with replication in Japanese independent cohort (959 cases and 2128 controls; $P = 0.035$)	Chinese Japanese	21095009
Lu et al. (2011) [86]	GWAS 1203 cases (high myopia; SE ≤ -6D) 955 controls (SE -0.50 D to +1.00 D)	Replication ($P = 2.17 \times 10^{-5}$) with a SNP in *CTNND2* region	Chinese	21911587
Wang et al. [87] (2011)	SNP ($n = 3$) look-up in 11q24.1 and 21q22.3 regions 1255 cases (complex myopia; SE < -10.00 D $<$SE ≤ -4.00 D) 563 cases (high myopia; SE $\le$-6.00 D) 1052 controls (-0.50 D $\le$ SE $\le +2.00$ D)	No statistically significant differences found for the genotype or allele frequencies of the three SNPs between the myopia cases and controls	Chinese	22194655
Yu et al. (2012) [88]	SNP ($n = 27$) look-up in 5p15 and 11q24 regions 321 cases (pathologic myopia; SE ≤ -6 D and AL $>$ 26 mm) 310 control	Significantly associated SNPs in the *CTNND2* gene and 11q24.1 region ($P = 0.0126$ and 0.0293, respectively) with pathological myopia, replicating previous findings for these loci	Chinese	22759899
Liu et al. (2014) [89]	Meta-analysis comprising the SNPs of all 5 previously published data on the *CTNND2* gene and 11q24.1 region association with myopia 6954 cases 9346 controls	Significant association of 11q24.1 region with myopia ($P = 0.013$). No significant association with myopia for the *CTNND2* gene (two SNPs tested: $P = 0.725$, $P = 0.065$)	Chinese Japanese	24672220
Li et al. (2011) [85]	GWAS 102 cases (high myopia; SE ≤ -8 D with retinal degeneration) 335 controls	The strongest association ($P = 7.70 \times 10^{-13}$) was in a gene desert within the *MYP11* region on 4q25	Chinese	21505071

Shi et al. (2011) [90]	GWAS 419 high myopia cases (≤−6D) 669 controls	The strongest association ($P = 1.91 \times 10^{-16}$) was in an intron within the *MIPEP* gene on 13q12	Han Chinese	21640322
Shi et al. (2013) [91]	GWAS 665 cases (high myopia; SE ≤ −6D) 960 controls	The strongest association ($P = 8.95 \times 10^{-14}$) was in the *VIPR2* gene within the MYP4 locus, followed by three other variants in LD of the *SNTB1* gene region ($P = 1.13 \times 10^{-8}$ to 2.13×10^{-11})	Han Chinese	23406873
Khor et al. (2013) [92]	GWAS meta-analysis of 4 Asian studies 1603 cases ("severe" myopia; SE ≤−6 D and AL ≥26 mm) 3427 controls	The *SNTB1* gene was confirmed and a novel variant within the *ZFHX1B* gene (also known as *ZEB2*) reached genome-wide significance ($P = 5.79 \times 10^{-10}$)	East-Asian	23933737
Hosada et al. (2018) [93]	GWAS meta-analysis of 5 Asian studies 828 cases 3624 controls	Discovery ($P = 1.46 \times 10^{-10}$) and replication ($P = 2.40 \times 10^{-6}$) of the CCDC102B locus.	East-Asian	29725004
Meng et al. (2012) [94]	GWAS 192 cases (high myopia; SE ≤−6 D) 1064 controls	Confirmation of SNPs 3kb downstream of *PPP1R3B* in vicinity of MYP10 on 8p23 ($P = 6.32 \times 10^{-7}$) and MYP15 on 10q21.1 ($P = 2.17 \times 10^{-5}$)	European	23049088
Pickrell et al. (2016) [95]	GWAS 106,086 cases (Myopia "yes"; questionnaire) 85,757 controls (Myopia "no"; questionnaire)	More than 100 novel loci associated with myopia	European	27182965

Table 5.4 Overview of the 37 novel loci found in 2013 by CREAM and 23andMe and subsequent replication

Locus #	Locus name	Discovery—*P* value HapMapII CREAM (2013)	Replication—*P* value HapMapII 23andMe (2013)	Replication—individual cohort (PMID)	Replication—*P* value 1000G CREAM&23 and Me (2018)
2	*BICC1*	2.06×10^{-13}	n/a	Simpson et al. (2014) [102] (25233373), Yoshikawa et al. (2014) [103] (25335978)	1.07×10^{-18}
3	*LAMA2*	1.79×10^{-12}	6.80×10^{-53}	Cheng et al. (2013) [104] (24144296), Simpson et al. (2014) [102] (25233373)	1.91×10^{-57}
4	*CD55*	3.05×10^{-12}	n/a	Cheng et al. (2013) [104] (24144296), Yoshikawa et al. (2014) [103] (25335978)	4.42×10^{-13}
5	*TOX/CA8*	3.99×10^{-12}	4.00×10^{-22}	Simpson et al. (2014) [102] (25233373)	4.64×10^{-31}
6	*RDH5*	4.44×10^{-12}	1.30×10^{-23}		4.06×10^{-43}
7	*CYP26A1*	1.03×10^{-11}	n/a	Yoshikawa et al. (2014) [103] (25335978)	7.49×10^{-10}
8	*RASGRF1*	4.25×10^{-11}	8.20×10^{-13}	Oishi et al. (2013) [105] (24150758), Yoshikawa et al. (2014) [103] (25335978)	4.24×10^{-23}
9	*CHRNG*	5.15×10^{-11}	n/a	Tideman et al. (2016) [106] (27611182)	1.16×10^{-24}
10	*SHISA6*	7.29×10^{-11}	5.20×10^{-15}		9.46×10^{-29}
11	*PRSS56*	7.86×10^{-11}	5.80×10^{-18}	Simpson et al. (2014) [102] (25233373)	2.25×10^{-29}
12	*MYO1D*	9.66×10^{-11}	n/a		2.91×10^{-16}
13	*ZMAT4/SFRP1*	3.69×10^{-10}	1.80×10^{-18}	Simpson et al. (2014) [102] (25233373), Yoshikawa et al. (2014) [103] (25335978)	1.02×10^{-27}
14	*A2BP/RBFOX1*	5.64×10^{-10}	4.10×10^{-26}	Simpson et al. (2014) [102] (25233373), Tideman et al. (2016) [106] (27611182)	1.13×10^{-42}
15	*KCNQ5*	4.18×10^{-9}	2.70×10^{-25}	Liao et al. (2017) [107] (28884119), Yoshikawa et al. (2014) [103] (25335978), Tideman et al. (2016) [106] (27611182)	5.43×10^{-48}
16	*PTPRR*	5.47×10^{-9}	n/a		1.81×10^{-13}
17	*GRIA4*	5.92×10^{-9}	n/a	Tideman et al. (2016) [106] (27611182), Yoshikawa et al. (2014) [103] (25335978)	8.84×10^{-12}

18	*TJP2*	7.26×10^{-9}	5.20×10^{-13}		1.35×10^{-21}
19	*SIX6*	1.00×10^{-8}	n/a		2.12×10^{-8}
20	*LOC100506035*	1.09×10^{-8}	n/a		1.56×10^{-15}
21	*BMP2*	1.57×10^{-8}	n/a	Tideman et al. (2016) [106] (27611182), Yoshikawa et al. (2014) [103] (25335978)	3.11×10^{-9}
22	*CHD7*	1.82×10^{-8}	n/a		1.94×10^{-7}
23	*PCCA*	2.11×10^{-8}	n/a		1.68×10^{-7}
24	*CACNA1D*	2.14×10^{-8}	n/a	Tideman et al. (2016) [106] (27611182)	4.10×10^{-10}
25	*KCNJ2*	2.79×10^{-8}	n/a		5.53×10^{-13}
26	*RORB*	4.15×10^{-8}	n/a		1.07×10^{-11}
27	*LRRC4C*	n/a	2.30×10^{-30}	Tideman et al. (2016) [106] (27611182), Yoshikawa et al. (2014) [103] (25335978)	4.43×10^{-42}
28	*PABPCP2*	n/a	1.50×10^{-14}		1.05×10^{-17}
29	*BMP3*	n/a	4.20×10^{-12}	Simpson et al. (2014) [102] (25233373)	2.08×10^{-20}
30	*RGR*	n/a	8.00×10^{-12}		9.26×10^{-17}
31	*DLG2*	n/a	1.70×10^{-11}		8.85×10^{-15}
32	*ZBTB38*	n/a	3.60×10^{-11}		1.23×10^{-15}
33	*PDE11A*	n/a	8.70×10^{-11}		1.30×10^{-15}
34	*DLX1*	n/a	1.40×10^{-10}		2.77×10^{-16}
35	*KCNMA1*	n/a	7.30×10^{-10}		2.36×10^{-16}
36	*BMP4*	n/a	1.10×10^{-9}	Yoshikawa et al. (2014) [103] (25335978)	1.09×10^{-12}
37	*ZIC2*	n/a	2.10×10^{-8}	Oishi et al. (2013) [105] (24150758), Simpson et al. (2014) [102] (25233373), Tideman et al. (2016) [106] (27611182)	2.80×10^{-15}
S-38*	*B4GALNT2*	n/a	8.30×10^{-7}	Yoshikawa et al. (2014) [103] (25335978)	2.68×10^{-10}
S-39*	*EHBP1L1*	n/a	2.10×10^{-7}	Yoshikawa et al. (2014) [103] (25335978)	1.07×10^{-9}

*These two loci were subthreshold (S) in the analysis in 2013, but exceeded genome-wide significance in 2018 using a larger sample size of age of spectacle wear in 55,177 participants of European ancestry. To the surprise of some in the field, the effect sizes and direction of the effects of the loci found by these two groups were concordant despite the difference in phenotype definition and in scale: dioptres for CREAM and hazard ratios for 23andMe [109]. Subsequently, replication studies provided validation for the associated loci and highlighted two other suggestive associations. At this point, the implicated loci explained 3% of the phenotypic variance in refractive error [108, 110].

The CREAM and 23andMe studies represented a large increase in sample size over the initial GWASs. Their meta-analysis approach was very effective in discovering new loci. This motivated joined efforts of CREAM and 23andMe, which resulted in a GWAS meta-analysis including 160,420 participants. Moreover, a denser imputation reference set was used (1000G phase 1 version 3), enabling better characterization of genetic variations. Although CREAM and 23andMe used different phenotypes (spherical equivalent and age at first spectacle wear, respectively) again the results were concordant and the new findings were replicated in an independent cohort with refractive error available (UK biobank, comprising 95,505 participants). Overall, this GWAS increased the number of risk loci to 161, explaining 7.8% of the phenotypic variance in refractive error. Very large sample sizes (millions) will be required to identify all of the loci contributing to myopia risk.

The genetic correlation was estimated to be 0.78 between European and Asian ancestry, suggesting that despite (1) large differences in the rate of myopia between these groups and (2) differences in the genetic ancestry of these groups, most of the genetic variation is in common. Figure 5.1 provides the chronological discovery of all associated loci and Fig. 5.2 shows the effect sizes of the established 161 loci.

Several "endophenotypes" have been considered for myopia: spherical equivalent, axial length, corneal curvature and age of diagnosis of myopia. Axial length is a well-studied "endophenotype" which correlates strongly with refractive error. The first GWAS of axial length considered 4944 Asian ancestry individuals and identified a locus at 1q41. A subsequent meta-analysis combining data on 12,531 European and 8216 Asian ancestry individuals uncovered a further eight genome-wide significant loci at *RSPO1*, *C3orf26*, *LAMA2*, *GJD2*, *ZNRF3*, *CD55*, *MIP*, *ALPPL2*, as well as confirming the 1q41 locus. Five of the axial length loci were also associated loci for refractive error. GWASs performed for corneal curvature [104, 111–114] identified the loci *FRAP1*, *CMPK1*, *RBP3* and *PDGFRA*; in the case of *PDGFRA*, associations have also been found with eye size. A study in 9804 Japanese individuals and replication in Chinese and European ancestry cohorts analysed three myopia-related traits (refractive error, axial length and corneal curvature). They replicated the association of *GJD2* and refractive error as well as the association of SNPs in *WNT7B* for axial length and corneal curvature [114, 115]

5.7 Pathway Analysis Approaches

GWAS approaches improve our understanding of the molecular basis of traits by map ping individual loci. However, it is possible to place such loci into a broader context by applying pathway analysis approaches. In myopia, a retina-to-sclera signaling cascade has been postulated, but the specific molecular components were unclear. Recent GWASs have uncovered genes which lie along this pathway [108, 110, 116]—genetic changes at individual loci only make small changes to phenotype but collectively these

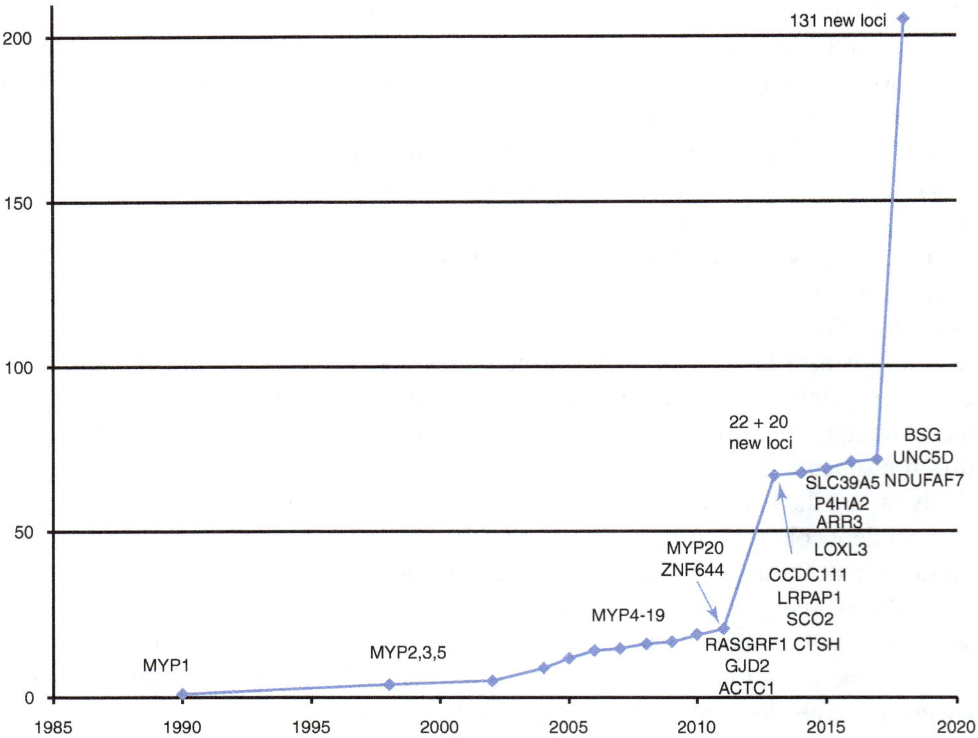

Fig. 5.1 Historic overview of myopia gene finding. Overview of myopia gene finding in historic perspective. Genes identified using whole exome sequencing are marked as purple. Other loci (linkage studies, GWAS) are marked as red

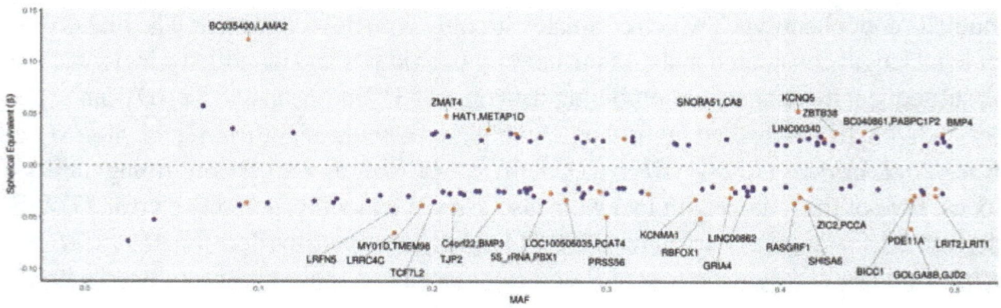

Fig. 5.2 Effect sizes of common and rare variants for myopia and refractive error. Overview of SNPs and annotated genes found in the most recent GWAS meta-analysis [18]. X-axis displays the minor allele frequency of each SNP; y-axis displays the effect size of per individual SNP. The blue dots represent the novel loci discovered by Tedja et al. [18] and the pink dots represent the loci found by Verhoeven et al. [108], which now have been replicated

perturbations are responsible for larger changes in the retina-to-sclera signaling cascade, ultimately explaining differences in refractive error from individual to individual.

Pathways inferred from the first large-scale CREAM GWAS [108, 110] included neurotransmission (*GRIA4*), ion transport (*KCNQ5*), retinoic acid metabolism (*RDH5*), extracellular matrix remodelling (*LAMA2*, *BMP2*) and eye development (*SIX6*, *PRSS56*). The 23andMe GWAS identified an overlapping set of pathways: neuronal development (*KCNMA1*, *RBFOX1*, *LRRC4C*, *NGL-1*, *DLG2*, *TJP2*),

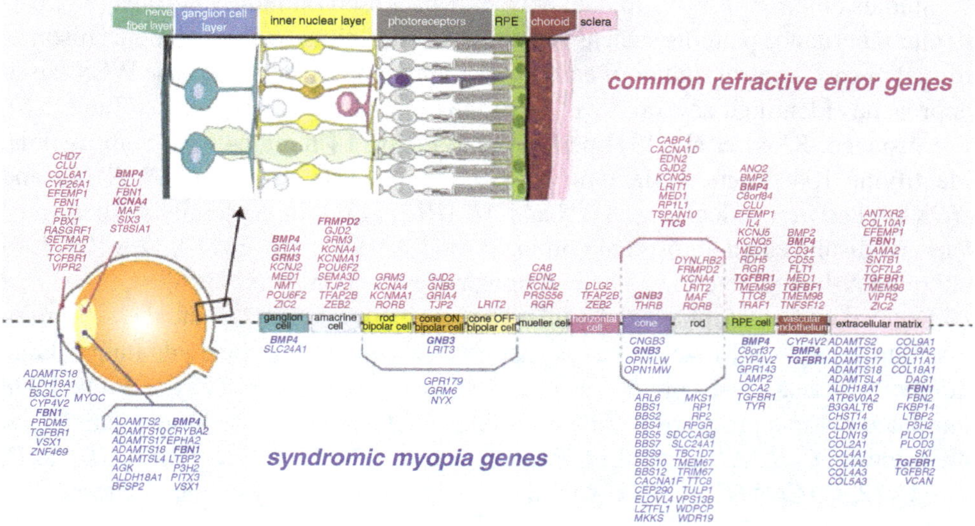

Fig. 5.3 Schematic overview of known function in retinal cell types of refractive error and syndromic myopia genes according to literature. Bold: genes identified for both common refractive error and in syndromic myopia

extracellular matrix remodelling (*ANTXR2*, *LAMA2*), the visual cycle (*RDH5*, *RGR*, *KCNQ5*), eye and body growth (*PRSS56*, *BMP4*, *ZBTB38*, *DLX1*) and retinal ganglion cell (*ZIC2*, *SFRP1*) [117]. When considered in the context of known protein–protein interactions, many genes in these pathways are related to growth and cell cycle pathways, such as the TGF-beta/SMAD and MAPK pathways [118].

The most recent meta-analysis combining data from CREAM and 23andMe data taken together confirmed previous findings and offered additional insights [18]. In a gene-set analysis, several pathways were highlighted including "abnormal photoreceptor inner segment morphology" (Mammalian Phenotype Ontology (MP) 0003730); "thin retinal outer nuclear layer" (MP 0008515); "nonmotile primary cilium" (Gene Ontology (GO) 0031513); "abnormal anterior-eye-segment morphology" (MP 0005193) and "detection of light stimulus" (GO 0009583). The genes implicated in this large-scale GWAS were distributed across all cell types in the retina-to-sclera signaling cascade (neurosensory retina, RPE, vascular endothelium and extracellular matrix, Fig. 5.3). The larger GWAS also suggested novel mechanisms, including angiogenesis, rod-and-cone bipolar synaptic neurotransmission and anterior-segment morphology. Interestingly, a novel association was found at the *DRD1* gene, supporting previous work linking the dopamine pathway to myopia.

5.8 Next Generation Sequencing

GWAS approaches have been highly effective in assessing the role of common variants in myopia but such methods cannot effectively characterize very rare genomic variants. Whole exome sequencing (WES) allows investigation of rare variants in exonic regions; due to cost, applications to date have primarily been in family studies or studies of early onset high myopia.

Studies employing WES to date have either focused on family designs (e.g. particular inheritance patterns such as X-linkage or conditions such as myopic anisometropia) or case-control studies of early onset high myopia [119–122]. The WES-based approaches identified several novel mutations in known myopia genes (Table 5.5). For instance, Kloss et al. [131] performed WES on 14 families with high myopia, identifying 104 genetic variants in both known MYP loci (e.g. *AGRN*, *EME1* and *HOXA2*) and in new loci (e.g. *ATL3* and *AKAP12*) [131]. In the family studies, most variants displayed an autosomal dominant mode of inheritance [119, 123, 124, 130] although X-linked heterozygous mutations were found in *ARR3* [126].

Both retinal dystrophies and ocular development disorders coincide with myopia. Sun et al. [132] investigated if there was a genetic link by evaluating a large number of retinal dystrophy genes in early onset high myopia. They examined 298 unrelated myopia probands and their families, identifying 29 potentially pathogenic mutations in *COL2A1*, *COL11A1*, *PRPH2*, *FBN1*, *GNAT1*, *OPA1*, *PAX2*, *GUCY2D*, *TSPAN12*, *CACNA1F* and *RPGR* with mainly an autosomal dominant pattern.

5.9 Environmental Influences Through Genetics

Although myopia is highly heritable within specific cohorts, dramatic changes in environment across many human populations have led to large changes in prevalence over time [133–136]. The role of changes in socioeconomic status, time spent outdoors, education and near-work are now well established as risk factors for myopia, based on observational studies [137–139]. Education has proven the most influential and consistent factor, with a doubling in myopia prevalence when attending higher education compared to finishing only primary education [140–142]. There are two main areas where genetic studies can inform our understanding of the role of environment. Firstly, gene–environment studies can highlight where interactions exist. Secondly, observational studies only establish association and not causation—in some circumstances genetic data can be used to strengthen the case for an environmental risk factor causally (or not) influencing myopia risk (Mendelian randomization).

Gene–environment (GxE) interaction analyses examine whether genes operate differently across varying environments. GxE studies in myopia have focused primarily on education. An early study in North American samples examined GxE for myopia and the matrix metalloproteinases genes (*MMP1-MMP10*): a subset of SNPs were only associated with refraction in the lower education level [58, 59]. A subsequent study in five Singapore cohorts found variants in *DNAH9*, *GJD2* and *ZMAT4*, which had a larger effect on myopia in a high education subset [143]. Subsequent efforts to examine GxE considered the aggregate effects of many SNPs together. A study in Europeans found that a genetic risk score comprising 26 genetic variants was most strongly associated with myopia in individuals with a university level education [144]. A study examining GxE in children considered near work and time outdoors in association with 39 SNPs and found weak evidence for an interaction with near work [144, 145]. Finally, a CREAM study was able to identify additional myopia risk loci by allowing for a GxE approach [19].

Mendelian randomization (MR) infers whether a risk factor is causally associated with a disease. MR exploits the fact that germline genotypes are randomly

Table 5.5 Overview of genes and their mutations found by next generation sequencing

Gene	Pathway	Method	Inheritance Pattern	Mutation type	Mutation	Author (Year)	PMID
CCDC111	DNA transcription	Targeted sequencing and exome sequencing	Autosomal dominant	Missense	c.265T>G:p.Y89D in *CCDC111*	Zhao et al. (2013) [120]	23579484
NDUFAF7	Mitochondrial function	Genotyping and WES	Autosomal dominant	Missense	c.798C>G:p.D266E in *NDUFAF7*	Wang et al. (2017) [121]	28837730
P4HA2	Collagen synthesis	WES	Autosomal dominant	Missense	c.1147A>G:p.(K383E) in *P4HA2*	Napolitano et al. (2018) [119]	29364500
SCO2	Mitochondrial function	WES	Autosomal dominant	Missense	c.334C>T:p.R112W; c.358C>T:p.R120W in *SCO2*	Jiang et al. (2014) [123]	25525168
SCO2	Mitochondrial function	WES	Autosomal dominant	Nonsense Missense	c.157C>T:p.Q53∗ in SCO2; c.341G>A:p.R114H; c.418G>A:p.E140K and c.776C>T:p.A259V) in *SCO2*	Tran-Viet et al. (2013) [124]	23643385
UNC5D	Cell signaling	WES	Autosomal dominant	Missense	c.1297C>T:p.R433C in *UNC5D*	Feng et al. (2017) [122]	28614238
BSG	Cell signaling	WES	Autosomal dominant	Missense Splicing Nonsense	c.889G>A:p.G297S; c.661C>T:p.P221S in *BSG* c.205C>T:p.Q69X in *BSG* c.415+1G>A in *BSG*	Jin et al. [125] (2017)	28373534
ARR3	Retina-specific signal transduction	WES	X-linked female-limited	Missense	c.893C>A:p.A298D; c.298C>T:p.R100∗ and c.239T>C:p.L80P in *ARR3*	Xiao et al. (2016) [126]	27829781

LOXL3	Transforming growth factor-beta pathway	WES	Autosomal recessive	Frameshift	c.39dup:p.L14Afs∗21; c.39dup:p.L14Afs∗21 and c.594delG:p.Q199Kfs∗35 in *LOXL3*	Li et al. [127] (2016)	26957899
SLC39A5	Transforming growth factor-beta pathway	WES	Autosome dominant Autosome dominant	Nonsense Missense	c.141C>G:p.Y47∗ in *SLC39A5* c.911T>C:p.M304T in *SLC39A5*	Guo et al. [128] (2014)	24891338
SLC39A5	Transforming growth factor-beta pathway	WES	Autosome dominant	Missense	c.1238G>C:p.G413A in *SLC39A5*	Jiang et al. (2014) [123]	25525168
LRPAP1	Transforming growth factor-beta pathway	WES	Autosomal recessive	Frameshift, truncating	N202Tfs∗8 and I288Rfs∗118 in *LRPAP1*	Aldahmesh [129] et al. (2013)	23830514
LRPAP1	Transforming growth factor-beta pathway	WES	Autosomal recessive	Truncating	c.199delC:p.Q67Sfs∗8 in *LRPAP1*	Jiang et al. (2014) [123]	25525168
CTSH	Degradation of proteins in lysosomes	WES	Autosomal recessive	Frameshift, truncating	c.485_488del in *CTSH*	Aldahmesh [129] et al. (2013)	23830514
ZNF644	DNA transcription	WES	Autosomal dominant	Missense	I587V, R680G, C699Y, 3′UTR+12 C>G, and 3′UTR+592 G>A in ZNF644	Shi et al. [130] (2011)	21695231
ZNF644	DNA transcription	WES	Autosomal dominant	Missense	c.2014A>G:p.S672G; c.2048G>C:p.R683T and c.2551G>C:p.D851H	Jiang et al. (2014) [123]	25525168
104 novel genetic variants (73 rare)	–	WES in 14 families	Autosomal dominant	Non synonymous	–	Kloss et al. (2017) [131]	28384719

assigned at meiosis, to enable a “natural” randomized controlled trial. Since the assigned genotypes are independent of non-genetic confounding and are unmodified by disease processes, MR offers a better assessment of causality than that available from observational studies [146, 147].

Two MR studies found a causal effect of education on the development of myopia. One of the MR studies tested for causality bi-directionally [148]. Both found a larger effect through MR than that estimated from observational studies suggesting that confounding in observational studies may have been obscuring the true relationship [149]. As expected, there was little evidence of myopia affecting education (−0.008 years/dioptre, $P = 0.6$). Another study focused on the causality of low vitamin D on myopia due to controversy in the literature [150]. The estimated effects of vitamin D on refractive error were so small (Caucasians: −0.02 [95% CI −0.09, 0.04] dioptres (D) per 10 nmol/l increase in vitamin D concentration; Asians: 0.01 [95% CI −0.17, 0.19] D per 10 nmol/l increase) that the authors concluded that the true contribution of vitamin D levels to degree of myopia is probably zero and that previous observational findings were likely confounded by the effects of time spent outdoors.

5.10 Epigenetics

Epigenetics in refractive error and myopia is postulated to be important due to the known effects of environmental factors on refractive error and myopia development. Nevertheless, this field is still developing and some characteristics of epigenetics render it a difficult issue to unravel. Epigenetic features can be influenced by environmental factors and are time dependent and tissue specific. This complicates the study of these effects, since myopia and refractive errors develop during childhood and young adolescence and obtaining eye tissue, preferably retinal and scleral would be unethical. Furthermore, although some epigenetic processes are conserved across species, this is not always the case: making animal studies not always translational to humans.

Non-Coding RNAs and Myopia The latest GWAS meta-analysis found 31 of 161 loci residing in or near regions transcribing (small) noncoding RNAs, thus hinting towards the importance of epigenetics [18, 151]. MicroRNAs, or miRNAs, are the best-characterized family of small non-coding RNAs. They are approximately 19–24 nucleotides in length in their mature form. They are able to bind to 3′ UTR regions on RNA polymers by sequence-specific post-transcriptional gene silencing; one miRNA can regulate the translation of many genes. MiRNAs have been a hot topic in the last years due to their potential clinical application: the accessibility of the retina for miRNA-based therapeutic delivery has great potential for the prevention and treatment of retinal pathologies [152]. Up to now, there have only been a handful of studies on miRNA and its role in myopiagenesis in humans, these are summarized in Table 5.6.

5.11 Implications for Clinical Management

Due to the high polygenicity of myopia and low explained phenotypic variance by genetic factors (7.8%), clinical applications derived from genetic analyses of myopia are currently limited. Risk predictions for myopia in children are based on family history, education level of the parents, the amount of outdoor exposure and the easily measurable refractive error and axial length.

Currently, we are able to make a distinction between high myopes and high hyperopes based on the polygenic risk scores derived from CREAM studies: persons in the highest decile for the polygenic risk score had a 40-fold-greater risk of myopia relative to those in the lowest decile.

A prediction model including age, sex and polygenic risk score achieved an AUC of 0.77 (95% CI = 0.75–0.79) for myopia versus hyperopia in adults (Rotterdam Study I–III) [18]. This AUC is similar to that achieved by modelling environmental factors only; the AUC for myopia incidence in a European child cohort was 0.78 considering parental myopia, 1 or more books read per week, time spent reading, no participation in sports, non-European ethnicity, less time spent outdoors and baseline AL-to-CR ratio [156]. To date, one study has assessed both environmental and

Table 5.6 Overview of microRNAs associated with myopia

MiRNA	SNP	Study design	Outcome	Author
MiR-328 binding site in 3′UTR of PAX6 gene	rs662702	High myopia case-control study (Ncase = 1083, ≤−6 D; Ncontrol 1096 ≥−1.5 D)	Down regulation effect on PAX6 expression with C allele, relative to T allele. OR for CC genotype 2.1 ($P = 0.007$). This effect was significant for extreme myopia (<−10 D) and not for high myopia	Liang et al. (2011) [153]
MiR-184	n.a.	MiR-184 region sequenced in 780 unrelated keratoconus patients and 96 unrelated Han southern Chinese patients with axial myopia under the hypothesis that axial myopia is associated with keratoconus, possibly under regulation of MiR-184	No miR-184 mutations were detected in the axial myopia cohort	Lechner et al. (2013) [154]
MiR-29a	rs157907	High myopia case-control study (Ncases = 254, ≤−6 D; Ncontrols = 300, −0.5 to 0.5 D). COL1A1 is possibly targeted by MiR-29a	The G allele of the rs157907 locus was significantly associated with decreased risk of severe myopia (<10 D; $P = 0.04$), compared to the A allele. rs157907 A/G might regulate miR-29a expression levels, but no functional studies have been conducted to confirm this hypothesis	Xie et al. (2016) [155]
Let-7i	rs10877885	High myopia case-control study (Ncases = 254, ≤−6 D; Ncontrols = 300, −0.5 to 0.5 D). COL1A1 is possibly targeted by Let-7i	No significant association with rs10877885 (C/T) was found with myopia risk	Xie et al. (2016) [155]

genetic factors together and showed that modelling both genes and environment improved prediction accuracy [157]. Although these efforts to improve prediction are promising, a prediction-based approach will only be beneficial if randomized controlled trials of atropine therapy show that children with persistent myopic progression benefit from an earlier and higher dose of atropine administration. The additional costs of genetic testing and potentially invasive regime (collecting blood from children) also need to be taken into account.

5.12 Concluding Remarks

The scientific community has discovered more than 200 loci associated with myopia and its endophenotypes with a variety of approaches (linkage, candidate gene, GWAS, post-GWAS gene-based associations, next generation sequencing approaches, gene environment interactions and epigenetic approaches). With the rise of large biobanks, such as the UK Biobank [158], further GWAS meta-analyses between large consortia and companies will enable identification of many more genes. This will allow full elucidation of the molecular mechanism of myopiagenesis. Whole genome sequencing approaches will replace both GWAS and WES, and will elucidate the genetic structure which regulates the function of the myopia risk variants.

To fully understand the underlying mechanisms, the focus should lie on unraveling the genetic and epigenetic architecture of myopia by exploring interactions and effects of other “omics” in relevant tissue, i.e. multi-omics. This concept includes incorporation of methylomics, transcriptomics, proteomics and metabolomics. Future projects should focus on gathering more omics data on eye tissue. Next to the multi-omics approach, modelling gene–environment effects will tell us more about the genetic key players which are also susceptible to the environment. Furthermore, future functional studies interrogating the candidate genes and loci will point us to therapeutic solutions for myopia management.

References

1. Tedja MS, et al. International Myopia Institute (IMI) - myopia genetics report. Investig Ophthalmol Vis Sci. 2019;60:M31–88.
2. Duke-Elder SS. The practice of refraction. Philadelphia: Blakiston; 1943.
3. Guggenheim JA. The heritability of high myopia: a reanalysis of Goldschmidt’s data. J Med Genet. 2000;37:227–31.
4. Sorsby A, Sheridan M, Leary GA. Refraction and its components in twins. Medical Research Council, Special Report Series No. 303; 1962.
5. Lin LL, Chen CJ. A twin study on myopia in Chinese school children. Acta Ophthalmol Suppl. 1988;185:51–3.
6. Wojciechowski R, et al. Heritability of refractive error and familial aggregation of myopia in an elderly American population. Invest Ophthalmol Vis Sci. 2005;46:1588–92.
7. Young FA, et al. The transmission of refractive errors within Eskimo families. Am J Optom Arch Am Acad Optom. 1969;46:676–85.
8. Angi MR, Clementi M, Sardei C, Piattelli E, Bisantis C. Heritability of myopic refractive errors in identical and fraternal twins. Graefes Arch Clin Exp Ophthalmol. 1993;231:580–5.
9. Teikari JM, Kaprio J, Koskenvuo MK, Vannas A. Heritability estimate for refractive errorsDOUBLEHYPHENa population-based sample of adult twins. Genet Epidemiol. 1988;5:171–81.

10. Lyhne N, Sjølie AK, Kyvik KO, Green A. The importance of genes and environment for ocular refraction and its determiners: a population based study among 20-45 year old twins. Br J Ophthalmol. 2001;85:1470–6.
11. Sanfilippo PG, Hewitt AW, Hammond CJ, Mackey DA. The heritability of ocular traits. Surv Ophthalmol. 2010;55:561–83.
12. OMIM - Online Mendelian Inheritance in Man. Available at https://www.omim.org/. Accessed 27 June 2018.
13. Hendriks M, et al. Development of refractive errors-what can we learn from inherited retinal dystrophies? Am J Ophthalmol. 2017;182:81–9.
14. Iglesias AI, et al. Cross-ancestry genome-wide association analysis of corneal thickness strengthens link between complex and Mendelian eye diseases. Nat Commun. 2018;9:1864.
15. Baratz KH, et al. E2-2 protein and Fuchs's corneal dystrophy. N Engl J Med. 2010;363:1016–24.
16. Mutti DO, et al. Candidate gene and locus analysis of myopia. Mol Vis. 2007;13:1012–9.
17. Metlapally R, et al. COL1A1 and COL2A1 genes and myopia susceptibility: evidence of association and suggestive linkage to the COL2A1 locus. Invest Ophthalmol Vis Sci. 2009;50:4080–6.
18. Tedja MS, et al. Genome-wide association meta-analysis highlights light-induced signaling as a driver for refractive error. Nat Genet. 2018;50:834–48.
19. Fan Q, et al. Meta-analysis of gene-environment-wide association scans accounting for education level identifies additional loci for refractive error. Nat Commun. 2016;7:11008.
20. Flitcroft DI, et al. Novel myopia genes and pathways identified from syndromic forms of myopia. Invest Ophthalmol Vis Sci. 2018;59:338–48.
21. Dawn Teare M, Barrett JH. Genetic linkage studies. Lancet. 2005;366:1036–44.
22. Wojciechowski R. Nature and nurture: the complex genetics of myopia and refractive error. Clin Genet. 2011;79:301–20.
23. Baird PN, Schäche M, Dirani M. The GEnes in Myopia (GEM) study in understanding the aetiology of refractive errors. Prog Retin Eye Res. 2010;29:520–42.
24. Hornbeak DM, Young TL. Myopia genetics: a review of current research and emerging trends. Curr Opin Ophthalmol. 2009;20:356–62.
25. Jacobi FK, Pusch CM. A decade in search of myopia genes. Front Biosci. 2010;15:359–72.
26. Zhang Q, et al. A new locus for autosomal dominant high myopia maps to 4q22-q27 between D4S1578 and D4S1612. Mol Vis. 2005;11:554–60.
27. Young TL, et al. A second locus for familial high myopia maps to chromosome 12q. Am J Hum Genet. 1998;63:1419–24.
28. Naiglin L, et al. A genome wide scan for familial high myopia suggests a novel locus on chromosome 7q36. J Med Genet. 2002;39:118–24.
29. Paluru P, et al. New locus for autosomal dominant high myopia maps to the long arm of chromosome 17. Invest Ophthalmol Vis Sci. 2003;44:1830–6.
30. Nallasamy S, et al. Genetic linkage study of high-grade myopia in a Hutterite population from South Dakota. Mol Vis. 2007;13:229–36.
31. Lam CY, et al. A genome-wide scan maps a novel high myopia locus to 5p15. Invest Ophthalmol Vis Sci. 2008;49:3768–78.
32. Stambolian D. Genetic susceptibility and mechanisms for refractive error. Clin Genet. 2013;84:102–8.
33. Stambolian D, et al. Genomewide linkage scan for myopia susceptibility loci among Ashkenazi Jewish families shows evidence of linkage on chromosome 22q12. Am J Hum Genet. 2004;75:448–59.
34. Wojciechowski R, et al. Genomewide scan in Ashkenazi Jewish families demonstrates evidence of linkage of ocular refraction to a QTL on chromosome 1p36. Hum Genet. 2006;119:389–99.
35. Wojciechowski R, et al. Genomewide linkage scans for ocular refraction and meta-analysis of four populations in the Myopia Family Study. Invest Ophthalmol Vis Sci. 2009;50:2024–32.
36. Hammond CJ, Andrew T, Mak YT, Spector TD. A susceptibility locus for myopia in the normal population is linked to the PAX6 gene region on chromosome 11: a genomewide scan of dizygotic twins. Am J Hum Genet. 2004;75:294–304.

37. Ciner E, et al. Genome-wide scan of African-American and white families for linkage to myopia. Am J Ophthalmol. 2009;147:512–517.e2.
38. Hawthorne FA, Young TL. Genetic contributions to myopic refractive error: insights from human studies and supporting evidence from animal models. Exp Eye Res. 2013;114:141–9.
39. Tkatchenko AV, Tkatchenko TV, Guggenheim JA, Verhoeven VJM, Hysi PG, Wojciechowski R, et al. APLP2 regulates refractive error and myopia development in mice and humans. PLoS Genet. 2015;11:e1005432.
40. Liu H-P, Lin Y-J, Lin W-Y, Wan L, Sheu JJ-C, Lin H-J, et al. A novel genetic variant of BMP2K contributes to high myopia. J Clin Lab Anal. 2009;23:362–7.
41. Lin H-J, Kung Y-J, Lin Y-J, Sheu JJC, Chen B-H, Lan Y-C, et al. Association of the lumican gene functional 3'-UTR polymorphism with high myopia. Invest Ophthalmol Vis Sci. 2010;51:96–102.
42. Lin H-J, Wan L, Tsai Y, Chen W-C, Tsai S-W, Tsai F-J. The association between lumican gene polymorphisms and high myopia. Eye. 2010;24:1093–101.
43. Lin H-J, Wan L, Tsai Y, Chen W-C, Tsai S-W, Tsai F-J. Muscarinic acetylcholine receptor 1 gene polymorphisms associated with high myopia. Mol Vis. 2009;15:1774–80.
44. Lin H-J, Wan L, Tsai Y, Liu S-C, Chen W-C, Tsai S-W, et al. Sclera-related gene polymorphisms in high myopia. Mol Vis. 2009;15:1655–63.
45. Khor CC, Grignani R, Ng DPK, Toh KY, Chia K-S, Tan D, et al. cMET and refractive error progression in children. Ophthalmology. 2009;116:1469–74. 1474.e1
46. Inamori Y, Ota M, Inoko H, Okada E, Nishizaki R, Shiota T, et al. The COL1A1 gene and high myopia susceptibility in Japanese. Hum Genet. 2007;122:151–7.
47. Metlapally R, Li Y-J, Tran-Viet K-N, Abbott D, Czaja GR, Malecaze F, et al. COL1A1 and COL2A1 genes and myopia susceptibility: evidence of association and suggestive linkage to the COL2A1 locus. Invest Ophthalmol Vis Sci. 2009;50:4080–6.
48. Mutti DO, Cooper ME, O'Brien S, Jones LA, Marazita ML, Murray JC, et al. Candidate gene and locus analysis of myopia. Mol Vis. 2007;13:1012–9.
49. Ho DWH, Yap MKH, Ng PW, Fung WY, Yip SP. Association of high myopia with crystallin beta A4 (CRYBA4) gene polymorphisms in the linkage-identified MYP6 locus. PLoS One. 2012;7:e40238.
50. Han W, Yap MKH, Wang J, Yip SP. Family-based association analysis of hepatocyte growth factor (HGF) gene polymorphisms in high myopia. Invest Ophthalmol Vis Sci. 2006;47:2291–9.
51. Veerappan S, Pertile KK, Islam AFM, Schäche M, Chen CY, Mitchell P, et al. Role of the hepatocyte growth factor gene in refractive error. Ophthalmology. 2010;117:239–45.e1–2.
52. Yanovitch T, Li Y-J, Metlapally R, Abbott D, Viet K-NT, Young TL. Hepatocyte growth factor and myopia: genetic association analyses in a Caucasian population. Mol Vis. 2009;15:1028–35.
53. Metlapally R, Ki C-S, Li Y-J, Tran-Viet K-N, Abbott D, Malecaze F, et al. Genetic association of insulin-like growth factor-1 polymorphisms with high-grade myopia in an international family cohort. Invest Ophthalmol Vis Sci. 2010;51:4476–9.
54. Zhao YY, Zhang FJ, Zhu SQ, Duan H, Li Y, Zhou ZJ, et al. The association of a single nucleotide polymorphism in the promoter region of the LAMA1 gene with susceptibility to Chinese high myopia. Mol Vis. 2011;17:1003–10.
55. Chen ZT-Y, Wang I-J, Shih Y-F, Lin LL-K. The association of haplotype at the lumican gene with high myopia susceptibility in Taiwanese patients. Ophthalmology. 2009;116:1920–7.
56. Wang I-J, Chiang T-H, Shih Y-F, Hsiao CK, Lu S-C, Hou Y-C, et al. The association of single nucleotide polymorphisms in the 5'-regulatory region of the lumican gene with susceptibility to high myopia in Taiwan. Mol Vis. 2006;12:852–7.
57. Andrew T, Maniatis N, Carbonaro F, Liew SHM, Lau W, Spector TD, et al. Identification and replication of three novel myopia common susceptibility gene loci on chromosome 3q26 using linkage and linkage disequilibrium mapping. PLoS Genet. 2008;4:e1000220.
58. Wojciechowski R, Bailey-Wilson JE, Stambolian D. Association of matrix metalloproteinase gene polymorphisms with refractive error in Amish and Ashkenazi families. Invest Ophthalmol Vis Sci. 2010;51:4989–95.
59. Wojciechowski R, Yee SS, Simpson CL, Bailey-Wilson JE, Stambolian D. Matrix metalloproteinases and educational attainment in refractive error: evidence of gene-environment

interactions in the Age-Related Eye Disease Study. Ophthalmology. 2013;120:298–305.
60. Hall NF, Gale CR, Ye S, Martyn CN. Myopia and polymorphisms in genes for matrix metalloproteinases. Invest Ophthalmol Vis Sci. 2009;50:2632–6.
61. Tang WC, Yip SP, Lo KK, Ng PW, Choi PS, Lee SY, et al. Linkage and association of myocilin (MYOC) polymorphisms with high myopia in a Chinese population. Mol Vis. 2007;13:534–44.
62. Vatavuk Z, Skunca Herman J, Bencić G, Andrijević Derk B, Lacmanović Loncar V, Petric Vicković I, et al. Common variant in myocilin gene is associated with high myopia in isolated population of Korcula Island, Croatia. Croat Med J. 2009;50:17–22.
63. Zayats T, Yanovitch T, Creer RC, McMahon G, Li Y-J, Young TL, et al. Myocilin polymorphisms and high myopia in subjects of European origin. Mol Vis. 2009;15:213–22.
64. Han W, Leung KH, Fung WY, Mak JYY, Li YM, Yap MKH, et al. Association of PAX6 polymorphisms with high myopia in Han Chinese nuclear families. Invest Ophthalmol Vis Sci. 2009;50:47–56.
65. Kanemaki N, Meguro A, Yamane T, Takeuchi M, Okada E, Iijima Y, et al. Study of association of PAX6 polymorphisms with susceptibility to high myopia in a Japanese population. Clin Ophthalmol. 2015;9:2005–11.
66. Miyake M, Yamashiro K, Nakanishi H, Nakata I, Akagi-Kurashige Y, Tsujikawa A, et al. Association of paired box 6 with high myopia in Japanese. Mol Vis. 2012;18:2726–35.
67. Ng TK, Lam CY, Lam DSC, Chiang SWY, Tam POS, Wang DY, et al. AC and AG dinucleotide repeats in the PAX6 P1 promoter are associated with high myopia. Mol Vis. 2009;15:2239–48.
68. Tsai Y-Y, Chiang C-C, Lin H-J, Lin J-M, Wan L, Tsai F-J. A PAX6 gene polymorphism is associated with genetic predisposition to extreme myopia. Eye. 2008;22:576–81.
69. Khor CC, Fan Q, Goh L, Tan D, Young TL, Li Y-J, et al. Support for TGFB1 as a susceptibility gene for high myopia in individuals of Chinese descent. Arch Ophthalmol. 2010;128:1081–4.
70. Lin H-J, Wan L, Tsai Y, Tsai Y-Y, Fan S-S, Tsai C-H, et al. The TGFbetal gene codon 10 polymorphism contributes to the genetic predisposition to high myopia. Mol Vis. 2006;12:698–703.
71. Rasool S, Ahmed I, Dar R, Ayub SG, Rashid S, Jan T, et al. Contribution of TGFβ1 codon 10 polymorphism to high myopia in an ethnic Kashmiri population from India. Biochem Genet. 2013;51:323–33.
72. Zha Y, Leung KH, Lo KK, Fung WY, Ng PW, Shi M-G, et al. TGFB1 as a susceptibility gene for high myopia: a replication study with new findings. Arch Ophthalmol. 2009;127:541–8.
73. Lam DSC, Lee WS, Leung YF, Tam POS, Fan DSP, Fan BJ, et al. TGFbeta-induced factor: a candidate gene for high myopia. Invest Ophthalmol Vis Sci. 2003;44:1012–5.
74. Ahmed I, Rasool S, Jan T, Qureshi T, Naykoo NA, Andrabi KI. TGIF1 is a potential candidate gene for high myopia in ethnic Kashmiri population. Curr Eye Res. 2014;39:282–90.
75. Nishizaki R, Ota M, Inoko H, Meguro A, Shiota T, Okada E, et al. New susceptibility locus for high myopia is linked to the uromodulin-like 1 (UMODL1) gene region on chromosome 21q22.3. Eye. 2009;23:222–9.
76. Tang SM, et al. PAX6 gene associated with high myopia: a meta-analysis. Optom Vis Sci. 2014;91:419–29.
77. Li M, et al. Lack of association between LUM rs3759223 polymorphism and high myopia. Optom Vis Sci. 2014;91:707–12.
78. Zhang D, et al. Association of IGF1 polymorphism rs6214 with high myopia: a systematic review and meta-analysis. Ophthalmic Genet. 2017;38:434–9.
79. Springelkamp H, et al. New insights into the genetics of primary open-angle glaucoma based on meta-analyses of intraocular pressure and optic disc characteristics. Hum Mol Genet. 2017;26:438–53.
80. Burdon KP, et al. Association of polymorphisms in the hepatocyte growth factor gene promoter with keratoconus. Invest Ophthalmol Vis Sci. 2011;52:8514–9.
81. Risch N, Merikangas K. The future of genetic studies of complex human diseases. Science. 1996;273:1516–7.
82. Ku CS, Loy EY, Pawitan Y, Chia KS. The pursuit of genome-wide association studies: where are we now? J Hum Genet. 2010;55:195–206.

83. Cordell HJ, Clayton DG. Genetic association studies. Lancet. 2005;366:1121–31.
84. Nakanishi H, et al. A genome-wide association analysis identified a novel susceptible locus for pathological myopia at 11q24.1. PLoS Genet. 2009;5:e1000660.
85. Li Y-J, et al. Genome-wide association studies reveal genetic variants in CTNND2 for high myopia in Singapore Chinese. Ophthalmology. 2011;118:368–75.
86. Lu B, et al. Replication study supports CTNND2 as a susceptibility gene for high myopia. Invest Ophthalmol Vis Sci. 2011;52:8258–61.
87. Wang Q, et al. Replication study of significant single nucleotide polymorphisms associated with myopia from two genome-wide association studies. Mol Vis. 2011;17:3290–9.
88. Yu Z, et al. Polymorphisms in theCTNND2Gene and 11q24.1 genomic region are associated with pathological myopia in a Chinese population. Ophthalmologica. 2012;228:123–9.
89. Liu J, Zhang H-X. Polymorphism in the 11q24.1 genomic region is associated with myopia: a comprehensive genetic study in Chinese and Japanese populations. Mol Vis. 2014;20:352–8.
90. Shi Y, et al. Genetic variants at 13q12.12 are associated with high myopia in the Han Chinese population. Am J Hum Genet. 2011;88:805–13.
91. Shi Y, et al. A genome-wide meta-analysis identifies two novel loci associated with high myopia in the Han Chinese population. Hum Mol Genet. 2013;22:2325–33.
92. Khor CC, et al. Genome-wide association study identifies ZFHX1B as a susceptibility locus for severe myopia. Hum Mol Genet. 2013;22:5288–94.
93. Hosoda Y, et al. CCDC102B confers risk of low vision and blindness in high myopia. Nat Commun. 2018;9:1782.
94. Meng W, et al. A genome-wide association study provides evidence for association of chromosome 8p23 (MYP10) and 10q21.1 (MYP15) with high myopia in the French population. Invest Ophthalmol Vis Sci. 2012;53:7983–8.
95. Pickrell JK, et al. Detection and interpretation of shared genetic influences on 42 human traits. Nat Genet. 2016;48:709–17.
96. Solouki AM, et al. A genome-wide association study identifies a susceptibility locus for refractive errors and myopia at 15q14. Nat Genet. 2010;42:897–901.
97. Hysi PG, et al. A genome-wide association study for myopia and refractive error identifies a susceptibility locus at 15q25. Nat Genet. 2010;42:902–5.
98. Stambolian D, et al. Meta-analysis of genome-wide association studies in five cohorts reveals common variants in RBFOX1, a regulator of tissue-specific splicing, associated with refractive error. Hum Mol Genet. 2013;22:2754–64.
99. Verhoeven VJM, et al. Large scale international replication and meta-analysis study confirms association of the 15q14 locus with myopia. The CREAM consortium. Hum Genet. 2012;131:1467–80.
100. Schache M, et al. Genetic association of refractive error and axial length with 15q14 but Not 15q25 in the Blue Mountains Eye Study cohort. Ophthalmology. 2013;120:292–7.
101. Simpson CL, et al. Regional replication of association with refractive error on 15q14 and 15q25 in the Age-Related Eye Disease Study cohort. Mol Vis. 2013;19:2173–86.
102. Simpson CL, Wojciechowski R, Oexle K, Murgia F, Portas L, Li X, et al. Genome-wide meta-analysis of myopia and hyperopia provides evidence for replication of 11 loci. PLoS One. 2014;9:e107110.
103. Yoshikawa M, Yamashiro K, Miyake M, Oishi M, Akagi-Kurashige Y, Kumagai K, et al. Comprehensive replication of the relationship between myopia-related genes and refractive errors in a large Japanese cohort. Invest Ophthalmol Vis Sci. 2014;55:7343–54.
104. Cheng C-Y, Schache M, Ikram MK, Young TL, Guggenheim JA, Vitart V, et al. Nine loci for ocular axial length identified through genome-wide association studies, including shared loci with refractive error. Am J Hum Genet. 2013;93:264–77.
105. Oishi M, Yamashiro K, Miyake M, Akagi-Kurashige Y, Kumagai K, Nakata I, et al. Association between ZIC2, RASGRF1, and SHISA6 genes and high myopia in Japanese subjects. Invest Ophthalmol Vis Sci. 2013;54:7492–7.
106. Tideman JWL, Fan Q, Polling JR, Guo X, Yazar S, Khawaja A, et al. When do myopia genes have their effect? Comparison of genetic risks between children and adults. Genet Epidemiol. 2016;40:756–66.
107. Liao X, Yap MKH, Leung KH, Kao PYP, Liu LQ, Yip SP. Genetic association study of

KCNQ5 polymorphisms with high myopia. Biomed Res Int. 2017;2017:3024156.
108. Verhoeven VJM, et al. Genome-wide meta-analyses of multiancestry cohorts identify multiple new susceptibility loci for refractive error and myopia. Nat Genet. 2013;45:314–8.
109. Wojciechowski R, Hysi PG. Focusing in on the complex genetics of myopia. PLoS Genet. 2013;9:e1003442.
110. Kiefer AK, et al. Genome-wide analysis points to roles for extracellular matrix remodeling, the visual cycle, and neuronal development in myopia. PLoS Genet. 2013;9:e1003299.
111. Mishra A, et al. Genetic variants near PDGFRA are associated with corneal curvature in Australians. Invest Ophthalmol Vis Sci. 2012;53:7131–6.
112. Guggenheim JA, et al. A genome-wide association study for corneal curvature identifies the platelet-derived growth factor receptor α gene as a quantitative trait locus for eye size in white Europeans. Mol Vis. 2013;19:243–53.
113. Han S, et al. Association of variants in FRAP1 and PDGFRA with corneal curvature in Asian populations from Singapore. Hum Mol Genet. 2011;20:3693–8.
114. Chen P, et al. CMPK1 and RBP3 are associated with corneal curvature in Asian populations. Hum Mol Genet. 2014;23:6129–36.
115. Miyake M, et al. Identification of myopia-associated WNT7B polymorphisms provides insights into the mechanism underlying the development of myopia. Nat Commun. 2015;6:6689.
116. Hysi PG, et al. Common mechanisms underlying refractive error identified in functional analysis of gene lists from genome-wide association study results in 2 European British cohorts. JAMA Ophthalmol. 2014;132:50–6.
117. Chandra A, Mitry D, Wright A, Campbell H, Charteris DG. Genome-wide association studies: applications and insights gained in ophthalmology. Eye. 2014;28:1066–79.
118. Hysi PG, Wojciechowski R, Rahi JS, Hammond CJ. Genome-wide association studies of refractive error and myopia, lessons learned, and implications for the future. Invest Ophthalmol Vis Sci. 2014;55:3344–51.
119. Napolitano F, et al. Autosomal-dominant myopia associated to a novel P4HA2 missense variant and defective collagen hydroxylation. Clin Genet. 2018;93:982–91.
120. Zhao F, et al. Exome sequencing reveals CCDC111 mutation associated with high myopia. Hum Genet. 2013;132:913–21.
121. Wang B, et al. A novel potentially causative variant of NDUFAF7 revealed by mutation screening in a Chinese family with pathologic myopia. Invest Ophthalmol Vis Sci. 2017;58:4182–92.
122. Feng L, et al. Exome sequencing identifies a novel UNC5D mutation in a severe myopic anisometropia family: a case report. Medicine. 2017;96:e7138.
123. Jiang D, et al. Detection of mutations in LRPAP1, CTSH, LEPREL1, ZNF644, SLC39A5, and SCO2 in 298 families with early-onset high myopia by exome sequencing. Invest Ophthalmol Vis Sci. 2014;56:339–45.
124. Tran-Viet K-N, et al. Mutations in SCO2 are associated with autosomal-dominant high-grade myopia. Am J Hum Genet. 2013;92:820–6.
125. Jin ZB, et al. Trio-based exome sequencing arrests de novo mutations in early-onset high myopia. Proc Natl Acad Sci U S A. 2017;114:4219–24.
126. Xiao X, Li S, Jia X, Guo X, Zhang Q. X-linked heterozygous mutations in cause female-limited early onset high myopia. Mol Vis. 2016;22:1257–66.
127. Li J, et al. Exome sequencing identified null mutations in LOXL3 associated with early-onset high myopia. Mol Vis. 2016;22:161–7.
128. Guo H, et al. SLC39A5 mutations interfering with the BMP/TGF-β1 pathway in non-syndromic high myopia. J Med Genet. 2014;51:518–25.
129. Aldahmesh MA, et al. Mutations in LRPAP1 are associated with severe myopia in humans. Am J Hum Genet. 2013;93:313–20.
130. Shi Y, et al. Exome sequencing identifies ZNF644 mutations in high myopia. PLoS Genet. 2011;7:e1002084.
131. Kloss BA, et al. Exome sequence analysis of 14 families with high myopia. Invest Ophthalmol Vis Sci. 2017;58:1982–90.
132. Sun W, et al. Exome sequencing on 298 probands with early-onset high myopia: approximately one-fourth show potential pathogenic mutations in RetNet genes. Invest Ophthalmol

Vis Sci. 2015;56:8365–72.
133. Morgan I, Rose K. How genetic is school myopia? Prog Retin Eye Res. 2005;24:1–38.
134. Morgan IG, Ohno-Matsui K, Saw S-M. Myopia. Lancet. 2012;379:1739–48.
135. Dolgin E. The myopia boom. Nature. 2015;519:276–8.
136. Williams KM, et al. Increasing prevalence of myopia in europe and the impact of education. Ophthalmology. 2015;122:1489–97.
137. Dirani M, Shekar SN, Baird PN. The role of educational attainment in refraction: the Genes in Myopia (GEM) twin study. Invest Ophthalmol Vis Sci. 2008;49:534–8.
138. Foster PJ, Jiang Y. Epidemiology of myopia. Eye. 2014;28:202–8.
139. Pan C-W, Ramamurthy D, Saw S-M. Worldwide prevalence and risk factors for myopia. Ophthalmic Physiol Opt. 2012;32:3–16.
140. Mirshahi A, et al. Myopia and level of education: results from the Gutenberg Health Study. Ophthalmology. 2014;121:2047–52.
141. Morgan IG, Rose KA. Myopia and international educational performance. Ophthalmic Physiol Opt. 2013;33:329–38.
142. Ramessur R, Williams KM, Hammond CJ. Risk factors for myopia in a discordant monozygotic twin study. Ophthalmic Physiol Opt. 2015;35:643–51.
143. Fan Q, et al. Education influences the association between genetic variants and refractive error: a meta-analysis of five Singapore studies. Hum Mol Genet. 2014;23:546–54.
144. Verhoeven VJM, et al. Education influences the role of genetics in myopia. Eur J Epidemiol. 2013;28:973–80.
145. Fan Q, et al. Childhood gene-environment interactions and age-dependent effects of genetic variants associated with refractive error and myopia: The CREAM Consortium. Sci Rep. 2016;6:25853.
146. Ebrahim S, Davey Smith G. Mendelian randomization: can genetic epidemiology help redress the failures of observational epidemiology? Hum Genet. 2008;123:15–33.
147. Smith GD, Ebrahim S. Mendelian randomization: prospects, potentials, and limitations. Int J Epidemiol. 2004;33:30–42.
148. Mountjoy E, et al. Education and myopia: assessing the direction of causality by mendelian randomisation. BMJ. 2018;362:k2932.
149. Cuellar-Partida G, et al. Assessing the genetic predisposition of education on myopia: A Mendelian Randomization Study. Genet Epidemiol. 2016;40:66–72.
150. Cuellar-Partida G, et al. Genetically low vitamin D concentrations and myopic refractive error: a Mendelian randomization study. Int J Epidemiol. 2017;46:1882–90.
151. Teperino R, Lempradl A, Pospisilik JA. Bridging epigenomics and complex disease: the basics. Cell Mol Life Sci. 2013;70:1609–21.
152. Jiang B, Huo Y, Gu Y, Wang J. The role of microRNAs in myopia. Graefes Arch Clin Exp Ophthalmol. 2017;255:7–13.
153. Liang CL, et al. A functional polymorphism at 3'UTR of the PAX6 gene may confer risk for extreme myopia in the Chinese. Invest Ophthalmol Vis Sci. 2011;52:3500–5.
154. Lechner J, et al. Mutational analysis of MIR184 in sporadic keratoconus and myopia. Invest Ophthalmol Vis Sci. 2013;54:5266–72.
155. Xie M, et al. Genetic variants in MiR-29a associated with high myopia. Ophthalmic Genet. 2016;37:456–8.
156. Tideman JWL, et al. Environmental factors explain socioeconomic prevalence differences in myopia in 6-year-old children. Br J Ophthalmol. 2018;102:243–7.
157. Ghorbani Mojarrad N, Williams C, Guggenheim JA. A genetic risk score and number of myopic parents independently predict myopia. Ophthalmic Physiol Opt. 2018;38(5):492–502. https://doi.org/10.1111/opo.12579.
158. Sudlow C, et al. UK biobank: an open access resource for identifying the causes of a wide range of complex diseases of middle and old age. PLoS Med. 2015;12:e1001779.

6

Myopia and its Diverse Risk Factors

Ian G. Morgan, Amanda N. French, and Kathryn A. Rose

Key Points

- Myopia commencing school myopia is found mainly is found mainly in developed societies, with only around 1% of any population affected by predominantly genetic forms of myopia.
- Exposure to environmental risk factors plays a significant role in the development of "school myopia" myopia, both within and between populations.
- Within populations, changes in exposure to environmental risk factors are primarily responsible for the emergence of an increasing prevalence of myopia.
- The major environmental risk factors identified are educational pressures, perhaps best characterized in terms of near work, and limited time outdoors during daylight hours.
- These risk factors suggest that strategies based on decreases in the amount of near work and increases in the amount of time spent outdoors during school hours are likely to be useful in the controlling the epidemic of myopia.

I. G. Morgan (✉)
Research School of Biological Science, Australian National University, Canberra, ACT, Australia
e-mail: ian.morgan@anu.edu.au

A. N. French · K. A. Rose
Discipline of Orthoptics, Graduate School of Health, University of Technology Sydney, Ultimo, NSW, Australia

It is now generally accepted that there is an environmental epidemic of myopia in several parts of East and Southeast Asia, namely Singapore, Japan, South Korea, China, including Hong Kong and Macau, as well as in Taiwan [1–8]. In these parts of the world, the prevalence of myopia in young adults who have completed 12 years of schooling, as most do, is now 70–90%, up from 20 to 30% two or three generations ago. In addition, the prevalence of high and potentially pathological myopia (more than 5 D or 6 D of myopia) is of the order of 10–20% [9–12]. The simple argument that the speed at which the prevalence of myopia has increased in these locations is not compatible with a predominant role for genetic determination of myopia [1, 2] has generally been accepted, even though genetic variation associated with myopia has been conclusively demonstrated [13]. This emphasizes the need to define the environmental exposures responsible for the rapid increases in prevalence, in order to design preventive interventions.

The term "an epidemic of myopia" covers two distinct, but related, issues. The first is an increase in the prevalence of myopia overall, with a characteristic increase in onset of myopia in children in the early school years, leading to a need to provide optical correction for a significant proportion of the population from an early age. The high prevalence of myopia observed in young adults will gradually become the norm for the entire adult population, as younger more myopic generations replace those who are older and less myopic.

The second issue is an increase in the prevalence of high myopia, which is associated with a higher prevalence of pathological outcomes. The cutoff values used to define high myopia are somewhat arbitrary (generally −5 D or −6 D), since the prevalence of pathological complications rises steeply with severity of myopia. The best cutoff to define high and potentially pathological myopia is one which distinguishes, as effectively as possible, between lower and higher risks of pathology, but no cutoff will do this perfectly [14]. The increase in more severe levels of myopia seems to arise from the fact that myopia has appeared at increasingly early ages as the epidemic has developed [11]. With subsequent progression, the myopic refractive error will increase toward the cutoff for high myopia, a tendency exacerbated by rapid progression in younger children [15]. In these circumstances, slowing the onset of myopia should lead to a disproportionate reduction in high myopia. An important question in this area is whether the risk factors for increased prevalence of myopia are similar to the risk factors for progression, or in practical terms whether increased time outdoors would help to limit progression directly, as well as by delaying the onset of myopia. It is certainly possible to slow the development of high myopia by clinically slowing progression rates, using optical or pharmaceutical interventions, and many of these interventions are now available [16].

This chapter reviews the scientific evidence on risk factors in all these areas, and relates this evidence to strategies for slowing the onset and progression of myopia. We will also mention a number of commonly believed risk factors for myopia that may not have a substantial scientific basis. Myopia is such a common condition in societies with well-developed education systems that there are many popular beliefs about the causes of myopia. These often remain influential, sometimes even when the scientific evidence is against them.

6.1 Key Issues When Studying Risk Factors for Myopia

In assessing the literature on risk factors for myopia, it is essential to be clear about a number of fundamental issues.

6.1.1 Myopia Is Etiologically Heterogeneous

It is now generally accepted that environmental factors have a major role to play in the development of myopia. Nevertheless, there are 100–200 clearly genetic forms of myopia documented in the Online Mendelian Inheritance in Man (OMIM) database (https://www.omim.org/, accessed Jan 30, 2019) that clearly run in families [17]. These are individually quite rare, but account collectively for myopia in around 1% of any population. In a recent detailed analysis, 119 genes were associated specifically with myopia, generally in association with other clinical features [17]. Most of these forms are therefore called syndromic, although in some, myopia seems to be the major clinical feature. The latter cases are often called nonsyndromic [18]. Environmental factors appear to play a rather limited role in these diseases, but their existence does not mean that all forms of myopia are similarly genetic—This issue is further discussed in Chapter 5 etc.

In addition to these genetic forms, in modern societies, myopia generally appears in association with schooling, as "school myopia." It is this form that has increased in the epidemics of myopia. Genetic variation has some role to play in this form of myopia, with the most recent genetic data identifying variants in over 160 genes associated with spherical equivalent refraction (SER). Many of these variants are associated with the genes involved in the more clearly genetic forms, suggesting that mutations in coding regions of the same genes can lead to highly genetic forms of myopia, or to more modest effects if the mutations affect regulatory regions [17].

Identified single nucleotide polymorphisms (SNPs) in samples of European ancestry account for less than 10% of the variance in refraction [13]. Measured as SNP-heritability, they may account for 20–35% of the phenotypic variance [19]. These values fall well short of the twin study heritability of 80–90% [20–22]—an example of the missing heritability seen with many complex traits [23]. The estimated SNP-heritability in East Asian samples is much lower at around 5% [13], as would be expected if the amount of phenotypic variation due to genetic variation had remained constant, but that induced by environmental factors had increased substantially in populations severely affected by the environmentally induced epidemic of myopia. We have recently reviewed this area, and readers can consult these reviews for more details [2, 24].

Given this picture, genetic variation may have little, if any, role to play in the rapid changes that have produced the current epidemic of myopia, but this does not mean that it has no role to play in the determination of variations in refractive error within a population. In fact, some myopia geneticists have argued that environmental factors are important between populations, but within populations, genetic factors are the primary determinants [5, 6, 8]. However, this argument does

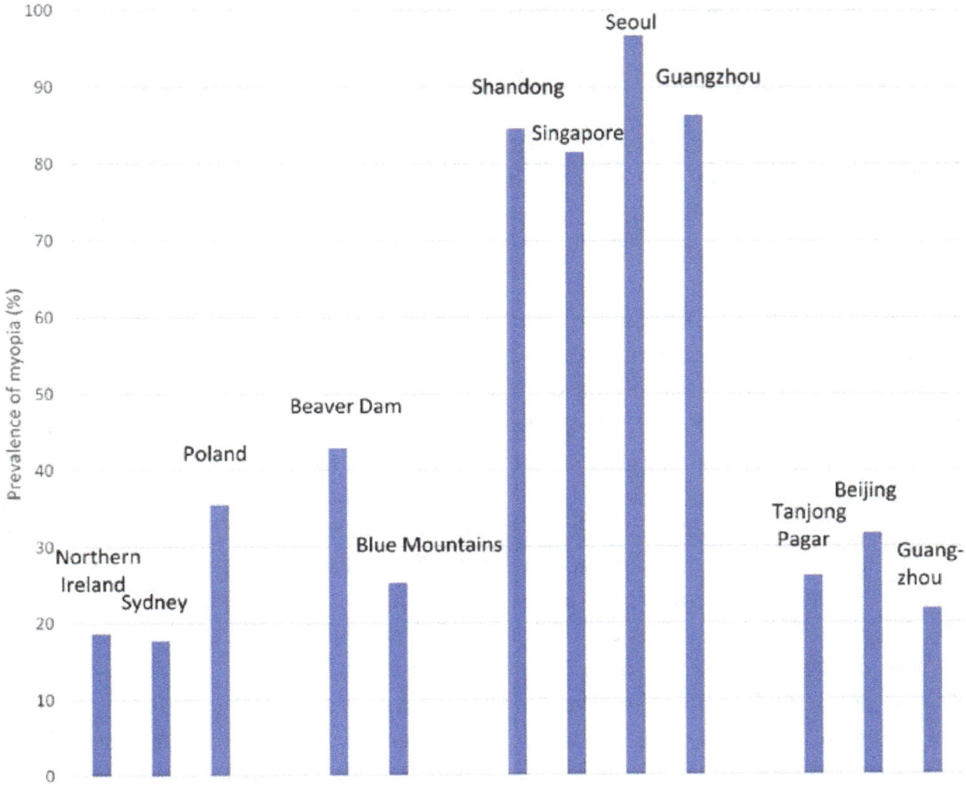

Fig. 6.1 Prevalence of myopia in older and more recent cohorts in older and more recent younger cohorts. Data taken from cohorts closest in age to 20 from Breslin et al. [66], French et al. [96], Czepita et al. [71] Wang et al. [58], Attebo et al. [59], Wu et al. [12], Koh et al. [10], Jung et al. [9], Wong et al. [60]. Xu et al. [198], and He et al. [140]

not make sense, because between-population differences have largely emerged due to selective changes within populations of the kind seen in East and Southeast Asia (Fig. 6.1). The key to understanding lies in the recognition that the balance between genetic and environmental factors is population-specific. In the case of myopia, the evidence suggests that there is little difference between ethnic groups in the levels of SNPs associated with myopia [13], although studies on a wider range of ethnic groups are required. However, environmental exposures can differ substantially between ethnic groups, and can change rapidly. Environmental factors are therefore far more likely to be involved in rapid intergenerational change, or in the rapid emergence of differences between societies—both features of the current epidemic.

This has an important implication; key insights into the epidemics are most likely to come from comparisons of societies with different prevalence of myopia, rather than from detailed studies within populations. Many epidemiologists are wary of this ecological approach, because of what is known as the "ecological fallacy"—the error that can be made if conclusions are based only upon ecological comparisons. But in the case of myopia, this is not an issue, because education and time outdoors clearly play a role both within and between populations.

6.1.2 Myopia Is a Developmental Condition

Developmental considerations also support the importance of etiological heterogeneity. Some forms of myopia appear in children before they start school. These are often severe forms, with a strong genetic etiology, and are called early onset myopia. In contrast, "school myopia" results from excessive elongation of the eye during the school years. Other ocular components, such as corneal and lens power, are within the normal age-specific range. Myopic refractions are also seen in two other conditions—keratoconus and cataract-related myopic shifts in older people. These conditions are etiologically quite distinct from "school myopia"—the first involving abnormal increases in corneal power, generally during the teen-age years, and the second involving abnormal increases in lens power in older adults. These forms are likely to have a different relationship to pathological myopia than "school myopia," because they do not involve excessive enlargement of the posterior pole of the eye.

Most children are born hyperopic, although premature children have a tendency toward more myopic refractions [25]. At birth, the distribution of refractions is close to Gaussian, and subsequent development involves clustering of refractions to produce a tighter distribution, combined with reduction in hyperopic refractions [26–28]. These changes are often called "emmetropisation" because, as a general rule, refractions move from hyperopic toward emmetropic. However, emmetropia is not the end point for human refractive development under normal conditions. Rather, the preferred end point appears to be a moderate level of hyperopia (1.0–1.3 D), provided that cycloplegic refraction is measured [29]. This mildly hyperopic state can be maintained even in adults in some environments [30]. However, in populations where the prevalence of myopia becomes high, the hyperopic clustering of refractions disappears.

This part of refractive development is consistent with animal studies on experimental myopia that suggest that hyperopic defocus induces faster axial elongation, thus reducing hyperopic refractive error, while myopic defocus can slow axial elongation, and thus might be expected to affect the progression of myopia [31]. Simple expectations from the animal models, namely that myopia would be a self-limiting condition, or that it would be dangerous to correct myopia since it would reduce the error signal, are not consistent with current evidence [32–34]. However, there is some evidence that early myopic errors can be cleared [35], and contact lenses designed to impose myopic appear to slow the progression of myopia [36]. Thus, these mechanisms can come into play in particular circumstances, but what these circumstances are is currently unclear.

6.1.3 Cycloplegia and Definitions of Myopia: Important Methodological Issues

It is now generally accepted that cycloplegia is the gold standard for studies with children, with the use of up to three drops of 1% cyclopentolate as a common practice, with monitoring of pupil diameter and the light reflex to assess adequacy of cycloplegia [37]. This issue is particularly important in young children, where the prevalence of myopia is low, and a small amount of pseudomyopia can significantly increase prevalence estimates. It is also important when comparing ethnic groups, because it is harder to achieve cycloplegia in children with darkly pigmented irises. Without cycloplegia, hyperopia is substantially underestimated, emmetropia may be overestimated, with a smaller but significant overestimation of the prevalence of myopia. Suboptimal cycloplegia is likely to lead to errors of lesser magnitude, but in the same direction.

In contrast to studies on children, cycloplegia has generally not been used in studies on adults. Adults over the age of 50 show minimal differences between cycloplegic and noncycloplegic refractions [37, 38], consistent with the evidence that by this age, accommodative capacity has essentially disappeared, resulting in the need for some form of correction for reading. However, in younger adults, cycloplegia is required for accurate refraction, yet it generally has not been used in the larger studies on adults, even if they included young adults.

This emphasis on cycloplegia poses problems, because gaining informed consent for cycloplegia appears to be becoming more difficult. It is worth considering alternatives, and biometric variables like axial length and the ratio of the axial length to corneal radius of curvature (AL/CR ratio) could be used [39–41]. Both correlate highly with myopia [42, 43]. Changes in lens power also play a major role in refractive development, but they do not correlate highly with refraction and cannot be measured directly [44]. The advantage of the first two parameters is that they can be measured noninvasively. Their disadvantage is that measurement requires relatively expensive modern equipment, and that there is only a very limited set of data for comparison. But where repeated measures of cycloplegic refraction are envisaged, the highly correlated biometric variables may provide a useful alternative.

It is also important to note that a range of definitions is used in the literature for both myopia and high myopia. Cutoff values for myopia range from −0.25 D to −1.0 D, with some variation in the use of less than, or less than or equal to. Results are sometimes reported in relation to the better eye, worse eye, either eye, or both eyes, depending, to some extent, on the aims of the study. The most common standard for epidemiology is at least −0.5 D in the right eye. Similarly, the prevalence of high myopia is sometimes reported in relation to a cutoff of −5 D or −6 D. Sometimes more stringent cutoffs (−8 D, −10 D or −12 D) are used, which is likely to concentrate more genetic forms of myopia in the sample. Cumberland et al. [45] have therefore called for the development of an approach that "serves research, policy and practice," but made no specific recommendations. However, standard definitions will be of little use without standardization of cycloplegia. While awaiting agreement in both these areas, if it ever comes, we suggest a pragmatic approach is to publish a distribution of refraction in all studies in sufficient detail that others can apply the cutoff they think is most relevant. Cumberland et al. [45] also emphasized the sensitivity of risk factor analysis to different definitions of myopia, and where appropriate, sensitivity analysis should be used to establish that conclusions are robust [46].

These issues are very relevant to several major studies on risk factors for myopia. Studies on childhood and adolescence, the period during which myopia develops, and on young adults, when myopia stabilizes, are particularly important, since exposures over this period can be most directly related to the development of myopia. In addition, studies on young adults give estimates of prevalence that can be most directly compared to assess whether and to what extent there is an epidemic of myopia. Table 6.1 lists some of the most important studies that used cycloplegia. In general, there is a dearth of systematic evidence on the prevalence of myopia in most populations, particularly in the critical period

Table 6.1 Major studies on childhood refraction that measured cycloplegic refraction

Detailed studies of risk factors for refractive errors in school-aged children using cycloplegic refraction	
Australia	
Study name	*Sydney Myopia Study (SMS) and Sydney Adolescent Vascular and Eye Disease Study (SAVES)*
Location	Sydney, Australia
Design	School based, with stratified randomized selection of schools. Large cohorts at baseline in Year 1 (1765, 6–7 year olds) and Year 7 (2353, 12–13 year olds), with 4–5 year follow-up
Methodology	Cycloplegic refraction (cyclopentolate plus tropicamide). Risk factor questionnaire, including near work and time outdoors
Europe	
Study name	*Northern Ireland Childhood Errors of Refraction (NICER)*
Location	Northern Ireland
Design	Stratified, random-cluster design with school-based assessment. Cohorts 6–7 years old (392) and 12–13 years old (661) at baseline, with 6 year follow-up
Methodology	Cycloplegic refraction (cyclopentolate). Risk factor questionnaire, not including near work and time outdoors
Study name	*Ireland Eye Study*
Location	Republic of Ireland
Design	School based with stratified randomized selection of schools. Cohorts of 6–7 year olds (681) and 12–13 year olds (745) at baseline
Methodology	Cycloplegic refraction (cyclopentolate). Lifestyle questionnaire
Study name	*Generation R Study*
Location	Rotterdam, The Netherlands
Design	Birth Cohort Study, with 4734 children examined at the age of 6 and 9
Methodology	Cycloplegic refraction (cyclopentolate) introduced for a large subsample at age 9. Risk factor questionnaire including near work and time outdoors
United States	
Study name	*Orinda Longitudinal Study of Myopia (OLSM)*
Location	Orinda, California
Design	Volunteer sample of 1246 children from the Orinda Union School District followed up longitudinally
Methodology	Cycloplegic refraction (tropicamide). Annual parent questionnaire on risk factors including education and time outdoors or on sports

(continued)

Table 6.1 (continued)

Study name	*Collaborative Longitudinal Evaluation of Ethnicity and Refractive Error (CLEERE)*
Location	Multi-Centre Study, with centers at Orinda (California), Eutaw (Alabama), Houston (Texas), Irvine (California), and Tucson (Arizona)
Design	Volunteer sample of 2583 with selective recruitment of children of different ethnicities from different centers, followed up longitudinally
Methodology	Cycloplegic refraction (tropicamide or cyclopentolate plus tropicamide). Risk factor questionnaire
Singapore	
Study name	*Singapore Cohort Study of the Risk Factors for Myopia (SCORM)*
Location	Singapore
Design	1979 children aged 7–9 recruited from three schools in Singapore, with longitudinal follow-up
Methodology	Cycloplegic refraction (cyclopentolate). Risk factor questionnaire, including near work and time outdoors
China	
Study name	*Anyang Childhood Eye Study*
Location	Anyang City, Hebei Province
Design	At baseline, cohorts recruited from Year 1 (2283) and Year 7 (1453), with longitudinal follow-up for 5 and 3 years respectively
Methodology	Cycloplegic refraction (cyclopentolate). Risk factor questionnaire including near work and time outdoors
Study name	*Guangzhou Twin Eye Study*
Location	Guangzhou City, Guangdong Province
Design	Population-based recruitment of over 1000 twin pairs aged from 7 to 15 at baseline from Guangzhou City, with annual longitudinal follow-up
Methodology	Cycloplegic refraction (cyclopentolate). Risk factor questionnaire including near work and time outdoors
Study name	*Mojiang Eye Study*
Location	Mojiang County, Yunnan Province
Design	At baseline, cohorts recruited from all students in Year 1 (2432) and Year 7 (1453), with annual follow-up for 5 and 3 years respectively
Methodology	Cycloplegic refraction (cyclopentolate). Risk factor questionnaire including near work and time outdoors
Study name	*Jiading Eye Study*
Location	Jiading District, Shanghai
Design	Cross-sectional study of 8267 students from randomly selected preschools and primary schools
Methodology	Cycloplegic refraction (cyclopentolate) and risk factor questionnaire

up to the emergence of young adults. Large studies have rarely been designed to look at refractive errors, and studies reporting on refractive errors from the 1958 British Birth Cohort Study [47], the Avon Longitudinal Study of Parents and Children (ALSPAC) [48–50], the British Twins Early Development Study (TEDS) [51], the US-based National Health and Nutrition Evaluation Survey (NHANES) [52], the Korean NHANES [53], the Gutenberg Health Survey [54], and the UK Biobank Study [55] measured noncycloplegic refractions. Data from the European Eye Epidemiology (E3) consortium suffers from the same bias [56,

57]. Major studies of eye diseases, including refractive errors, such as the Beaver Dam Eye Study [58], the Blue Mountains Eye Study [59], and the Tanjong Pagar Eye Study [60] also measured noncycloplegic refractions. However, the Tehran Eye Study measured both cycloplegic and noncycloplegic refractions over a wide age range [61].

In general, studies designed to look specifically at refractive errors in school age children, such as the pioneering studies from Taiwan [11], the RESC (Refractive Error Study in Children) Studies [62], the Singapore Cohort Study of the Risk Factors for Myopia (SCORM) Study [63], the Orinda [64] and Collaborative Longitudinal Evaluation of Ethnicity and Refractive Error (CLEERE) [34] Studies in the United States, the Sydney Myopia Study and the Sydney Adolescent Vascular and Eye Study (SMS and SAVES) [65], the Northern Ireland Childhood Errors of Refraction Study [66], the Ireland Eye Study [67], several studies from China [12, 58, 68, 69] and Poland [70, 71], have measured cycloplegic refractions. The Generation R birth cohort study [72] introduced cycloplegic refractions at an early stage, but after the initial data collection. Studies on pediatric and preschool samples are more limited, but cycloplegia has generally been used [27, 28, 35, 73–77]. Cycloplegia needs to be carefully controlled in these studies, because when the prevalence of myopia is low, even a small amount of pseudomyopia may have a significant effect on the apparent prevalence.

6.1.4 Myopia: The Importance of Causal Pathways

The aim of identifying risk factors is to generate preventive interventions. This requires identification of modifiable causal risk factors, not just associations. Observational epidemiological studies can only establish associations, but far too often, papers on cross-sectional associations conclude with a limitation that conclusions about causality cannot be drawn. This seems to imply that longitudinal data can establish causality, but this is not correct. Parallel longitudinal changes are equally ambiguous, and this makes understanding the epidemic of myopia difficult since many parameters, such as industrialization, urbanization, pollution, incomes, nutrition, and education, have changed over the same period.

Strictly, randomized intervention studies are required to establish causality, but often studies of this kind would be regarded as unethical. In many cases, we therefore have to rely on the nonrandomized trials that occur as a part of social development. For example, it would be unethical to offer differential educational opportunities to children in a randomly selected fashion, but social differences often lead to differential educational opportunities, and these can be highly informative, although they lack randomization. The high prevalence of myopia seen in Jewish males who received an intensive religious education, compared to their sisters who received a less intensive religious education, as well as boys and girls who received a less intensive secular education [78], provides rather compelling evidence of causality. In some cases, Mendelian randomization analysis can be used. Although there are strict limitations on its use [79, 80], it has already been usefully applied to the problem of myopia [81–83].

While the limitations of cross-sectional or longitudinal data are clear, avoiding discussing causality misses the point, because whether the association is potentially causal is crucial. Causality is therefore an important issue to discuss. Unfortunately, journals often discourage speculation, both explicitly and through tight word and reference limits. We recognize that wild speculation is not useful—Curtin's description of the ophthalmologist waking after a sleepless night with "a new and usually more bizarre" hypothesis often rings true [84]. But evidence-based speculation should be encouraged, and subjected to critical review.

A related issue is the distinction between proximal and distal risk factors. Proximal risk factors are those closest to having a direct impact on eye growth, whereas distal factors will modulate the magnitude of more proximal factors. A plausible causal chain leads from education (excessive near work and limited time outdoors) to control of dopamine release and changes in axial elongation. Parental socioeconomic status, increases in the accessibility to education, and social attitudes to education may all increase involvement in education and/or result in reduced time outdoors, changing the prevalence of myopia through a common pathway that probably involves regulation of dopamine release and certainly involves regulation of axial elongation.

6.1.5 Statistical Analysis

There are also some associated considerations in relation to statistical analysis. A very common approach in analysis of risk factors is to identify significant associations in univariate analysis, then put the significant associations into multivariate regression analysis, labeling those factors that remain significant as "independent" risk factors. Often this appears to be done without serious consideration of whether the risk factors make sense in terms of causal pathways, whether they are modifiable, whether they are accurately measureable, whether they are likely to be collinear, whether they could result from reverse causality, and how complete the list of variables is. All these considerations can affect the validity of regression analysis.

Statistical analysis can be used more scientifically to address specific hypotheses about mediation by associated factors [85]. For example, in considering the relationship between myopia, education, and socioeconomic status (SES), it is possible to include SES and then the SES and education to see if there is a reduction in the strength of the association. This would be a sign that education mediates the influence of SES. In general, stepwise procedures need to be increasingly used in analysis. The quality of the variables is also important—whether they are continuous or categorical variables, and whether they can be accurately measured. Even if one factor is entirely mediated by another, if either variable is poorly measured, adjustment may only reduce rather than largely eliminate the effect of the other variable. Thus, the concept of independent risk factors is somewhat problematic [86].

Some of the variables are intrinsically complex. Education, for example, can be assessed in adults as a set of categories (primary school, high school, and university completed) or as a continuous variable (years of education). But intensity of education is also important, since children who obtain higher academic grades at a given level of schooling are more likely to be myopic. No variable captures both duration and intensity effectively. Myopia is associated with both intelligence quotient (IQ) [87] and school results [88]. Both are sometimes included in analyses to measure "innate" potential. But this approach is problematic since IQ shows complex changes over time [89, 90], and like myopia, combines significant twin heritability, considerable missing heritability, and social malleability [91]. There are both phenotypic and genetic correlations between myopia and IQ [92], as well as strong environmental effects. Inclusion of past performance or IQ in analyses as indicators of "innate potential," may, if these measures are influenced by the same environmental factors that influence myopia, obscure their role.

Regression analyses that combine variables that are more or less proximal also pose a problem. It is well known that axial elongation is the biological basis of myopic shifts in refraction, and thus it correlates highly with SER. If axial length is included in a regression analysis with more distal factors, it will tend to obscure the associations of these more distal factors with refraction.

In summary, there are a number of conceptual and methodological issues that need careful consideration in seeking to tease out the risk factors for myopia. Further progress in the analysis of risk factors for myopia requires more critical approaches in several areas.

6.2 The Main Risk Factors for "School Myopia": Education and Time Outdoors

We have recently reviewed this topic in detail, and these reviews can be consulted for more detailed references [1, 2, 4, 24]. In one of them, we distinguish between societies where the provision of education is limited and the prevalence of myopia is low (operationally, less than 10% myopia in young adults), at an age when 12 years of schooling would be the norm in the developed world, societies with western style education where the prevalence is between 10 and 60%, and developed countries in East and Southeast Asia, where education is intense, time outdoors is low, and the prevalence of myopia is high at 70–90%, particularly in urban areas.

It seems likely that the gradual transition from a very low prevalence in societies with little formal education to that typical of modern western societies with widespread education is predominantly due to the expansion of educational provision to cover all children, combined with increases in educational standards. Many of the countries in the first group are currently well short of the UN Sustainable Development Goals in Education for 2030 (https://sustainabledevelopment.un.org/sdg4, accessed January 30, 2019). The prevalence of myopia is unlikely to increase in these countries until progress is made in achieving these goals. In contrast, the very high prevalence rates now typical of developed countries in East and Southeast Asia compared to the much more moderate prevalence rates observed in western countries cannot be attributed to more years of education, but are probably related to more intense education, early onset of high homework loads, and much less time outdoors.

Because of the common observation in societies with significant educational provision that the prevalence of myopia increases with age, there is now a widespread assumption that myopia is affected by chronological age. However, the low prevalence of myopia in societies where educational opportunities are limited, suggests that it is not chronological age, but cumulative experience of schooling that is important, because without schooling most children do not become myopic. For this reason, it is often a useful sampling strategy to obtain a large sample of a given age, rather than smaller age-specific samples over a range of ages.

In adults, years of schooling is often used as a variable to look at associations with myopia. Consistent with the preceding arguments, those who have completed university education are more likely to be myopic than those who have completed secondary education, or primary education [55, 93]. Data from the UK Biobank dataset was recently used to address the issue of causality in relation to years of schooling and myopia [83]. The authors used two sets of genetic data—one on SNPs that associated with years of education, the other on SNPs associated with myopia. It was found that people with SNPs associated with more years of education were more likely to be myopic, whereas those with SNPs associated with more myopia did not have more years of education. This provides a clear direction of causation from years of education to myopia. It is important to note that this does not mean that variables such as years of education or myopia are predominantly genetically determined. The percentage of variation in the two parameters explained by identified SNPs was low in both cases.

Rapid historical increases in years of schooling cannot be explained by genetic change but must depend on more distal social changes that made mass education more available, and linked employment and salary to increased skill levels, creating a strong incentive for parents to extend the education of their children. In the west, the expansion of mass education paralleled industrialization and the rise of modern capitalism, and later the introduction of new technologies. Data suggesting that the prevalence of myopia has increased can in fact be traced back to the early years of last century in the United States [94]. In contrast, the rapid economic development of countries in East and Southeast Asia has been based on industrialization supported by rapid development of a skilled work force. This, combined with recent experiences of rural poverty and Confucian concepts of familial obligation and work ethic, appears to have taken educational intensity to a much higher level, producing the epidemic of myopia.

Intensity of schooling shows up in measures of achievements during schooling. There is a general association of higher school performance with more myopia, for a given number of years of schooling [88], with associations of more myopia with involvement in accelerated learning streams within or between schools [95–97], and use of after-school tutoring [98]. These factors seem to be associated with the strong international performance of school systems in the countries with high prevalence of myopia [99], and may point to possible control measures. For example, if involvement in accelerated learning streams starts early, this provides an incentive for parents to impose intensive study regimes on children early in life so that they get into the higher level streams, leading to early onset myopia and rapid progression. A possible reform would therefore be to delay the onset of myopia with policies designed to control the early introduction of accelerated or elite streams within or between schools, while controlling intensive academic streams in private schools, private tutorial colleges, or cram schools.

Analysis of the results of the E3 consortium suggested that education was not the whole story [56]. This is not surprising, since the role of time outdoors, discussed below, has been demonstrated. But the analysis rests on an implicit assumption that completion of primary education (defined in this paper as 16 years) posed the same educational load across the many decades of development of education systems. Putting to one side the rather unusual definition of primary school education, it is very unlikely that this is the case. Educational standards at the end of primary school when most children completed schooling to work as unskilled laborers or homemakers were almost certainly lower than they are today, when most children complete many further years of education, and a significant percentage engage in tertiary studies.

Two potentially more proximal factors that may be related to educational intensity have also been considered—reading distance and reading duration without breaks [100]. The first has a long history, dating back to Cohn, who supported the use of headrests to maintain head position while reading. These were abandoned, but it is not clear if that was because they were not effective, or because children refused to use with them. Some studies report a strong independent association of reading distance with myopia, but it is not clear whether the relationship is causal, or whether children decrease their reading distance as they become myopic. The use of headrests has been reintroduced in some schools in China, and many products are available online to control head position. Longitudinal studies are required to establish if close reading positions are adopted prior to, or in parallel with the development of myopia, and randomized trials are required to assess whether controlling reading position does reduce myopia. Reading without breaks has also often been regarded as a risk factor, and the rule of a 10 min break every 30 min forms part of myopia prevention in both Taiwan and mainland China. An intervention study is also important in this area.

6.2.1 The Search for Causal Mechanisms for Education

While there can be no doubt about the causal relationship between education and myopia, the causal pathways are less clear. Near work was generally considered to be a likely mediating factor; however, the evidence on near work has been rather inconsistent, although meta-analyses indicate that there is a relatively small effect [101]. Part of the problem may be that near work is generally estimated from questionnaire responses which are intrinsically not particularly reliable. It is also difficult because the slow development of myopia means that near work estimates need to cover periods of at least some months if not years to be related to significant changes in axial length or refraction. Recent development of instruments for objectively measuring near work may provide better estimates, although considerable thought will need to be given to the sampling frames, given the marked daily, weekly, and seasonal variations in near work demands.

Initial thinking about the causal connection invoked accommodation as the probable driver, but this idea has been increasingly called into question. Some of the important negative evidence came from animal experimentation, which showed that refractive development was not drastically affected by cutting the ciliary nerve [102], and that animals that had no accommodative capacity showed normal patterns of refractive development [103, 104]. The ability of atropine to block axial elongation was initially interpreted as supporting the hypothesis, but this judgment had to be reevaluated, since atropine was effective, even in animals such as chickens where control of accommodation involves nicotinic rather than muscarinic pathways.

Attention therefore shifted to the possibility of control by defocus on the retina, given the clear role for defocus signals in controlling axial elongation demonstrated in animal models [31]. The link to education was provided by the hypothesis that lags in accommodation would result in residual hyperopia, which could stimulate axial elongation. Testing this hypothesis has led to inconsistent results, and Mutti et al. have shown that accommodative lag may be a consequence rather than a cause [105]. There is thus no clear pattern of support for the hypothesis.

It has also been suggested that peripheral rather than central defocus may play the dominant role in controlling eye growth [106]. This hypothesis developed from evidence that trainee pilots with eye shapes that created peripheral hyperopia were more likely to become myopic [107], leading to the idea that peripheral hyperopia leads to the development of myopia. Elegant animal experiments then demonstrated that eyes could normally regulate eye growth, even if the central retina was ablated [108]. However, this hypothesis has not been supported by several lines of evidence. The interpretation of the original evidence on development of myopia has been questioned [109], and while there is a general trend for eyes to develop from more oblate to more prolate, the relationship between eye shape and refraction has been quite variable tend to appear [110]. It remains possible that peripheral hyperopic defocus might drive myopic progression but attempts to control myopic correction by reducing peripheral hyperopic have not been particularly successful. However, selective imposition of myopic defocus in the periphery may provide a method for controlling myopia [111].

A clear causal mechanism linking education to myopia has therefore not been identified, but the causal relationship nevertheless appears to be solid. A recent hypothesis is that the problem may be associated with the predominant use of black text on white background [112]. This hypothesis proposes that the problem lies in the balance of stimulation of ON and OFF visual pathways, with natural scenes leading to balanced stimulation, with black text on white heavily overstimulating OFF pathways. Given that ON-bipolar pathways stimulate release of dopamine from amacrine cells [113], and dopamine agonists can inhibit axial elongation in animal models [114, 115], this is a promising link.

6.2.2 Protection by Time Outdoors

In contrast to the long history of speculation and research about near work, solid evidence that time outdoors was an important factor only became available about 10 years ago. However, since the first presentation of the evidence at the 2006 ARVO meeting, a large amount of evidence supporting the idea has been accumulated [2, 116], and a recent meta-analysis has confirmed the association [117]. Two key pieces of evidence are shown in Figs. 6.2 and 6.3 [118, 119]. The first shows that increased time outdoors can override the impact of increased near work, the second that increased time outdoors can override the impact of parental myopia. There are some reports that have failed to find this association, but these have generally been in situations where the amount of time spent outdoors is low and may be subthreshold for protection. The evidence now includes successful school-based intervention trials that have shown that increases in time outdoors of 40–80 min per day produced significant reductions in incident myopia [46, 120, 121], consistent with expectations from the epidemiological data.

Rose et al. [118] postulated that the mechanism was probably that the brighter light outdoors during daylight hours led to more dopamine release, which in turn inhibited axial elongation. This hypothesis was confirmed by laboratory experiments that demonstrated the inhibitory effects of bright light on myopia, and the protective effect was shown to involve D2-dopamine receptors [122–126]. The plausible possibility that lower vitamin D levels, observed in children who spend less time outdoors, played a causal role has not been supported by further analysis [81, 82, 127]. The hypothesis that the protective effects might be due to a different balance of hyperopic and myopia defocus outdoors as compared to indoors [14], while plausible in terms of the results of animal experimentation, also seems unlikely, given that increasing light intensity alone blocks experimental myopia.

The question of causality has been settled with the randomized intervention trials in children. However, some issues are still unclear. The initial studies were based on distinctions between time spent outdoors and indoors, and were later linked to an operational definition of outdoors as involving light intensities over 1000 lux.

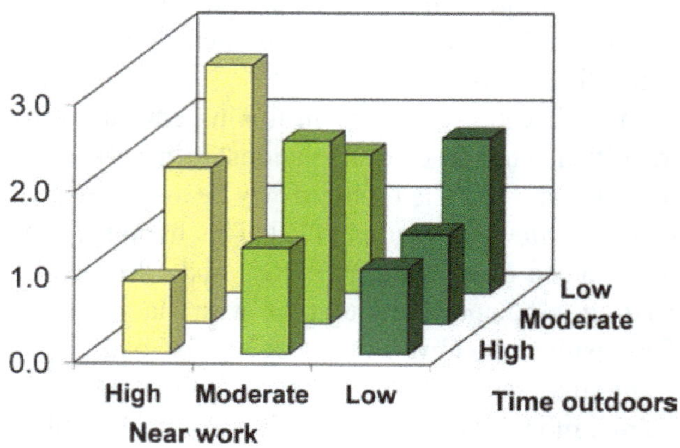

Fig. 6.2 Impacts of tertiles of near work and time outdoors on the odds ratio for myopia. Figure reproduced from Rose et al. [118]

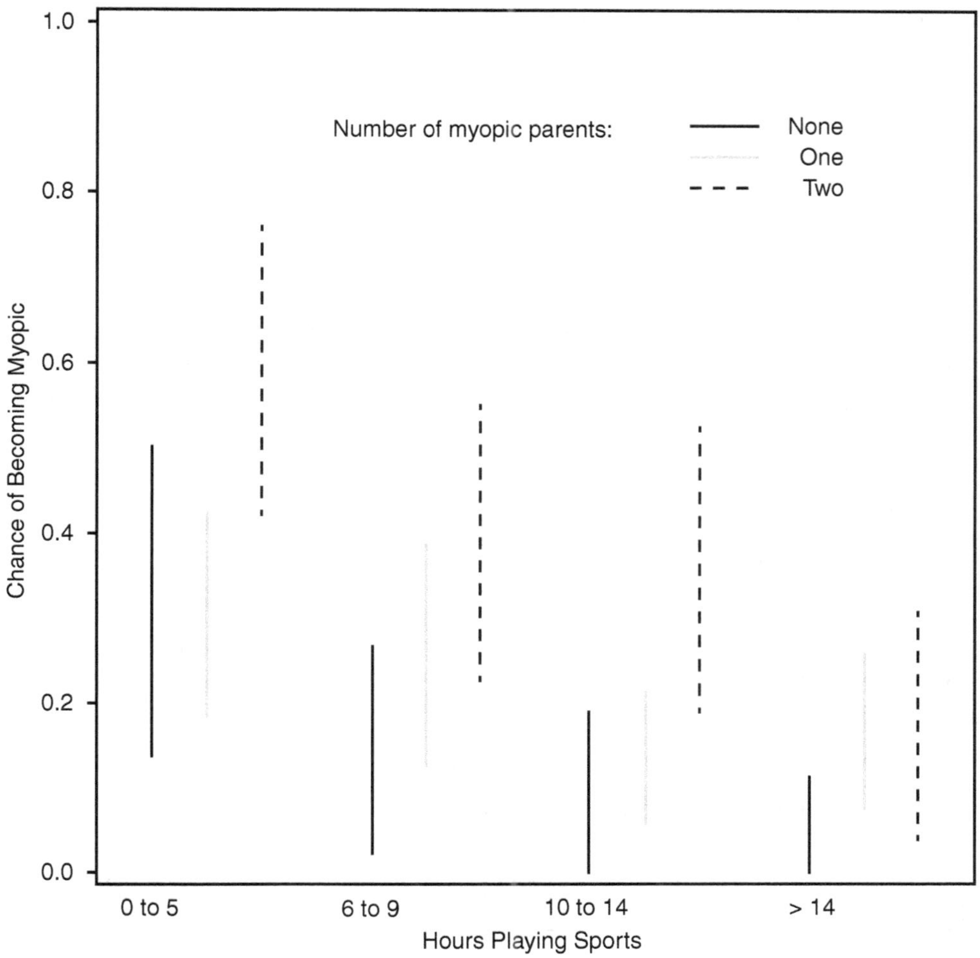

Fig. 6.3 Impact of hours playing sport (and outdoor activity) on the risk of myopia against number of myopic parents. Figure reproduced with permission from Jones et al. [119]

Animal studies suggested that light intensities considerably higher, at least 10,000 lux, might be required to produce significant effects, but there is suggestive evidence that lower light intensities might be effective in humans [120, 128]. One intervention trial has even suggested that modest increases in classroom lighting strongly inhibit the development of myopia [129], and this study requires urgent replication. A school-based intervention trial in Taiwan has reported that more modest outdoor light exposures might also reduce incident myopia and, in fact, some research using objective measurements of light suggests that effective exposures of over a few thousand lux are rare outdoors, even though light appears to be regulating axial elongation. It would not be surprising if animal experimentation overestimated the light exposures required for protection, given that the stimulus for eye growth is strong and constant, whereas signals in humans may be more intermittent. It has also been suggested that the timing of the exposures, or their frequency, and parameters such as spectral composition may be important. There is limited and so far inconsistent support for these ideas, but the uncertainty around them does not matter when the simple intervention, increased time outdoors, is considered. These factors may become important if increased time outdoors needs to be supplemented or even replaced by artificial light exposures.

There is also controversy over whether increased time outdoors reduces progression as well as onset of myopia. The initial work did not support this possibility [118, 119, 130], but even at that time, there was considerable evidence that there were seasonal differences in progression that suggested that progression rates were slower in summer than in winter, suggesting regulation of progression consistent with the documented effects of near work and time outdoors [131–135]. More recent reports have provided evidence that more time outdoors may slow progression [120, 136], but more definitive work in this area is required.

6.3 Other Possible Risk Factors for Myopia

A range of other "independent" risk factors that are less obviously related to education have been documented. As well as summarizing the evidence for them, we will discuss whether they are likely to be mediated by exposures associated with education and time outdoors (Table 6.2).

Table 6.2 Summary of probable mechanisms for risk factors for myopia

Risk factor	Possibly mediated by environmental exposures	Independent biological pathways	Genetic basis
Digital screen time	X		
Ethnicity	X		
Sex	X		
Parental myopia	X		
Urban/rural differences	X		
Pollution	X		
Housing	X		
Height	X		
Diet	X		
Sleep	X		
Smoking		X	
Birth order	X	X	
Season of birth	X		
Allergic rhinoconjunctivitis		X	X
Childhood febrile diseases		X	X

While the evidence is not conclusive, most of the reported independent risk factors for myopia might be mediated by environmental exposure to educational pressures and limited time outdoors. Systematic use of mediation analysis is required to test independence

6.3.1 Use of Computers and Smart Phones

In the last few years, use of computers and smart phones has become a routine part of daily life, with digital devices integrated into schooling in advanced countries. Increased digital screen time is often invoked to explain claimed continuing increases in the prevalence and severity of myopia, or at least as explanations for the increasingly early onset of myopia. Somewhat in advance of the available evidence, Taiwan has introduced laws controlling the amount of digital screen time that children of preschool age are allowed, although how regulations of this kind could be enforced is not clear. Dirani et al. [137] have recently asked whether increased digital screen time might be "the single modifiable risk factor for myopia," accounting for "increased near-work activity and decreased outdoor activity."

We suggest that this is unlikely, since the epidemic of myopia appeared well before the common use of these electronic devices. The prevalence of myopia was already high in Taiwan and Singapore for children born in the early 1960s, whereas the internet did not become available to the general public until 1993. Early analysis in the Sydney Myopia Study found that use of devices such as Nintendos and Game Boys was associated with less myopia, perhaps because they were predominantly used by academically underperforming boys. It is certainly possible that digital devices have now come to constitute a significant form of near work, and will correlate more closely with education and myopia, and some recent studies have documented significant associations between myopia and digital screen time [51, 138].

However, the historical perspective is important in considering preventive interventions. If limits are placed on the use of digital devices, children may simply revert to older forms of near work, such as reading books. And if digital devices encourage even more time indoors, active steps may need to be taken to get children to break with established behavior patterns and spend more time outdoors. We believe overemphasis on digital screen time may in fact have negative consequences if it leads to neglect of the other important factors. There is currently no evidence that time using digital devices is more dangerous than a similar amount of time reading. However, digital devices may make near work more pervasive and favor indoor lifestyles.

6.3.2 Sex

Many studies have compared the prevalence of myopia in males and females. Older studies have some tendency to report higher prevalence in males, whereas more recent studies more commonly report higher prevalence in females. For example, the Blue Mountains Eye Study reported that older male adults were more myopic than females [59], but the situation was reversed in the Sydney Myopia Study on children [42, 43, 96, 139]. Similarly, the Liwan Eye Study reported that sex differences in older adults were marginal [140], but in younger cohorts, girls were more likely to be myopic than boys [141]. The massive difference between the prevalence of myopia in girls and boys in Orthodox Jewish communities in Israel, where the boys undergo very intensive education from an early age, provides an extreme inverted example of this trend [78]. This variability does not suggest a direct biological link between sex and myopia, but rather suggests that the links may be mediated by social factors such as access to education for girls, which have changed considerably in many places in recent decades.

6.3.3 Ethnicity

Ethnicity or race has often been proposed as a risk factor for myopia, and indeed as evidence for genetic determination of myopia. It is however important to note that ethnicity and race covers both genetic differences, which are small in magnitude compared to the commonalities that make us human, and cultural differences that are often hard to quantify. Epidemiological evidence clearly shows major differences between ethnic groups in the prevalence of myopia, but more detailed analysis shows that these are predominantly due to environmental exposures. For example, the prevalence of myopia is high in the three major ethnic groups in Singapore, Chinese, Indian, and Malay, but in India and Malaysia, the prevalence is much lower [1, 4, 24]. This suggests that it is the environment of Singapore, perhaps most of all the education system and the limited time spent outdoors, that is crucial.

6.3.4 Parental Myopia

One of the best documented risk factors for myopia that is not directly linked to education is having myopic parents. Although shared attitudes to education are just as plausible, it is often assumed that this must be a genetic phenomenon, which is clearly true for the very genetic, highly familial forms of myopia. But the impact of parental myopia is also seen for "school myopia." Consistently, studies covering a range of different ethnic groups have shown that having one or two myopic parents increases the risk of myopia [142–147], although the risk is inevitably lower in populations with a high prevalence of myopia. Wu and Edwards have shown the impact of parental myopia over three generations in China [148].

The effect of parental myopia is often cited as evidence for a genetic contribution to myopia, on the grounds that parents and children share genes. But they also share environments, and the possibility that myopic parents provide their children with environments more conducive for developing myopia, perhaps by placing more emphasis on education, has not been excluded, although early analyses did not support this hypothesis. However, recent studies have shown that children with myopic parents do not have a significantly greater level of myopia-associated SNPs [149], undermining the genetic argument. A more detailed analysis of environmental risk factors with objective measures of near work and time outdoors may be required to explain this association.

6.3.5 Intelligence

Higher intelligence or IQ, and some other cognitive measures, are generally associated with myopia. However, whether they are factors independent of education and time outdoors is not clear. While there are some genetic influences on these factors, as noted previously, like myopia, they are socially malleable, rather than genetically determined [89, 90]. In the SCORM Study, both academic grades and IQ scores appear to be independently associated with myopia [87, 88], and the same result has been obtained in a very large study of Israeli conscripts [150]. But the causal chains are very obscure, with a number of questions to be answered. For example, Are the links explained by the genetic correlations of the phenotypes? Do people with high IQs do more near work? Or is part of their high IQ achieved by more time reading and indoors? Do people with higher IQs need less effort to achieve high grades? Whatever the answer to these questions, reducing intelligence does not provide a route to prevention.

6.3.6 Urban/Rural Differences

Another consistent association of myopia is with urban residence, with children growing up in more rural areas generally being less myopic. In general, educational outcomes for children from rural areas are lower, and they often report less near work and more time outdoors. It is hard to see a direct link between axial elongation and postcode, and we suggest that urban/rural differences are likely to be based on differences in near work and time outdoors.

Population density has been invoked as one factor [151], but a major study in China has found that while there was a positive association of myopia with increased population density [152], even in the area with the lowest population density studied, the prevalence of myopia was still very high. This suggests other factors were more important. Access to green space has also been linked to lower use of spectacles [153].

6.3.7 Pollution

Pollution is one of the factors that has increased markedly since the Second World War in parts of East and Southeast Asia. There are many forms of pollution. Speculation about this factor has been fueled by the high levels of air pollution seem in some parts of China, but in fact, in international terms, Chinese cities rank well behind many cities in South Asia and the Middle East, where the prevalence of myopia is much lower than in Chinese cities (https://www.who.int/airpollution/data/cities/en/, accessed Jan 30, 2019). Increased use of spectacles, presumably for myopia, has been associated with traffic-related pollution [154], but this may in fact be related to the association between urban residence and more myopia, as well as links to socioeconomic status, area of residence, and education [153].

6.3.8 Housing

Nature of housing has also been invoked as a factor. However, the results in this area are currently quite contradictory. In Singapore, more spacious housing was associated with more myopia, possibly because of a causal chain involving socioeconomic status and its associations with education [60, 95]. In contrast, in both Sydney [151] and Hong Kong [155], small apartment dwelling has been associated with more myopia. A causal chain is not as obvious in this case and more complex pathways may need to be considered.

6.3.9 Height

Height has often been considered as a potential risk factor for myopia, and indeed, there have been substantial increases in height in populations over the last 150 years. These increases in height have been generally attributed to more adequate nutrition. It has also been argued that associations between height and myopia might be expected, given that taller people have longer axial lengths, but this argument does not take into account the "emmetropisation" mechanisms that produce substantial convergence of refractive status, despite differences in body stature. While several papers have reported that height is a risk factor for myopia [9, 156], the evidence on this is very inconsistent. Rosner et al. [157] reported that Israeli male military conscripts, who were not myopic, were taller and weighed more than those who were not myopic—the reverse of expectations. Another inconsistency lies in the difference in prevalence of myopia between males and females, with a higher prevalence of myopia being commonly reported in girls in recent studies. If there were a tight biological link between height and refraction, a more consistent relationship would be expected. Social factors affecting nutrition and education may therefore be important. Given the differences in height between the sexes, studies need to be carried out with population stratification wherever possible.

Rahi and colleagues reported that maternal height (and age) was associated with more myopia [47]. In the United Kingdom, height differs by socioeconomic status, with greater heights (and also maternal age) in higher SES groups [158]. Since children from higher SES groups are generally more myopic, these associations need to be tested for mediation by social factors.

6.3.10 Diet

Diets in East and Southeast Asia have changed significantly since the Second World War, and Cordain et al. argued that dietary change could have contributed to the increased prevalence of myopia, backed up by a plausible hypothesis linking insulin resistance, chronic hyperinsulinemia, increased circulating insulin-like growth factor (IGF-1), decreased circulating growth hormone, and decreased retinoid receptor signaling to increases in scleral growth [159]. But in other ways, this hypothesis has gained little support, and expected associations of height, weight, body mass index (BMI) and obesity with myopia have not been consistently observed. Improved diet is associated with greater height and axial length, but it does not appear to have produced increased refraction, consistent with the powerful eye growth control mechanisms that have been reported. It is also worth noting that international variations in overweight and obesity do not parallel the international distribution of myopia, with none of the countries with a high prevalence of myopia making the list of the top 20 countries ranked by percentage of obesity (https://www.who.int/gho/ncd/risk_factors/overweight/en/, accessed Jan 30, 2019) and thus there is little support for a tight biological link between diet and myopia.

6.3.11 Sleep

Associations between sleep and myopia have also been reported, but the evidence is quite inconsistent [160–162]. It is clear that children who have heavy study loads after school are likely to get less sleep, both because there is less time available, but also because mental activity close to bed time can disrupt sleep. Lack of sleep is more likely to be a problem in the senior years of school, when homework loads in many parts of East and Southeast Asia are very high. However, sleep deprivation is likely to be less common in the early primary years, when myopia first appears, which reduces the likelihood that it is a major risk factor. Kearney et al. [163] have recently reported that myopes in the Northern Ireland Childhood Errors of Refraction (NICER) Study have lower levels of serum melatonin, which could be linked to disruption of circadian rhythms, which have sometimes been linked to myopia [164], or could be linked to reduced light exposures and dopaminergic function.

6.3.12 Smoking

Maternal smoking was associated with a lower risk of myopia in the SCORM Study from Singapore, but there was no association with paternal smoking, and the number of mothers who smoked was small [165]. In the subsequent Strabismus, Amblyopia and Refractive Error in young Singaporean Children Study (STARS) Study, a stronger negative association with maternal and paternal smoking was reported [166]. A similar protective relationship was reported in a sample from a pediatric ophthalmology clinic, which largely persisted after adjustment for a range of factors including child's near work activity and parental myopia and education [167]. A detailed study from South Korea reported consistent results for exposure to passive smoke estimated from urinary cotinine level [168], supporting the suggestion that nicotinic pathways are involved in the regulation of eye growth. In contrast, Rahi et al. reported a positive association between maternal smoking in early pregnancy and more myopia [47]. Although some of the associations reported are substantial, given the associations of smoking with SES and education, and lower gestational weight, these studies need to be carefully controlled for confounding.

6.3.13 Birth Order

Associations between myopia and birth order were reported with first-born children tending to be more myopic [49]. However, in educational studies, it is well documented that first-born children generally get more education [169]. A subsequent study on the UK Biobank dataset, adjusted for education, showed that the association between myopia and birth order was reduced but not eliminated [170]. In addition, in China, children from one child families are also more myopic than other children with siblings, and this was attributed to greater parental support for their child's education [171]. However, the sociology of these differences is very complex, and more work needs to be done to establish that birth order is an independent risk factor.

6.3.14 Season of Birth

Season of birth has also been associated with myopia in several studies, with children born in summer tending to be more myopic [51, 172, 173]. No plausible pathway has been suggested for a direct link. Instead, it has been suggested that children born in summer often start school up to a year younger than their peers born in spring. This could mean first exposure to education and less time outdoors at an age when myopic shifts in refraction, including myopic progression, are larger, resulting in more myopia.

6.3.15 Allergic Conjunctivitis: Hay Fever and Kawasaki Disease

In 2011, Herbort et al. proposed a general association of myopia with inflammatory conditions affecting the choriocapillaris [174]. An association between ocular inflammatory conditions such as uveitis was subsequently demonstrated [175]. Later, a higher risk of myopia was associated with allergic conjunctivitis, and less so allergic rhinitis, atopic dermatitis, and asthma [176]. A large population-based study using the NHANES dataset showed that hay fever was also associated with a higher prevalence of high myopia [177]. A recent report has also associated increased myopia with Kawasaki disease [178], which has conjunctivitis as one of its core diagnostic criteria. This association needs further study.

These studies provide a persuasive case for some link between ocular allergic responses and the development of myopia, and using an animal model. Wei et al. have proposed a mechanism involving increased tumor necrosis factor (TNF)-alpha and interleukins. It does not seem likely that a link between ocular inflammation and myopia can explain the epidemic of myopia in East and Southeast Asia, since there is no parallel between the international distribution myopia and that of allergic rhinoconjunctivitis in children [179]. One possibility is that eye rubbing may lead to myopic refractions through corneal changes, as may be the case with keratoconus [180], but the US study on hay fever ruled out a role for them. The possibility that children with these conditions tend to spend less time outside should be examined. It also seems possible that allergic conditions might add to the incidence and progression of myopia, without being the primary determinant.

6.3.16 Febrile Diseases

Using data from the UK Biobank, Guggenheim et al. reported associations between several childhood diseases and myopia. From a list including pneumonia, encephalitis, meningitis, rheumatic fever, measles, rubella, mumps, diphtheria, and pertussis, rubella, mumps and pertussis were associated with myopia, while measles, rubella, and pertussis were associated with high myopia [181]. The authors argued against a link to educational disruption or limited time outdoors, since not all serious childhood diseases were linked to myopia, but this link, whatever its causes, cannot explain the emergence of the epidemic of myopia. But these findings may have clinical implications that need to be explored.

6.3.17 Fertility Treatment

The British TEDS Study has documented a standard range of social variables, with level of maternal education, summer birth, hours spent playing computer games surviving full multivariate regression analysis, with associations with socioeconomic status, educational attainment, reading enjoyment, and cognitive variables showing associations at multiple stages in the life-course analysis. A unique feature of the analysis was the protective associations of fertility treatment detected in the final analysis [51]. The authors ruled out associations with parental education, and the causes are currently obscure.

6.4 Popular Beliefs About the Causes of Myopia

There are many popular beliefs in the causes of myopia around the world, which have presumably arisen because the development of myopia and its progression is often observed by parents, who naturally seek explanations. In the western world, a common belief is that reading in dim light, or under the bed clothes causes vision to deteriorate, but this outcome, and these behaviors might indeed be common in those who like reading books, and there is some evidence that reading for pleasure is a risk factor for myopia. We have not attempted a systematic survey in this area, but in China, there seem to be many beliefs of this kind, perhaps because the prevalence of myopia has increased so conspicuously. One commonly encountered belief is that myopia is associated with reading and writing postures that violate the "foot, fist, inch" rule, that is the eyes should be one foot from the book, the chest should be one fist from the desk, and the fingers should be 1 inch from the nib of the pen. This is a variant on the idea that bad posture while reading leads to the development of myopia, which has widespread currency, but has never been proven. A similar common belief is that reading while riding on public transport is dangerous, but again this has never been tested. Other, intuitively unlikely ideas include the development of myopia in children who read on their back, or their front, or who read extracurricular books with font sizes greater than standard textbooks. These have occasionally been looked at in scientific papers, and associations have sometimes been reported. These proposed factors need to be rigorously tested epidemiologically, and if they survive that sort of testing, they need to be subjected to standard Randomised Control Trial (RCT) testing. Unfortunately, without any positive evidence, two of these have been written into China's National Myopia Prevention Plan.

6.5 Comparing Genetic and Environmental Effects

Comparing the impact of genetic to environmental effects is difficult, because they are often quantified in different ways, with genetic effects generally determined in relation to variation in refraction, while evidence on the impact of environmental effects is generally related to prevalence of myopia. Genetic studies have identified myopia-associated SNPs that account for slightly less than 10% of the variance in refraction, although these factors are very precisely measured [13]. Compared to the possibly misplaced expectations from twin studies with heritability estimates in the range of 80–90%, there is obviously a large amount of what has come to be called missing heritability, although it is actually the identified genetic variation which is missing. Use of the SNP-heritability approach suggests that Genome-Wide Association Study (GWAS) has the potential to explain more like 20–35% of the variance [19]. It is often suggested that improvements in methodology and increases in sample size may help to close the gap, although there is a law of diminishing returns with increased sample sizes. There is little evidence that other forms of genetic variation such as copy number variations or rare genetic effects of large size have a role to play.

In contrast, the measurement of risk factor exposures is much less precise, largely involving estimates derived from questionnaires. These questionnaires not only suffer from the general problem of recall bias, but in relation to near work and time outdoors, they also ask for a very difficult task to be performed, namely estimating average exposures. Not surprisingly, such questionnaires are more accurate when estimates of recent exposures over a limited time frame are compared to measurements obtained using objective instruments, but even then, discrepancies are significant. We are therefore not yet in a position to calculate individual environmental risk factor effect sizes. This may explain why attempts to quantify the associations between estimates of near work and time outdoors on the one hand and myopia on the other explain only low percentages of the variance [19], despite the evidence that changes in them appear to be responsible for the major increases in prevalence of myopia seen recently.

We suggest that while awaiting more quantitative data on environmental risk exposures, the change in mean SER from the age of 5–6 to the end of schooling may be taken to represent the cumulative effect of relevant environmental exposures over this time. This assumption seems reasonable, given that children exposed to only limited schooling generally develop little myopia. The only exception that we have found to this statement is the increase in prevalence of myopia in Eskimo and Inuit children after exposure to rudimentary schooling in extreme northern latitudes [182–184]. This may be an exception due to the limited light exposures available during winter, combined with reductions in the amount of time spent outdoors.

The data from the RESC Study in Nepal, where there is little development of myopia and limited schooling, appears to be an average shift of −0.02 D/year with minimal schooling [185]. This figure is about −0.16 D/year of schooling in the Sydney Myopia Study. East Asian studies suggest a total change that is much greater. In the Guangzhou RESC Study, refraction changed by at least −3.00 D over 10 years, or a change of −0.3 D/year [141]. In the Shandong Eye Study [12], the change was closer to −4.00 D over 10 years, or −0.4 D/year. One limitation of this simple analysis is that it assumes linear changes across the years of schooling, which may not be the case. These values compare with estimates from the UK Biobank Study on refractive shifts associated with years of schooling, which suggest shifts from epidemiological analysis of −0.16 D/year, while the Mendelian randomization analysis gives a change of −0.28 D/year [83]. It is encouraging that these figures are in the same ballpark when children have been exposed to schooling, but it needs to be recognized that these figures are only first approximations.

Accepting these estimates as the best currently available, we can then attempt to use them to understand the onset of myopia. Age of onset may be a very significant parameter, since it has decreased markedly during the emergence of the myopia epidemics [11], appears to have similar genetic associations to the final level of myopia in adults [13, 186], and appears to be a good predictor of final myopia [187].

In several studies that have used rigorous cycloplegia, refractions at the age of 5–7 are concentrated in the range of 1.0–1.3 D. This range has been documented for children in East Asia [12, 46, 75, 188] and in western societies [43, 76, 96]. The similarity of the values reported for children of East Asian and European backgrounds is striking, given the massively different prevalence rates that emerge later. In other reports, mean SER has been lower, and we suggest that, in many of these cases, inadequate cycloplegia may be involved. This means that the challenge is to explain how genetic factors and environmental factors can produce myopic shifts of 1.5 D or more to reach the threshold for myopia of −0.5 D. The steps involved in moving from this baseline value to the threshold for myopia and onto final SER at the age of 20 are summarized in Fig. 6.4.

In the ALSPAC Study [149] on average, participants carried around 130 risk alleles, with most of the distribution fitting within ±15 alleles [149]. If the average number of risk alleles corresponds to a mean SER of +1.0 to 1.3 D, with an average effect size of −0.1 D/risk allele, few participants would reach the myopia cutoff of −0.5 D on purely genetic grounds, and several years of schooling would be required to reach the threshold. Modeling by Ghorbani-Mojarrad et al. [149] also suggests that additive genetic effects are unlikely to produce "school myopia," without additional contributions from environmental factors. In contrast, in East Asian environments, 2–4 years of schooling would bring many children past the myopia cutoff. This is likely to happen more rapidly for those who are already at risk genetically.

This picture is based on a number of assumptions and needs extensive further development in relation to the size and linearity of effects, but it provides a

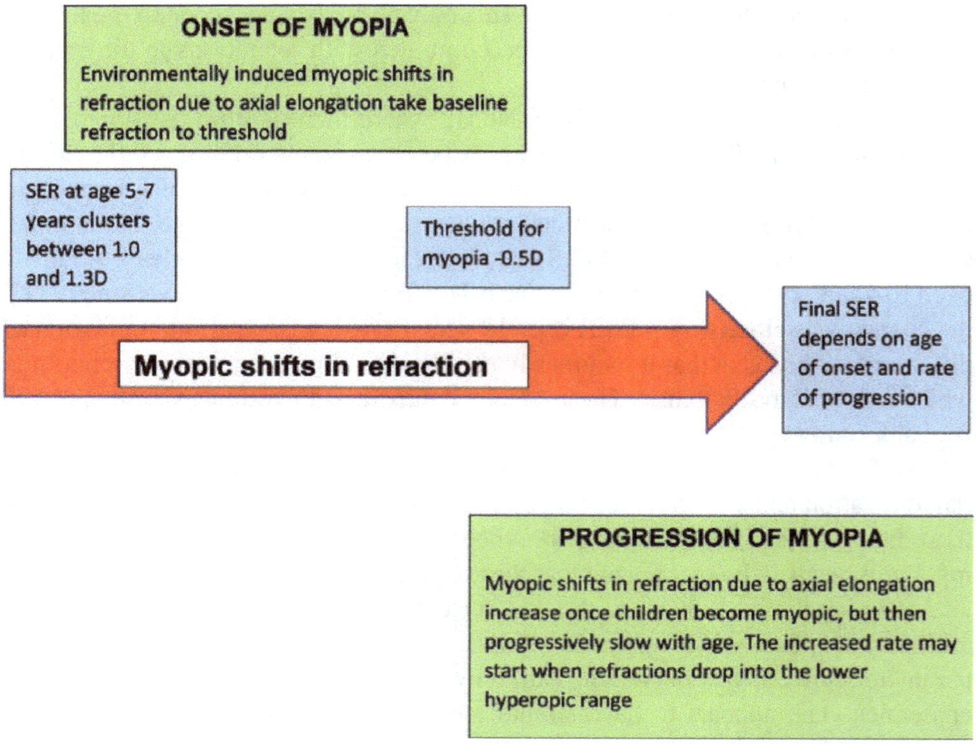

Fig. 6.4 Environmentally driven axial elongation and myopic shifts in refraction lead to final refraction. Rate of axial elongation and myopia shifts in refraction increase prior to the onset of myopia, and remain elevated but decline with age [199, 200]. This increase may begin when SER reaches the low hyperopic range [201]. The earlier the onset, the greater the progression

framework for understanding one of the distinctive characteristics of the current epidemic of "school myopia," the importance of environmental exposures and the modest impact of genetic risk. It also suggests that more work needs to be done on the determinants of spherical equivalent at the age of 5–7 years, and determinants of the age of onset of myopia, because the latter is a significant predictor of subsequent progression and final myopia [187].

Gene–environment interactions also need to be taken into account. It must be remembered that simple environmental regulation of gene expression is not an example of gene–environment interactions. Gene–environment interactions are characterized by situations in which genetic risk and environmental risk combine to produce impacts which are greater or less than expected from their individual effects—or in other words that expression of different alleles of a given gene are differentially affected by different environments. Verhoeven et al. [189] have examined the specific case of the interaction of genetic risk and educational risk, reporting major interactions, with the combination of high genetic risk and high educational risk producing very high risk greater than the arithmetic sum of the individual risks, using the synergy analyses of Rothman [190–192]. Cortina-Borjas et al. [193] have argued that this method produces many false cases of gene–environment interactions, in part because when using odds ratios, risks are more likely to be multiplicative. From our analysis of the data in the paper by Verhoeven et al., the interactions in this paper are close to multiplicative, and we suggest that a more detailed analysis is required. A search for more specific cases has produced some more specific examples of gene–environment interactions [194–197], but the cases reported appear to be rare. More work is clearly needed in this complex area.

6.6 Conclusions

Our overview of risk factors for myopia has identified education and limited time outdoors as the major risk factors for myopia. We suggest that the evidence on these two risk factors is now very strong. These two factors both suggest evidence-based approaches to control of myopia, such as increased time outdoors and decreased near work time. These two factors then appear to converge to regulate eye growth, through cellular and biological pathways that require further definition, but appear to involve regulation of the rate of dopamine release as one component, and axial elongation as another.

Many other risk factors for myopia have been proposed. Many of them may be more distal social factors such as parental and social attitudes to education, provision of educational opportunities, and organization of school systems and schools, and may be mediated by the educational and time outdoor exposures that children receive.

We suggest that future studies in this area need to become more rigorous in several ways. Cycloplegia needs to the required standard in new studies. Mediation analysis needs to become a standard part of risk factor analysis, used to define causal pathways. As a minimum, new studies also need to collect data on educational exposures and time outdoors, increasingly using the new methods for collection of objective data that are becoming available. These higher standards need to be enforced by more rigorous review and publication processes.

While there are many aspects of the risk factors for myopia that require further analysis, the picture that we currently have provides important insight into the characteristics of the current epidemics. In particular, we can now see why genetic effects on "school myopia" are so slight, despite the evidence for a large number of SNPs of small effect size associated with myopia.

The evidence for a major role of education and time outdoors has given us insight into effective means of control, some of which are currently being implemented in myopia control rather than school myopia programs, such as programs aimed to increase time outdoors. Many other interventions at more distal levels also can be envisaged that might reduce early competition for privileged places in schools. When these are combined with clinical interventions to control myopia progression, and there are now many available, in principle, we now understand how to turn back the epidemic of myopia.

But understanding does not automatically lead to success in prevention; after all we have known how to correct refractive errors for some time, but uncorrected refractive error is still a major cause of visual impairment. Research into more effective means of preventing the onset and progression of myopia needs to, and will undoubtedly continue. But the next big challenge may already be to identify and overcome the barriers to implementation, so that we can ensure that we achieve what increasingly appears to be a realizable goal—the prevention of "school myopia."

References

1. Morgan I, Rose K. How genetic is 'school myopia'? Prog Retin Eye Res. 2005;24:1–38.
2. Morgan IG, French AN, Ashby RS, Guo X, Ding X, He M, et al. The epidemics of myopia: aetiology and prevention. Prog Retin Eye Res. 2018;62:134–49.
3. Morgan IG, He M, Rose KA. Epidemic of pathological myopia: what can laboratory studies and epidemiology tell us? Retina. 2017;37:989–97.
4. Morgan IG, Ohno-Matsui K, Saw SM. Myopia. Lancet. 2012;379:1739–48.
5. Hysi PG, Wojciechowski R, Rahi JS, Hammond CJ. Genome-wide association studies of refractive error and myopia, lessons learned, and implications for the future. Invest Ophthalmol Vis Sci. 2014;55:3344–51.
6. Wojciechowski R. Nature and nurture: the complex genetics of myopia and refractive error. Clin Genet. 2011;79:301–20.
7. Wojciechowski R, Cheng CY. Involvement of multiple molecular pathways in the genetics of ocular refraction and myopia. Retina. 2017;38:91–101.
8. Wojciechowski R, Hysi PG. Focusing in on the complex genetics of myopia. PLoS Genet. 2013;9:e1003442.
9. Jung SK, Lee JH, Kakizaki H, Jee D. Prevalence of myopia and its association with body stature and educational level in 19-year-old male conscripts in Seoul, South Korea. Invest Ophthalmol Vis Sci. 2012;53:5579–83.
10. Koh V, Yang A, Saw SM, Chan YH, Lin ST, Tan MM, et al. Differences in prevalence of refractive errors in young Asian males in Singapore between 1996-1997 and 2009-2010. Ophthalmic Epidemiol. 2014;21:247–55.
11. Lin LL, Shih YF, Hsiao CK, Chen CJ. Prevalence of myopia in Taiwanese schoolchildren: 1983 to 2000. Ann Acad Med Singap. 2004;33:27–33.
12. Wu JF, Bi HS, Wang SM, Hu YY, Wu H, Sun W, et al. Refractive error, visual acuity and causes of vision loss in children in Shandong, China. The Shandong Children Eye Study. PLoS One. 2013;8:e82763.
13. Tedja MS, Wojciechowski R, Hysi PG, Eriksson N, Furlotte NA, Verhoeven VJM, et al. Genome-wide association meta-analysis highlights light-induced signaling as a driver for refractive error. Nat Genet. 2018;50:834–48.
14. Flitcroft DI. The complex interactions of retinal, optical and environmental factors in myopia aetiology. Prog Retin Eye Res. 2012;31:622–60.
15. Sankaridurg PR, Holden BA. Practical applications to modify and control the development of ametropia. Eye. 2014;28:134–41.
16. Huang J, Wen D, Wang Q, McAlinden C, Flitcroft I, Chen H, et al. Efficacy comparison of 16 interventions for myopia control in children: a network meta-analysis. Ophthalmology. 2016;123:697–708.
17. Flitcroft DI, Loughman J, Wildsoet CF, Williams C, Guggenheim JA, Consortium C. Novel myopia genes and pathways identified from syndromic forms of myopia. Invest Ophthalmol Vis Sci. 2018;59:338–48.
18. Young TL. Molecular genetics of human myopia: an update. Optom Vis Sci. 2009;86:E8–E22.
19. Guggenheim JA, St Pourcain B, McMahon G, Timpson NJ, Evans DM, Williams C. Assumption-free estimation of the genetic contribution to refractive error across childhood. Mol Vis. 2015;21:621–32.

20. Baird PN, Schache M, Dirani M. The GEnes in Myopia (GEM) study in understanding the aetiology of refractive errors. Prog Retin Eye Res. 2010;29:520–42.
21. Hammond CJ, Snieder H, Gilbert CE, Spector TD. Genes and environment in refractive error: the twin eye study. Invest Ophthalmol Vis Sci. 2001;42:1232–6.
22. Lyhne N, Sjolie AK, Kyvik KO, Green A. The importance of genes and environment for ocular refraction and its determiners: a population based study among 20-45 year old twins. Br J Ophthalmol. 2001;85:1470–6.
23. Manolio TA, Collins FS, Cox NJ, Goldstein DB, Hindorff LA, Hunter DJ, et al. Finding the missing heritability of complex diseases. Nature. 2009;461:747–53.
24. Morgan IG, Rose KA. Myopia: is the nature-nurture debate finally over? Clin Exp Optom. 2019;102:3–17.
25. Varughese S, Varghese RM, Gupta N, Ojha R, Sreenivas V, Puliyel JM. Refractive error at birth and its relation to gestational age. Curr Eye Res. 2005;30:423–8.
26. Cook RC, Glasscock RE. Refractive and ocular findings in the newborn. Am J Ophthalmol. 1951;34:1407–13.
27. Mayer DL, Hansen RM, Moore BD, Kim S, Fulton AB. Cycloplegic refractions in healthy children aged 1 through 48 months. Arch Ophthalmol. 2001;119:1625–8.
28. Mutti DO, Mitchell GL, Jones LA, Friedman NE, Frane SL, Lin WK, et al. Axial growth and changes in lenticular and corneal power during emmetropization in infants. Invest Ophthalmol Vis Sci. 2005;46:3074–80.
29. Morgan IG, Rose KA, Ellwein LB, Refractive Error Study in Children Survey G. Is emmetropia the natural endpoint for human refractive development? An analysis of population-based data from the refractive error study in children (RESC). Acta Ophthalmol. 2010;88:877–84.
30. Sorsby A, Sheridan M, Leary GA, Benjamin B. Vision, visual acuity, and ocular refraction of young men: findings in a sample of 1,033 subjects. Br Med J. 1960;1:1394–8.
31. Wallman J, Winawer J. Homeostasis of eye growth and the question of myopia. Neuron. 2004;43:447–68.
32. French AN, Morgan IG, Mitchell P, Rose KA. Risk factors for incident myopia in Australian schoolchildren: the Sydney adolescent vascular and eye study. Ophthalmology. 2013;120:2100–8.
33. Ma X, Congdon N, Yi H, Zhou Z, Pang X, Meltzer ME, et al. Safety of spectacles for children's vision: a cluster-randomized controlled trial. Am J Ophthalmol. 2015;160:897–904.
34. Zadnik K, Sinnott LT, Cotter SA, Jones-Jordan LA, Kleinstein RN, Manny RE, et al. Prediction of juvenile-onset myopia. JAMA Ophthalmol. 2015;133:683–9.
35. Ehrlich DL, Atkinson J, Braddick O, Bobier W, Durden K. Reduction of infant myopia: a longitudinal cycloplegic study. Vis Res. 1995;35:1313–24.
36. Lam CS, Tang WC, Tse DY, Tang YY, To CH. Defocus incorporated soft contact (DISC) lens slows myopia progression in Hong Kong Chinese schoolchildren: a 2-year randomised clinical trial. Br J Ophthalmol. 2014;98:40–5.
37. Morgan IG, Iribarren R, Fotouhi A, Grzybowski A. Cycloplegic refraction is the gold standard for epidemiological studies. Acta Ophthalmol. 2015;93:581–5.
38. Fotouhi A, Morgan IG, Iribarren R, Khabazkhoob M, Hashemi H. Validity of noncycloplegic refraction in the assessment of refractive errors: the Tehran Eye Study. Acta Ophthalmol. 2012;90:380–6.
39. He X, Zou H, Lu L, Zhao R, Zhao H, Li Q, et al. Axial length/corneal radius ratio: association with refractive state and role on myopia detection combined with visual acuity in Chinese school children. PLoS One. 2015;10:e0111766.
40. Tideman JWL, Polling JR, Vingerling JR, Jaddoe VWV, Williams C, Guggenheim JA, et al. Axial length growth and the risk of developing myopia in European children. Acta Ophthalmol. 2018;96:301–9.
41. Guo Y, Liu LJ, Tang P, Lv YY, Feng Y, Xu L, et al. Outdoor activity and myopia progression in 4-year follow-up of Chinese primary school children: The Beijing Children Eye Study. PLoS One. 2017;12:e0175921.

42. Ip JM, Huynh SC, Robaei D, Kifley A, Rose KA, Morgan IG, et al. Ethnic differences in refraction and ocular biometry in a population-based sample of 11-15-year-old Australian children. Eye. 2008;22:649–56.
43. Ojaimi E, Rose KA, Morgan IG, Smith W, Martin FJ, Kifley A, et al. Distribution of ocular biometric parameters and refraction in a population-based study of Australian children. Invest Ophthalmol Vis Sci. 2005;46:2748–54.
44. Iribarren R. Crystalline lens and refractive development. Prog Retin Eye Res. 2015;47:86–106.
45. Cumberland PM, Bountziouka V, Rahi JS. Impact of varying the definition of myopia on estimates of prevalence and associations with risk factors: time for an approach that serves research, practice and policy. Br J Ophthalmol. 2018;102:1407–12.
46. He M, Xiang F, Zeng Y, Mai J, Chen Q, Zhang J, et al. Effect of time spent outdoors at school on the development of myopia among children in China: a randomized clinical trial. JAMA. 2015;314:1142–8.
47. Rahi JS, Cumberland PM, Peckham CS. Myopia over the lifecourse: prevalence and early life influences in the 1958 British birth cohort. Ophthalmology. 2011;118:797–804.
48. Deere K, Williams C, Leary S, Mattocks C, Ness A, Blair SN, et al. Myopia and later physical activity in adolescence: a prospective study. Br J Sports Med. 2009;43:542–4.
49. Guggenheim JA, McMahon G, Northstone K, Mandel Y, Kaiserman I, Stone RA, et al. Birth order and myopia. Ophthalmic Epidemiol. 2013;20:375–84.
50. Guggenheim JA, Northstone K, McMahon G, Ness AR, Deere K, Mattocks C, et al. Time outdoors and physical activity as predictors of incident myopia in childhood: a prospective cohort study. Invest Ophthalmol Vis Sci. 2012;53:2856–65.
51. Williams KM, Kraphol E, Yonova-Doing E, Hysi PG, Plomin R, Hammond CJ. Early life factors for myopia in the British Twins Early Development Study. Br J Ophthalmol. 2019. https://doi.org/10.1136/bjophthalmol-2018-312439.
52. Vitale S, Ellwein L, Cotch MF, Ferris FL, Sperduto R. Prevalence of refractive error in the United States, 1999-2004. Arch Ophthalmol. 2008;126:1111–9.
53. Kim EC, Morgan IG, Kakizaki H, Kang S, Jee D. Prevalence and risk factors for refractive errors: Korean National Health and Nutrition Examination Survey 2008-2011. PLoS One. 2013;8:e80361.
54. Wolfram C, Hohn R, Kottler U, Wild P, Blettner M, Buhren J, et al. Prevalence of refractive errors in the European adult population: the Gutenberg Health Study (GHS). Br J Ophthalmol. 2014;98:857–61.
55. Cumberland PM, Bao Y, Hysi PG, Foster PJ, Hammond CJ, Rahi JS, et al. Frequency and distribution of refractive error in adult life: methodology and findings of the UK Biobank Study. PLoS One. 2015;10:e0139780.
56. Williams KM, Bertelsen G, Cumberland P, Wolfram C, Verhoeven VJ, Anastasopoulos E, et al. Increasing prevalence of myopia in Europe and the impact of education. Ophthalmology. 2015;122:1489–97.
57. Williams KM, Verhoeven VJ, Cumberland P, Bertelsen G, Wolfram C, Buitendijk GH, et al. Prevalence of refractive error in Europe: the European Eye Epidemiology (E(3)) Consortium. Eur J Epidemiol. 2015;30:305–15.
58. Wang Q, Klein BE, Klein R, Moss SE. Refractive status in the Beaver Dam Eye Study. Invest Ophthalmol Vis Sci. 1994;35:4344–7.
59. Attebo K, Ivers RQ, Mitchell P. Refractive errors in an older population: the Blue Mountains Eye Study. Ophthalmology. 1999;106:1066–72.
60. Wong TY, Foster PJ, Hee J, Ng TP, Tielsch JM, Chew SJ, et al. Prevalence and risk factors for refractive errors in adult Chinese in Singapore. Invest Ophthalmol Vis Sci. 2000;41:2486–94.
61. Hashemi H, Fotouhi A, Mohammad K. The age- and gender-specific prevalences of refractive errors in Tehran: the Tehran Eye Study. Ophthalmic Epidemiol. 2004;11:213–25.
62. Negrel AD, Maul E, Pokharel GP, Zhao J, Ellwein LB. Refractive error study in children: sampling and measurement methods for a multi-country survey. Am J Ophthalmol. 2000;129:421–6.

63. Saw SM, Carkeet A, Chia KS, Stone RA, Tan DT. Component dependent risk factors for ocular parameters in Singapore Chinese children. Ophthalmology. 2002;109:2065–71.
64. Zadnik K. The Glenn A. Fry Award Lecture (1995). Myopia development in childhood. Optom Vis Sci. 1997;74:603–8.
65. Ojaimi E, Rose KA, Smith W, Morgan IG, Martin FJ, Mitchell P. Methods for a population-based study of myopia and other eye conditions in school children: the Sydney Myopia Study. Ophthalmic Epidemiol. 2005;12:59–69.
66. Breslin KM, O'Donoghue L, Saunders KJ. A prospective study of spherical refractive error and ocular components among Northern Irish schoolchildren (the NICER study). Invest Ophthalmol Vis Sci. 2013;54:4843–50.
67. Harrington SC, Stack J, Saunders K, O'Dwyer V. Refractive error and visual impairment in Ireland school children. Br J Ophthalmol. 2019. https://doi.org/10.1136/bjophthalmol-2018-312573.
68. Li SM, Liu LR, Li SY, Ji YZ, Fu J, Wang Y, et al. Design, methodology and baseline data of a school-based cohort study in Central China: the Anyang Childhood Eye Study. Ophthalmic Epidemiol. 2013;20:348–59.
69. Zheng Y, Ding X, Chen Y, He M. The Guangzhou twin project: an update. Twin Res Hum Genet. 2013;16:73–8.
70. Czepita D, Mojsa A, Zejmo M. Prevalence of myopia and hyperopia among urban and rural schoolchildren in Poland. Ann Acad Med Stetin. 2008;54:17–21.
71. Czepita D, Zejmo M, Mojsa A. Prevalence of myopia and hyperopia in a population of Polish school children. Ophthalmic Physiol Opt. 2007;27:60–5.
72. Tideman JWL, Polling JR, Jaddoe VWV, Vingerling JR, Klaver CCW. Environmental risk factors can reduce axial length elongation and myopia incidence in 6- to 9-year-old children. Ophthalmology. 2019;126:127–36.
73. Ehrlich DL, Braddick OJ, Atkinson J, Anker S, Weeks F, Hartley T, et al. Infant emmetropization: longitudinal changes in refraction components from nine to twenty months of age. Optom Vis Sci. 1997;74:822–43.
74. Giordano L, Friedman DS, Repka MX, Katz J, Ibironke J, Hawes P, et al. Prevalence of refractive error among preschool children in an urban population: the Baltimore Pediatric Eye Disease Study. Ophthalmology. 2009;116:739–46.
75. Guo X, Fu M, Ding X, Morgan IG, Zeng Y, He M. Significant axial elongation with minimal change in refraction in 3- to 6-year-old chinese preschoolers: the Shenzhen Kindergarten Eye Study. Ophthalmology. 2017;124:1826–38.
76. Mutti DO, Sinnott LT, Lynn Mitchell G, Jordan LA, Friedman NE, Frane SL, et al. Ocular component development during infancy and early childhood. Optom Vis Sci. 2018;95:976–85.
77. Wen G, Tarczy-Hornoch K, McKean-Cowdin R, Cotter SA, Borchert M, Lin J, et al. Prevalence of myopia, hyperopia, and astigmatism in non-Hispanic white and Asian children: multi-ethnic pediatric eye disease study. Ophthalmology. 2013;120:2109–16.
78. Zylbermann R, Landau D, Berson D. The influence of study habits on myopia in Jewish teenagers. J Pediatr Ophthalmol Strabismus. 1993;30:319–22.
79. Paternoster L, Tilling K, Smith GD. Genetic epidemiology and Mendelian randomization for informing disease therapeutics: conceptual and methodological challenges. PLoS Genet. 2017;13:e1006944.
80. Smith GD, Ebrahim S. Mendelian randomization: prospects, potentials, and limitations. Int J Epidemiol. 2004;33:30–42.
81. Cuellar-Partida G, Lu Y, Kho PF, Hewitt AW, Wichmann HE, Yazar S, et al. Assessing the genetic predisposition of education on myopia: a Mendelian randomization study. Genet Epidemiol. 2016;40:66–72.
82. Cuellar-Partida G, Williams KM, Yazar S, Guggenheim JA, Hewitt AW, Williams C, et al. Genetically low vitamin D concentrations and myopic refractive error: a Mendelian randomization study. Int J Epidemiol. 2017;46:1882–90.
83. Mountjoy E, Davies N, Plotnikov D, Davey Smith G, Rodriguez S, Williams C, Guggenheim J, Atan D. Education and myopia: a Mendelian randomisation study. BMJ. 2018;361:k2022.

84. Curtin BJ. The myopias: basic science and clinical management. Philadelphia: Harper and Row; 1985.
85. Lee H, Herbert RD, McAuley JH. Mediation analysis. JAMA. 2019;321(7):697–8.
86. Brotman DJ, Walker E, Lauer MS, O'Brien RG. In search of fewer independent risk factors. Arch Intern Med. 2005;165:138–45.
87. Saw SM, Tan SB, Fung D, Chia KS, Koh D, Tan DT, et al. IQ and the association with myopia in children. Invest Ophthalmol Vis Sci. 2004;45:2943–8.
88. Saw SM, Cheng A, Fong A, Gazzard G, Tan DT, Morgan I. School grades and myopia. Ophthalmic Physiol Opt. 2007;27:126–9.
89. Shayer M, Ginsburg D. Thirty years on--a large anti-Flynn effect? (II): 13- and 14-year-olds. Piagetian tests of formal operations norms 1976-2006/7. Br J Educ Psychol. 2009;79: 409–18.
90. Shayer M, Ginsburg D, Coe R. Thirty years on - a large anti-Flynn effect? The Piagetian test volume & heaviness norms 1975-2003. Br J Educ Psychol. 2007;77:25–41.
91. Sauce B, Matzel LD. The paradox of intelligence: heritability and malleability coexist in hidden gene-environment interplay. Psychol Bull. 2018;144:26–47.
92. Williams KM, Hysi PG, Yonova-Doing E, Mahroo OA, Snieder H, Hammond CJ. Phenotypic and genotypic correlation between myopia and intelligence. Sci Rep. 2017;7:45977.
93. Au Eong KG, Tay TH, Lim MK. Education and myopia in 110,236 young Singaporean males. Singap Med J. 1993;34:489–92.
94. Lee KE, Klein BE, Klein R, Wong TY. Changes in refraction over 10 years in an adult population: the Beaver Dam Eye study. Invest Ophthalmol Vis Sci. 2002;43:2566–71.
95. Quek TP, Chua CG, Chong CS, Chong JH, Hey HW, Lee J, et al. Prevalence of refractive errors in teenage high school students in Singapore. Ophthalmic Physiol Opt. 2004;24:47–55.
96. French AN, Morgan IG, Burlutsky G, Mitchell P, Rose KA. Prevalence and 5- to 6-year incidence and progression of myopia and hyperopia in Australian schoolchildren. Ophthalmology. 2013;120:1482–91.
97. Ma Y, Qu X, Zhu X, Xu X, Zhu J, Sankaridurg P, et al. Age-specific prevalence of visual impairment and refractive error in children aged 3-10 years in Shanghai, China. Invest Ophthalmol Vis Sci. 2016;57:6188–96.
98. Tsai DC, Fang SY, Huang N, Hsu CC, Chen SY, Chiu AW, et al. Myopia development among young schoolchildren: the myopia investigation study in Taipei. Invest Ophthalmol Vis Sci. 2016;57:6852–60.
99. Morgan IG, Rose KA. Myopia and international educational performance. Ophthalmic Physiol Opt. 2013;33:329–38.
100. Ip JM, Saw SM, Rose KA, Morgan IG, Kifley A, Wang JJ, et al. Role of near work in myopia: findings in a sample of Australian school children. Invest Ophthalmol Vis Sci. 2008;49:2903–10.
101. Huang HM, Chang DS, Wu PC. The association between near work activities and myopia in children-a systematic review and meta-analysis. PLoS One. 2015;10:e0140419.
102. Wildsoet C. Neural pathways subserving negative lens-induced emmetropization in chicks--insights from selective lesions of the optic nerve and ciliary nerve. Curr Eye Res. 2003;27:371–85.
103. McBrien NA, Moghaddam HO, New R, Williams LR. Experimental myopia in a diurnal mammal (Sciurus carolinensis) with no accommodative ability. J Physiol. 1993;469: 427–41.
104. McBrien NA, Moghaddam HO, Reeder AP. Atropine reduces experimental myopia and eye enlargement via a nonaccommodative mechanism. Invest Ophthalmol Vis Sci. 1993;34:205–15.
105. Mutti DO, Mitchell GL, Hayes JR, Jones LA, Moeschberger ML, Cotter SA, et al. Accommodative lag before and after the onset of myopia. Invest Ophthalmol Vis Sci. 2006;47:837–46.
106. Smith EL. Prentice award lecture 2010: a case for peripheral optical treatment strategies for myopia. Optom Vis Sci. 2011;88:1029–44.

107. Hoogerheide J, Rempt F, Hoogenboom WP. Acquired myopia in young pilots. Ophthalmologica. 1971;163:209–15.
108. Smith EL, Hung LF, Huang J. Relative peripheral hyperopic defocus alters central refractive development in infant monkeys. Vis Res. 2009;49:2386–92.
109. Atchison DA, Rosen R. The possible role of peripheral refraction in development of myopia. Optom Vis Sci. 2016;93:1042–4.
110. Sng CC, Lin XY, Gazzard G, Chang B, Dirani M, Lim L, et al. Change in peripheral refraction over time in Singapore Chinese children. Invest Ophthalmol Vis Sci. 2011;52:7880–7.
111. Smith EL, Hung LF, Huang J, Arumugam B. Effects of local myopic defocus on refractive development in monkeys. Optom Vis Sci. 2013;90:1176–86.
112. Aleman AC, Wang M, Schaeffel F. Reading and myopia: contrast polarity matters. Sci Rep. 2018;8:10840.
113. Boelen MK, Boelen MG, Marshak DW. Light-stimulated release of dopamine from the primate retina is blocked by 1-2-amino-4-phosphonobutyric acid (APB). Vis Neurosci. 1998;15:97–103.
114. Iuvone PM, Tigges M, Stone RA, Lambert S, Laties AM. Effects of apomorphine, a dopamine receptor agonist, on ocular refraction and axial elongation in a primate model of myopia. Invest Ophthalmol Vis Sci. 1991;32:1674–7.
115. McCarthy CS, Megaw P, Devadas M, Morgan IG. Dopaminergic agents affect the ability of brief periods of normal vision to prevent form-deprivation myopia. Exp Eye Res. 2007;84:100–7.
116. French AN, Ashby RS, Morgan IG, Rose KA. Time outdoors and the prevention of myopia. Exp Eye Res. 2013;114:58–68.
117. Xiong S, Sankaridurg P, Naduvilath T, Zang J, Zou H, Zhu J, et al. Time spent in outdoor activities in relation to myopia prevention and control: a meta-analysis and systematic review. Acta Ophthalmol. 2017;95:551–66.
118. Rose KA, Morgan IG, Ip J, Kifley A, Huynh S, Smith W, et al. Outdoor activity reduces the prevalence of myopia in children. Ophthalmology. 2008;115:1279–85.
119. Jones LA, Sinnott LT, Mutti DO, Mitchell GL, Moeschberger ML, Zadnik K. Parental history of myopia, sports and outdoor activities, and future myopia. Invest Ophthalmol Vis Sci. 2007;48:3524–32.
120. Wu PC, Chen CT, Lin KK, Sun CC, Kuo CN, Huang HM, et al. Myopia prevention and outdoor light intensity in a school-based cluster randomized trial. Ophthalmology. 2018;125:1239–50.
121. Wu PC, Tsai CL, Hu CH, Yang YH. Effects of outdoor activities on myopia among rural school children in Taiwan. Ophthalmic Epidemiol. 2010;17:338–42.
122. Ashby R, Ohlendorf A, Schaeffel F. The effect of ambient illuminance on the development of deprivation myopia in chicks. Invest Ophthalmol Vis Sci. 2009;50:5348–54.
123. Ashby RS, Schaeffel F. The effect of bright light on lens compensation in chicks. Invest Ophthalmol Vis Sci. 2010;51:5247–53.
124. Karouta C, Ashby RS. Correlation between light levels and the development of deprivation myopia. Invest Ophthalmol Vis Sci. 2015;56:299–309.
125. Smith EL, Hung LF, Arumugam B, Huang J. Negative lens-induced myopia in infant monkeys: effects of high ambient lighting. Invest Ophthalmol Vis Sci. 2013;54:2959–69.
126. Smith EL, Hung LF, Huang J. Protective effects of high ambient lighting on the development of form-deprivation myopia in rhesus monkeys. Invest Ophthalmol Vis Sci. 2012;53:421–8.
127. Guggenheim JA, Williams C, Northstone K, Howe LD, Tilling K, St Pourcain B, et al. Does vitamin D mediate the protective effects of time outdoors on myopia? Findings from a prospective birth cohort. Invest Ophthalmol Vis Sci. 2014;55:8550–8.
128. Read SA, Collins MJ, Vincent SJ. Light exposure and eye growth in childhood. Invest Ophthalmol Vis Sci. 2015;56:6779–87.
129. Hua WJ, Jin JX, Wu XY, Yang JW, Jiang X, Gao GP, et al. Elevated light levels in schools have a protective effect on myopia. Ophthalmic Physiol Opt. 2015;35:252–62.

130. Jones-Jordan LA, Sinnott LT, Cotter SA, Kleinstein RN, Manny RE, Mutti DO, et al. Time outdoors, visual activity, and myopia progression in juvenile-onset myopes. Invest Ophthalmol Vis Sci. 2012;53:7169–75.
131. Cui D, Trier K, Munk R-MS. Effect of day length on eye growth, myopia progression, and change of corneal power in myopic children. Ophthalmology. 2013;120:1074–9.
132. Deng L, Gwiazda J, Thorn F. Children's refractions and visual activities in the school year and summer. Optom Vis Sci. 2010;87:406–13.
133. Deng L, Pang Y. The role of outdoor activity in myopia prevention. Eye Sci. 2015;30: 137–9.
134. Donovan L, Sankaridurg P, Ho A, Chen X, Lin Z, Thomas V, et al. Myopia progression in Chinese children is slower in summer than in winter. Optom Vis Sci. 2012;89:1196–202.
135. Gwiazda J, Deng L, Manny R, Norton TT, Group CS. Seasonal variations in the progression of myopia in children enrolled in the correction of myopia evaluation trial. Invest Ophthalmol Vis Sci. 2014;55:752–8.
136. Sanchez-Tocino H, Villanueva Gomez A, Gordon Bolanos C, Alonso Alonso I, Vallelado Alvarez A, Garcia Zamora M, et al. The effect of light and outdoor activity in natural lighting on the progression of myopia in children. J Fr Ophtalmol. 2019;42:2–10.
137. Dirani M, Crowston JG, Wong TY. From reading books to increased smart device screen time. Br J Ophthalmol. 2019;103:1–2.
138. Saxena R, Vashist P, Tandon R, Pandey RM, Bhardawaj A, Gupta V, et al. Incidence and progression of myopia and associated factors in urban school children in Delhi: The North India Myopia Study (NIM Study). PLoS One. 2017;12:e0189774.
139. Ojaimi E, Robaei D, Rochtchina E, Rose KA, Morgan IG, Mitchell P. Impact of birth parameters on eye size in a population-based study of 6-year-old Australian children. Am J Ophthalmol. 2005;140:535–7.
140. He M, Huang W, Li Y, Zheng Y, Yin Q, Foster PJ. Refractive error and biometry in older Chinese adults: the Liwan eye study. Invest Ophthalmol Vis Sci. 2009;50:5130–6.
141. He M, Zeng J, Liu Y, Xu J, Pokharel GP, Ellwein LB. Refractive error and visual impairment in urban children in Southern China. Invest Ophthalmol Vis Sci. 2004;45:793–9.
142. Edwards MH. Effect of parental myopia on the development of myopia in Hong Kong Chinese. Ophthalmic Physiol Opt. 1998;18:477–83.
143. Ip JM, Huynh SC, Robaei D, Rose KA, Morgan IG, Smith W, et al. Ethnic differences in the impact of parental myopia: findings from a population-based study of 12-year-old Australian children. Invest Ophthalmol Vis Sci. 2007;48:2520–8.
144. Liang CL, Yen E, Su JY, Liu C, Chang TY, Park N, et al. Impact of family history of high myopia on level and onset of myopia. Invest Ophthalmol Vis Sci. 2004;45:3446–52.
145. Mutti DO, Mitchell GL, Moeschberger ML, Jones LA, Zadnik K. Parental myopia, near work, school achievement, and children's refractive error. Invest Ophthalmol Vis Sci. 2002;43:3633–40.
146. Xiang F, He M, Morgan IG. The impact of parental myopia on myopia in Chinese children: population-based evidence. Optom Vis Sci. 2012;89:1487–96.
147. Xiang F, He M, Morgan IG. The impact of severity of parental myopia on myopia in Chinese children. Optom Vis Sci. 2012;89:884–91.
148. Wu MM, Edwards MH. The effect of having myopic parents: an analysis of myopia in three generations. Optom Vis Sci. 1999;76:387–92.
149. Ghorbani Mojarrad N, Williams C, Guggenheim JA. A genetic risk score and number of myopic parents independently predict myopia. Ophthalmic Physiol Opt. 2018;38:492–502.
150. Rosner M, Belkin M. Intelligence, education, and myopia in males. Arch Ophthalmol. 1987;105:1508–11.
151. Ip JM, Rose KA, Morgan IG, Burlutsky G, Mitchell P. Myopia and the urban environment: findings in a sample of 12-year-old Australian school children. Invest Ophthalmol Vis Sci. 2008;49:3858–63.
152. Zhang M, Li L, Chen L, Lee J, Wu J, Yang A, et al. Population density and refractive error among Chinese children. Invest Ophthalmol Vis Sci. 2010;51:4969–76.

153. Dadvand P, Sunyer J, Alvarez-Pedrerol M, Dalmau-Bueno A, Esnaola M, Gascon M, et al. Green spaces and spectacles use in schoolchildren in Barcelona. Environ Res. 2017;152:256–62.
154. Dadvand P, Nieuwenhuijsen MJ, Basagana X, Alvarez-Pedrerol M, Dalmau-Bueno A, Cirach M, et al. Traffic-related air pollution and spectacles use in schoolchildren. PLoS One. 2017;12:e0167046.
155. Choi KY, Yu WY, Lam CHI, Li ZC, Chin MP, Lakshmanan Y, et al. Childhood exposure to constricted living space: a possible environmental threat for myopia development. Ophthalmic Physiol Opt. 2017;37:568–75.
156. Saw SM, Chua WH, Hong CY, Wu HM, Chia KS, Stone RA, et al. Height and its relationship to refraction and biometry parameters in Singapore Chinese children. Invest Ophthalmol Vis Sci. 2002;43:1408–13.
157. Rosner M, Laor A, Belkin M. Myopia and stature: findings in a population of 106,926 males. Eur J Ophthalmol. 1995;5:1–6.
158. Bann D, Johnson W, Li L, Kuh D, Hardy R. Socioeconomic inequalities in childhood and adolescent body-mass index, weight, and height from 1953 to 2015: an analysis of four longitudinal, observational, British birth cohort studies. Lancet Public Health. 2018;3: e194–203.
159. Cordain L, Eaton SB, Brand Miller J, Lindeberg S, Jensen C. An evolutionary analysis of the aetiology and pathogenesis of juvenile-onset myopia. Acta Ophthalmol Scand. 2002;80:125–35.
160. Jee D, Morgan IG, Kim EC. Inverse relationship between sleep duration and myopia. Acta Ophthalmol. 2016;94:e204–10.
161. Zhou Z, Morgan IG, Chen Q, Jin L, He M, Congdon N. Disordered sleep and myopia risk among Chinese children. PLoS One. 2015;10:e0121796.
162. Ayaki M, Torii H, Tsubota K, Negishi K. Decreased sleep quality in high myopia children. Sci Rep. 2016;6:33902.
163. Kearney S, O'Donoghue L, Pourshahidi LK, Cobice D, Saunders KJ. Myopes have significantly higher serum melatonin concentrations than non-myopes. Ophthalmic Physiol Opt. 2017;37:557–67.
164. Chakraborty R, Ostrin LA, Nickla DL, Iuvone PM, Pardue MT, Stone RA. Circadian rhythms, refractive development, and myopia. Ophthalmic Physiol Opt. 2018;38:217–45.
165. Saw SM, Chia KS, Lindstrom JM, Tan DT, Stone RA. Childhood myopia and parental smoking. Br J Ophthalmol. 2004;88:934–7.
166. Iyer JV, Low WC, Dirani M, Saw SM. Parental smoking and childhood refractive error: the STARS study. Eye. 2012;26:1324–8.
167. Stone RA, Wilson LB, Ying GS, Liu C, Criss JS, Orlow J, et al. Associations between childhood refraction and parental smoking. Invest Ophthalmol Vis Sci. 2006;47:4277–87.
168. Nam GE, Hwang BE, Lee YC, Paik JS, Yang SW, Chun YH, et al. Lower urinary cotinine level is associated with a trend toward more myopic refractive errors in Korean adolescents. Eye. 2017;31:1060–7.
169. Booth AJ, Kee HJ. Birth order matters. The effect of family size and birth order on educational attainment. J Popul Econ. 2009;22:367–97.
170. Guggenheim JA, Williams C, UK Biobank Eye and Vision Consortium. Role of educational exposure in the association between myopia and birth order. JAMA Ophthalmol. 2015;133:1408–14.
171. Zhao L, Zhou M. Do only children have poor vision? Evidence from China's one-child policy. Health Econ. 2018;27:1131–46.
172. Mandel Y, Grotto I, El-Yaniv R, Belkin M, Israeli E, Polat U, et al. Season of birth, natural light, and myopia. Ophthalmology. 2008;115:686–92.
173. McMahon G, Zayats T, Chen YP, Prashar A, Williams C, Guggenheim JA. Season of birth, daylight hours at birth, and high myopia. Ophthalmology. 2009;116:468–73.
174. Herbort CP, Papadia M, Neri P. Myopia and inflammation. J Ophthalmic Vis Res. 2011;6:270–83.

175. Lin HJ, Wei CC, Chang CY, Chen TH, Hsu YA, Hsieh YC, et al. Role of chronic inflammation in myopia progression: clinical evidence and experimental validation. EBioMedicine. 2016;10:269–81.
176. Wei CC, Kung YJ, Chen CS, Chang CY, Lin CJ, Tien PT, et al. Allergic conjunctivitis-induced retinal inflammation promotes myopia progression. EBioMedicine. 2018;28:274–86.
177. Shafer BM, Qiu M, Rapuano CJ, Shields CL. Association between hay fever and high myopia in United States adolescents and adults. Eye Contact Lens. 2017;43:186–91.
178. Kung YJ, Wei CC, Chen LA, Chen JY, Chang CY, Lin CJ, et al. Kawasaki disease increases the incidence of myopia. Biomed Res Int. 2017;2017:2657913.
179. Ait-Khaled N, Pearce N, Anderson HR, Ellwood P, Montefort S, Shah J, et al. Global map of the prevalence of symptoms of rhinoconjunctivitis in children: The International Study of Asthma and Allergies in Childhood (ISAAC) phase three. Allergy. 2009;64:123–48.
180. Gordon-Shaag A, Millodot M, Kaiserman I, Sela T, Barnett Itzhaki G, Zerbib Y, et al. Risk factors for keratoconus in Israel: a case-control study. Ophthalmic Physiol Opt. 2015;35:673–81.
181. Guggenheim JA, Williams C, Eye UKB, Vision C. Childhood febrile illness and the risk of myopia in UK Biobank participants. Eye. 2016;30:608–14.
182. Morgan RW, Munro M. Refractive problems in Northern natives. Can J Ophthalmol. 1973;8:226–8.
183. Morgan RW, Speakman JS, Grimshaw SE. Inuit myopia: an environmentally induced "epidemic"? Can Med Assoc J. 1975;112:575–7.
184. Young FA, Leary GA, Baldwin WR, West DC, Box RA, Harris E, et al. The transmission of refractive errors within eskimo families. Am J Optom Arch Am Acad Optom. 1969;46:676–85.
185. Pokharel GP, Negrel AD, Munoz SR, Ellwein LB. Refractive error study in children: results from Mechi zone, Nepal. Am J Ophthalmol. 2000;129:436–44.
186. Verhoeven VJ, Hysi PG, Wojciechowski R, Fan Q, Guggenheim JA, Hohn R, et al. Genome-wide meta-analyses of multiancestry cohorts identify multiple new susceptibility loci for refractive error and myopia. Nat Genet. 2013;45:314–8.
187. Chua SY, Sabanayagam C, Cheung YB, Chia A, Valenzuela RK, Tan D, et al. Age of onset of myopia predicts risk of high myopia in later childhood in myopic Singapore children. Ophthalmic Physiol Opt. 2016;36:388–94.
188. Lan W, Zhao F, Lin L, Li Z, Zeng J, Yang Z, et al. Refractive errors in 3-6 year-old Chinese children: a very low prevalence of myopia? PLoS One. 2013;8:e78003.
189. Verhoeven VJ, Buitendijk GH, Consortium for Refractive E, Myopia, Rivadeneira F, Uitterlinden AG, et al. Education influences the role of genetics in myopia. Eur J Epidemiol. 2013;28:973–80.
190. Rothman KJ. Synergy and antagonism in cause-effect relationships. Am J Epidemiol. 1974;99:385–8.
191. Rothman KJ. The estimation of synergy or antagonism. Am J Epidemiol. 1976;103:506–11.
192. Rothman KJ. Estimation versus detection in the assessment of synergy. Am J Epidemiol. 1978;108:9–11.
193. Cortina-Borja M, Smith AD, Combarros O, Lehmann DJ. The synergy factor: a statistic to measure interactions in complex diseases. BMC Res Notes. 2009;2:105.
194. Fan Q, Guo X, Tideman JW, Williams KM, Yazar S, Hosseini SM, et al. Childhood gene-environment interactions and age-dependent effects of genetic variants associated with refractive error and myopia: The CREAM Consortium. Sci Rep. 2016;6:25853.
195. Fan Q, Verhoeven VJ, Wojciechowski R, Barathi VA, Hysi PG, Guggenheim JA, et al. Meta-analysis of gene-environment-wide association scans accounting for education level identifies additional loci for refractive error. Nat Commun. 2016;7:11008.
196. Fan Q, Wojciechowski R, Kamran Ikram M, Cheng CY, Chen P, Zhou X, et al. Education influences the association between genetic variants and refractive error: a meta-analysis of five Singapore studies. Hum Mol Genet. 2014;23:546–54.
197. Tkatchenko AV, Tkatchenko TV, Guggenheim JA, Verhoeven VJ, Hysi PG, Wojciechowski R, et al. APLP2 regulates refractive error and myopia development in mice and humans. PLoS Genet. 2015;11:e1005432.

198. Xu L, Li J, Cui T, Hu A, Fan G, Zhang R, et al. Refractive error in urban and rural adult Chinese in Beijing. Ophthalmology. 2005;112(10):1676–83.
199. Mutti DO, Sinnott LT, Mitchell GL, Jones-Jordan LA, Moeschberger ML, Cotter SA, et al. Relative peripheral refractive error and the risk of onset and progression of myopia in children. Invest Ophthalmol Vis Sci. 2011;52(1):199–205.
200. Xiang F, He M, Morgan IG. Annual changes in refractive errors and ocular components before and after the onset of myopia in Chinese children. Ophthalmology. 2012;119(7):1478–84.
201. Thorn F, Gwiazda J, Held R. Myopia progression is specified by a double exponential growth function. Optom Vis Sci. 2005;82(4):286–97.

7

Onset of Myopia: Strategies of Prevention and Delay

Mingguang He, Yanxian Chen, and Yin Hu

Key Points

- Time spent outdoors is well recognized as a factor preventing the development of myopia onset, and measures including adding an outdoor class, locking classroom doors during class recess, or glassed roof and walls incorporated in a classroom have been developed. But promotion to increase time spent outdoors as a school-based intervention program remains challenging especially in East Asia.
- Near work activity has been suggested as a risk factor for myopia although the evidence is not entirely consistent. The total duration of near work activity may not be as important as the type of near work activity. Core techniques to implementing interventions of near work activities include effective measures of near work-related parameters, real-time data analyses, and alert systems.

M. He (✉)
Centre for Eye Research Australia, Royal Victorian Eye and Ear Hospital, Melbourne, VIC, Australia

Ophthalmology, Department of Surgery, University of Melbourne, Melbourne, VIC, Australia

State Key Laboratory of Ophthalmology, National Clinical Research Center, Zhongshan Ophthalmic Center, Sun Yat-sen University, Guangzhou, China

Y. Chen
Shenzhen Key Laboratory of Ophthalmology, Shenzhen Eye Hospital, Shenzhen University, School of Medicine, Shenzhen, China

Y. Hu
State Key Laboratory of Ophthalmology, National Clinical Research Center, Zhongshan Ophthalmic Center, Sun Yat-sen University, Guangzhou, China

- School children growing up in myopigenic environments are likely to benefit from optical interventions designed to induce myopic defocus. The lens with multiple segments of defocus showed promising effect on slowing progression of myopia.
- The Chinese eye exercises of acupoints advocated in mainland China and Taiwan were designed to relieve ocular fatigue and reduce the development and progression of myopia. But clinical significance of its efficacy has not been established according to available data.
- Maximizing the utility of time outdoors is still the priority in the prevention of myopia onset. The role of screen time in myopia development is still ambiguous, the restriction may enable more time for children to go outdoors. Other approaches to prevent myopia onset still require further investigations, such as imposed myopic defocus, low-dose atropine, or some novel pharmacological agents for non-myopes.

7.1 Introduction

Over recent decades, the prevalence of myopia in school-aged children has been increasing significantly in East Asia. Up to 80% of junior high school students have myopia, of which 20% have high myopia in mainland China [1, 2], Hong Kong [3], Taiwan [4], South Korea [5], Japan [6], and Singapore [7]. Longitudinal data suggests that the incidence of myopia is around 10–20% per year among school-aged children [8–11]. If the onset of myopia can be delayed, the prevalence of myopia as well as high myopia in school-aged children will likely reduce. This chapter focuses on the clinical strategy to prevent or delay the onset of myopia among school-aged children, summarizing the interventions currently available, and takes a glance at future perspectives.

7.2 Onset of Myopia

The vast majority of literature suggests that most cases of myopia develop during the school-going age in children. The prevalence of myopia among preschool children is relatively low [12–15]; furthermore, a longitudinal study in Shunyi Beijing demonstrates that the annual incidence of myopia among 5-year-old children is below 5% [16]. After the age of 6 years, the prevalence of myopia starts to rise [6, 16–19]. The highest annual incidence of myopia is reported among school children from urban mainland China [18] and Taiwan [20], ranging from 20% to 30% through ages 7–14 years with earlier onset of myopia also being identified [6]. A study in Japan showed that while the prevalence of myopia has been increasing from 1984 to 1996, the prevalence among children aged 6 or younger has remained unchanged. This suggests that the majority of increased myopia onset is secondary to increased educational intensity and develops when children reach school age (Fig. 7.1) [6].

A long-term longitudinal study has demonstrated that there is a steady shift in refraction toward myopia, before the actual onset of myopia. Rates of progression increase dramatically the year of onset and this has been suggested by spherical equivalent refraction and axial length (Fig. 7.2) [21]. After the first detection of

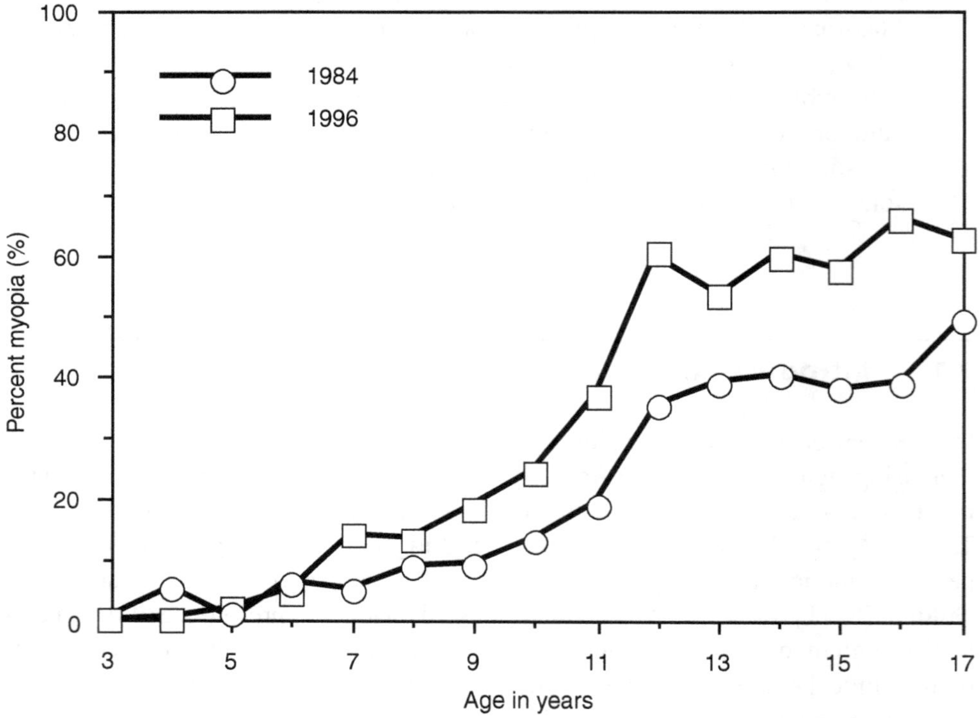

Fig. 7.1 Age-specific prevalence of myopia in Japan in 1984 and 1996. © Matsumura et al. [6]

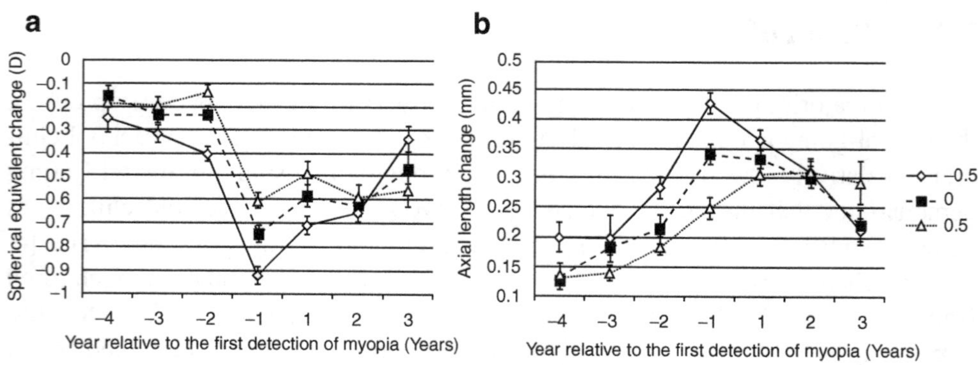

Fig. 7.2 Changes in spherical equivalent refractions (**a**) and axial lengths (**b**) before and after myopia onset. © Xiang et al. [21]

myopia, this acceleration is reduced (Fig. 7.2) [21, 22]. Myopic refractions tend to stabilize in late adolescent but can remain progressive until adulthood. The mean age at myopia stabilization is 15.6 years but this can vary among children of different ethnicities [23].

Several factors have been found to be associated with the development of incident myopia in school. Asian ethnicity [19, 24], parental history of myopia [25, 26], reduced time outdoors [26], and level of near work activity [27, 28] are risk factors for incident myopia, although the evidence can be seen as controversial in some instances. Some studies have also suggested that non-myopic children with less hyperopic refractions and greater axial length/corneal radius of curvature ratios are more predisposed to develop myopia [18, 19]. The impact of gender to the development of myopia varies among populations. In Chinese school children, females have a greater chance of progressing to myopia [18]; while in multiethnic populations, gender seems to be less impactful [19, 24, 27].

Attempts have been made to establish tools to identify children at risk of developing myopia or high myopia. Among numerous associated factors, spherical equivalent refraction is the most promising predictor. By using a single measurement of refraction alone, future myopia onset of non-myopic children can be accurately predicted [29]. Moreover, children at risk of developing high myopia in adulthood can also be identified, with reasonably good sensitivity and specificity, when using an age-specific 5th percentile curve of refraction of the population (Fig. 7.3) as a cutoff [30]. Other promising tools for the prediction of future high myopia include the age of myopia onset [31] and age-specific annual refraction progression of children with myopia (Fig. 7.4) [32]. Information on age of myopia onset alone can predict high myopia with 85% accuracy using a receiver operating curve (ROC) [31].

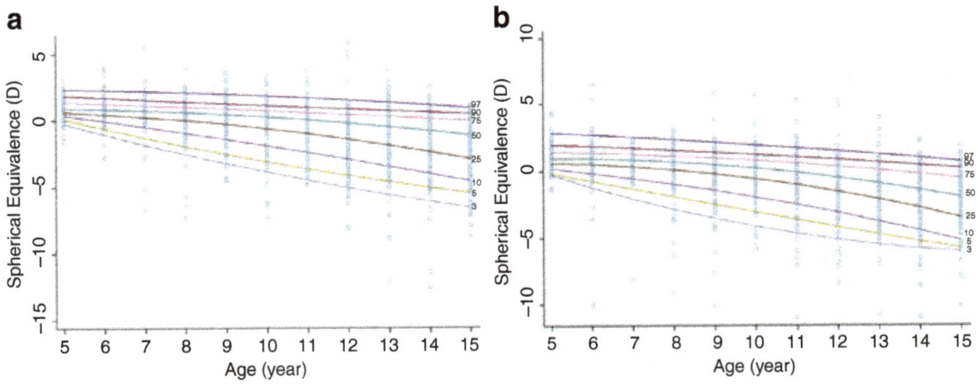

Fig. 7.3 Percentile curves of refractions for urban Chinese boys (**a**) and girls (**b**). © Chen et al. [30]

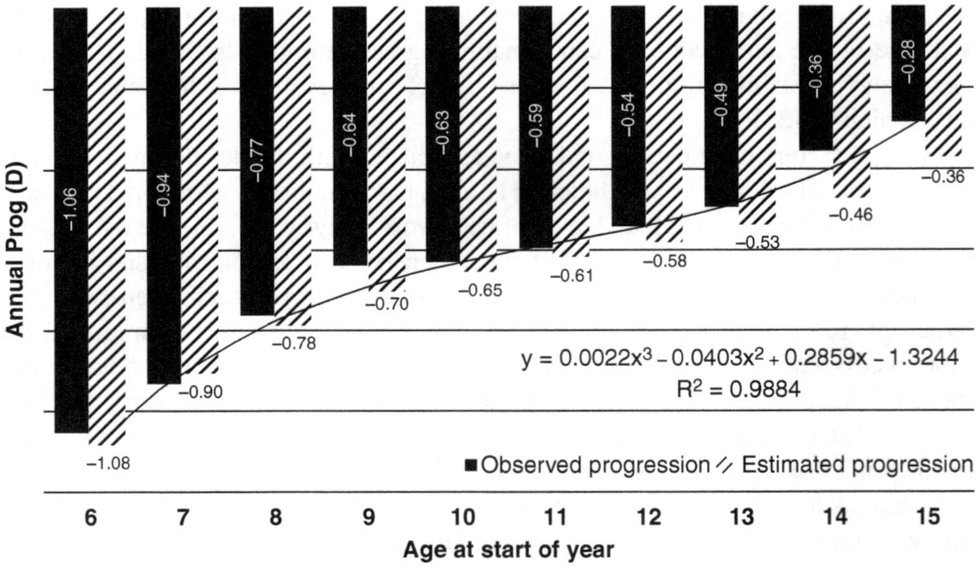

Fig. 7.4 Age-specific annual progression of refraction in children with myopia. © Sankaridurg et al. [32]

7.3 Increased Time Outdoors as an Intervention

Time spent outdoors is well recognized as a factor preventing the development of myopia onset. Evidence of this was first presented in a three-year follow-up study of myopia in school children, showing that those who spent more time outdoors were less likely to progress [33]. Consistent results were reported in various studies, such as the Sydney Myopia Study, Orinda study as well as the Singapore Cohort Study of Risk Factors for Myopia [34–36]. This led to the commencement of several clinical trials, which confirmed the protective effect against myopia and indicated a dose-dependent effect, among them is the randomized clinical trial in Guangzhou which reported that an additional 40 min of outdoor activity can reduce the incidence of myopia by 23%. Additionally, the trial in Taiwan suggested that an extra 80 min may further reduce incidence by 50% [10, 37].

The mechanism of increased outdoor time as an intervention is not completely clear. Spending time outdoors itself, instead of physical activities outdoors, has been suggested to be the major protective factor [38]. Results from animal experiments indicated that protection due to bright light may be mediated by dopamine [39]. Some believe that ultraviolet light also plays an important role [40], with evidence suggesting that there is an association between vitamin D level and myopia [41–43], but data from a population-based cohort did not support this idea [44]. Alternatively, patterns of defocus on the retina by three-dimensional structures of the environment have also been proposed as a possible mechanism of protection from outdoor activities [45].

As an economically feasible intervention, getting children outside the classroom has been promoted in many public health programs such as Taiwan's "Daily 120." However, promotion to increase time spent outdoors as a school-based intervention program remains challenging. First, what is an effective amount of time outdoors? Population-based data suggest that 2–3 h a day would be beneficial [26, 35], however, this is difficult to achieve in some East Asian countries where the education system is very intensive. Some programs recommend adding an outdoor class into the curriculum, while others recommend prohibiting being inside during recess by locking classroom doors. Another group of researchers proposed a classroom design that incorporates a glassed roof and walls that enable maximize light intensity while students study indoors (Fig. 7.5) [46]. The protective effect of this bright classroom is now under investigation. Second, what is the appropriate location for outdoor activities? The ideal location appears to be in an area with bright light more than 10,000 lux, suggested by evidence from animal experiments [47, 48]. But the most recent results from Wu et al.'s study indicated that less bright light exposure, 1000-lux or 3000-lux for instance, is sufficient enough to generate a protective effect (Fig. 7.6) [49]. These findings seem to suggest that an environment such as the shade of a tree or building, the hallway, or playground could still work with an advantage to avoid sunburn or other side effects from UV exposure.

Another concern is how do we measure outdoor activities? Traditionally, questionnaires have been commonly used to measure time outdoors but are less accurate due to recall bias. Objective measures can provide more precise real-time data. Wearable detectors have been developed to record light intensity and time outdoors, and even track the patterns of outdoor activities, including HOBO light meters, Nike+ Fuel Band, and others. Other measures have been used to estimate exposure to natural light such as conjunctival ultraviolet autofluorescence and skin photodamage, but these are more appropriate when measuring the cumulative light dosage or UV exposure [50, 51].

If increased time spent outdoors can prevent or delay the onset of myopia, it would ultimately reduce the prevalence of myopia or even high myopia among

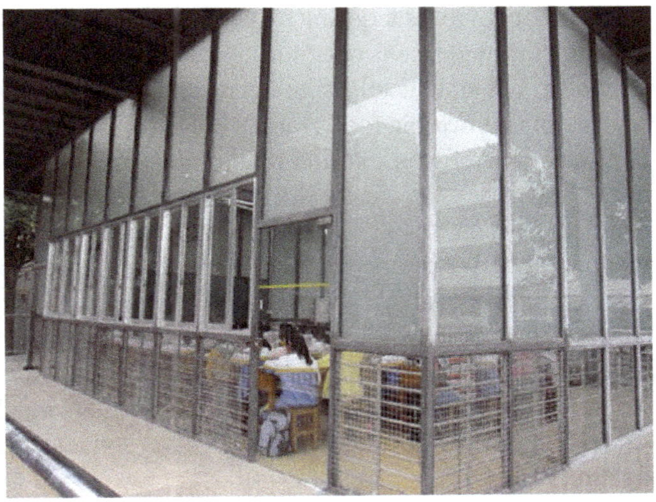

Fig. 7.5 Classroom constructed with glass in China. ©Zhou et al. [46]

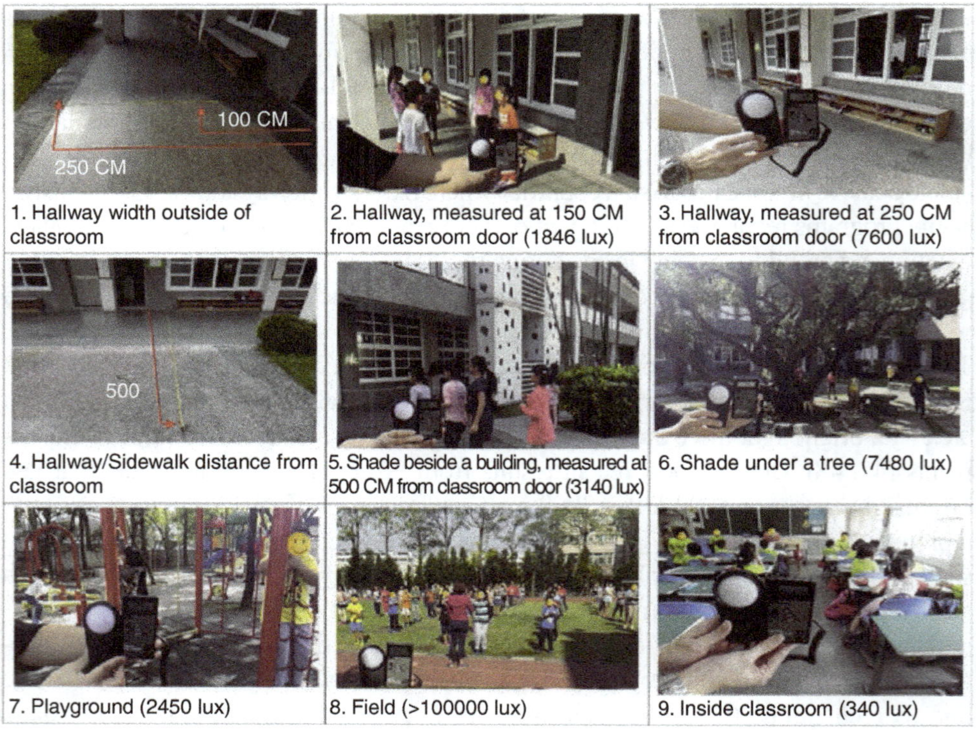

Fig. 7.6 Light intensity of different locations in the school. ©Wu et al. [49]

school-aged children. Documentation on the impact of time spent outdoors on the prevalence of myopia is of public health importance.

7.4 Reduced Near Work Intensity as an Intervention

Near work activity as a risk factor for myopia has been documented in some studies, although the evidence is not entirely consistent. A recent meta-analysis has reported a modest, but statistically significant, association between time spent performing near work and myopia (odds ratio, 1.14) [28].

It has been argued that the total duration of near work activity may not be as important as the type of near work activity. Studies have found that continuous reading of more than 30–45 min is associated with the presence of myopia and greater myopic refractive errors [52, 53]. Interestingly, after prolonged continuous reading, children are more likely to take up their preferred relaxed postures [54], such as close reading distance [53] and head tilt [52], both of which have been reported to be associated with the presence of myopia. Other factors that have been proposed to potentially contribute to the development of myopia include close nib-to-finger distance [52], downward angle of gaze [55, 56] and inadequate desk [52], or classroom lighting [56].

Efforts have been dedicated to developing novel devices to detect and correct inadequate near work behaviors. In mainland China, pens for myopia prevention has been invented. The pens are capable of detecting close reading distances (China Invention Patent, 200620010200.6) or nib-to-finger distances (China Invention Patent, 201020640746.6). Real-time retraction of the nib will occur when the eyes are too close to the reading materials or the nib-to-finger distance is inadequate, compelling children to adopt correct postures. The effect of the pens on preventing myopia onset is to be examined by future clinical trials.

Core techniques to implementing interventions of near work activities include effective measures of near work-related parameters, real-time data analyses, and alert systems. Wearable devices that possess these techniques have emerged in the last decade. A head-mounted instrument (Fig. 7.7) was built in Hong Kong for continuous logging of near work distance [57]. Measurements have proved to be accurate and repeatable over a range of distances and angles [57]. The Clouclip (Fig. 7.8) is another novel device developed in mainland China, primarily for the use of

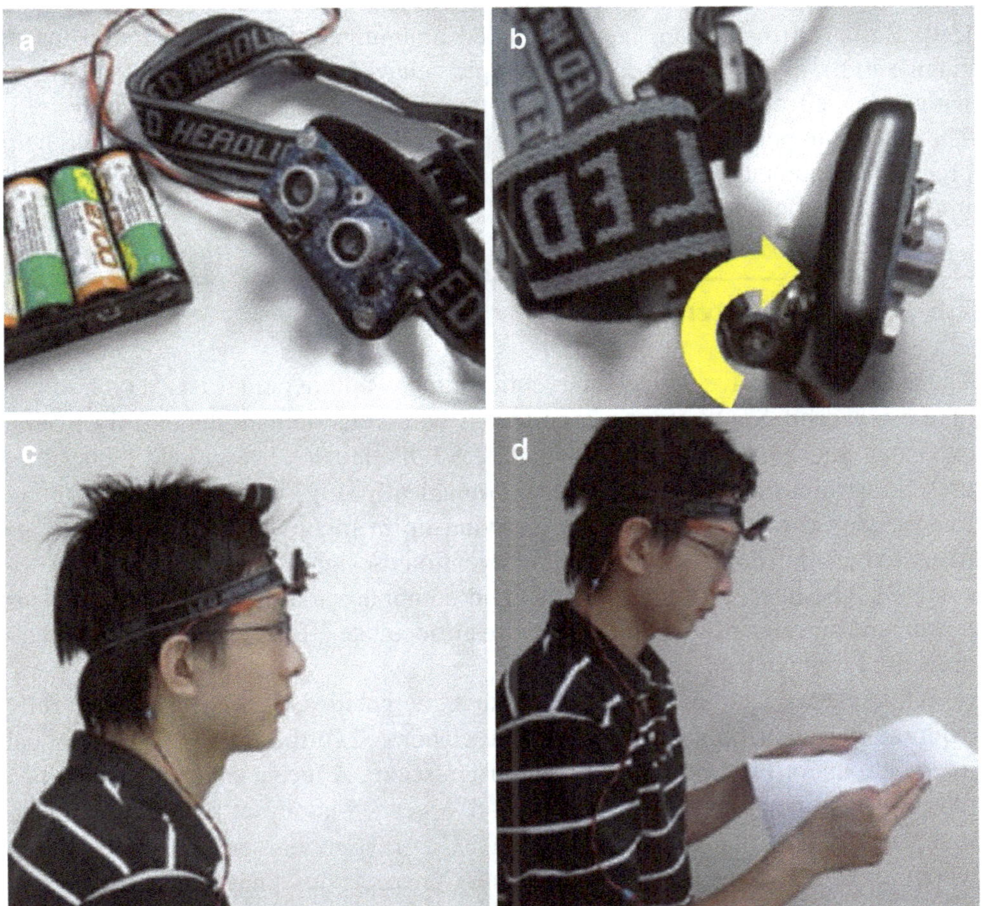

Fig. 7.7 Front view (**a**) and side view (**b**) of the near work analyzer for logging near work distance and its alignment in a straight-ahead position (**c**) and reading position (**d**). © Leung et al. [57]

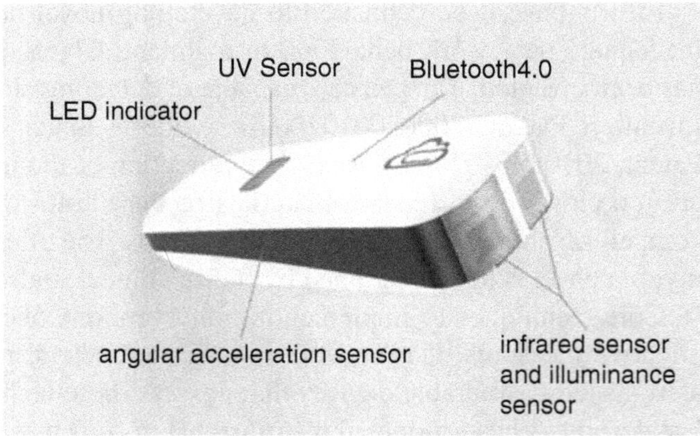

Fig. 7.8 Clouclip to monitor near work time. © Wen et al. [58]

myopic children [58]. The device can measure reading distances and ambient illuminance, perform real-time data analyses, and feedback to children and parents (www.clouclip.com). This group of researchers used Clouclip to track reading distance and eye-level illuminance of children over a representative period of time [59]. Based on these data, they developed a summative index and found that a change in the index toward a more myopic behavior was significantly associated with increased myopic refractive errors in a preliminary longitudinal study [59]. The attempt to generate a simplified, summative index for risk estimation will help provide comprehensive information on near work-related behaviors and may help improve the efficacy of interventions.

7.5 Optical Interventions

The use of noninvasive optical interventions to prevent myopia is based on findings of the powerful STOP signals reported in numerous animal studies. By briefly exposing chickens to myopic defocus (the STOP signals), eye growth induced by presenting minus lenses can be slowed dramatically (Fig. 7.9) [60, 61]. It is therefore suggested that school children growing up in myopigenic environments are likely to benefit from routine optical interventions designed to induce myopic defocus [62]. The intervention regimen should combine variables including age, lens power, and duration of exposure to achieve an adequate effect on delaying the development of myopia [62].

While these optical interventions are an attractive idea, they have not been fully explored in human subjects—this will be elaborated further in Chap. 13 (Optical interventions for Prevention of Myopia Progression). A recent study has prescribed plus lenses to non-myopic children aged 5–8 years who are at risk of developing myopia [63]. The plus lenses imposed a 1.0 D myopic defocus and the children wore the correction the entire day. No cases of myopia onset have been observed in this group of children during the follow-up period (ranging from 3 to 9 years) [63]. The robustness of these study findings needs to be examined by future investigations.

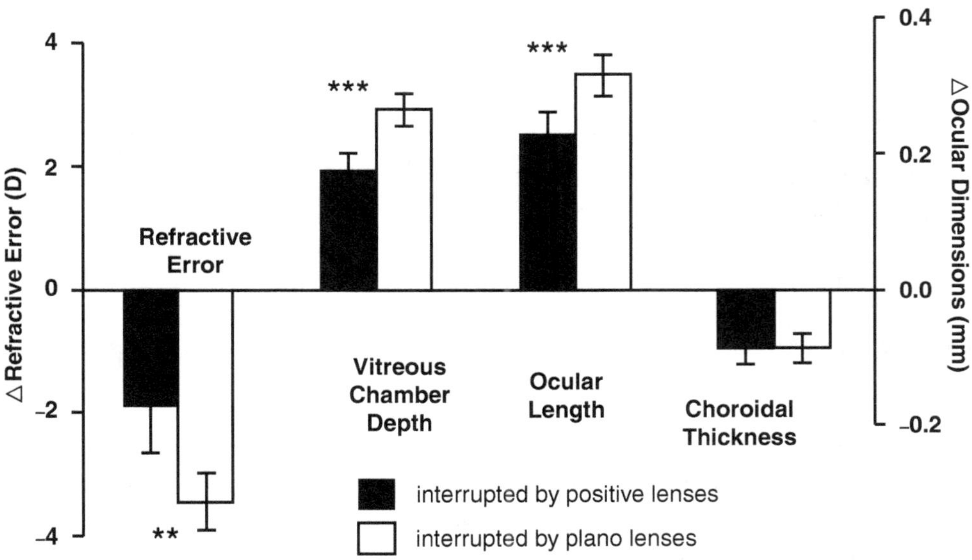

Fig. 7.9 Changes in refractions and ocular biometric parameters over 3 days of binocular negative lens wear interrupted by brief periods of positive lens wear on one eye and plano lens wear on the other eye. $**P < 0.01$; $***P < 0.001$. © Zhu et al. [61]

The Defocus Incorporated Multiple Segments Lens (DIMS Lens) is a novel spectacle lens primarily designed for use in myopic children. The lens is composed of a central zone for optical correction of refractive error and an annular peripheral zone to induce myopic defocus. Interestingly, the lens peripheral zone contains numerous well-arranged small plus lenses, separated by small non-defocus areas. By using this design, myopic defocus is induced and visual quality is well reserved at the same time (presentation at the 16th International Myopia Conference [IMC]). In a pilot study conducted among school children, the DIMS lens slowed progression of myopia by 59% (presentation at the 16th IMC). The lens may also be promising for preventing myopia onset if adaptation can be successfully made for non-myopic children.

7.6 Eye Exercises of Acupoints

The eye exercises of acupoints are a set of bilateral acupoint self-massages designed to relieve ocular fatigue and reduce the development and progression of myopia. These eye exercises were introduced by the Chinese National Education Commission and have been advocated since the 1960s in mainland China and Taiwan. Children in primary and junior middle schools are required to perform the eye exercises twice a day. The 5-min exercises include: (1) knead Tianying (Ashi); (2) press and squeeze Jingming (BL1); (3) press and knead Sibai (ST2); and (4) press Taiyang (EX-HN5) and scrape Cuanzhu (BL2), Yuyao (EX-HN4), Sizhukong (TE23), Tongziliao (GB1), Chengqi (ST1) (Fig. 7.10).

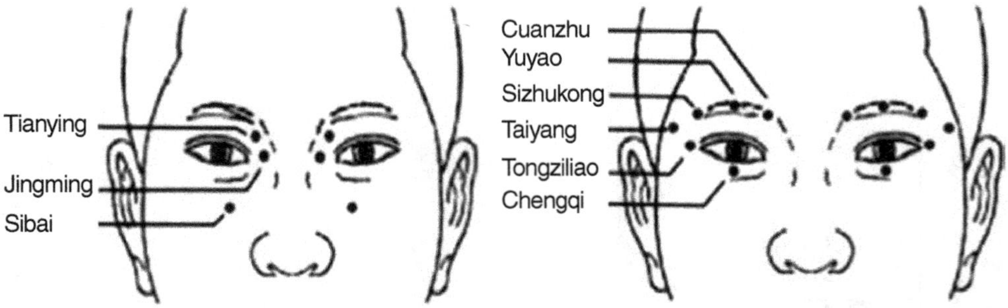

Fig. 7.10 Schematic diagram demonstrating the positions of acupoints used in Chinese eye exercises. © Lin et al. [67]

The efficacy of the Chinese eye exercises is believed to be from the theory of Traditional Chinese Medicine. By massaging the acupoints, Chi can be achieved and help relieve eye strain and recover ocular functions. Peak systolic velocity in the central retinal and ophthalmic arteries is observed after the eye exercises [64], which might provide some evidences to support this theory. Accommodative lag decreases significantly by 0.1 D after 5 min of performing the eye exercises [65].

Clinical significance has never been established in the published literature thus far. Cross-sectional studies have assessed the association between Chinese eye exercises and myopia with varied results [66–69]. The inconsistency can be explained by the different settings studied (rural vs. urban), failure to adjust for potential confounders (including parental myopia, time outdoors, and near work) and the lack of representative populations in some studies. In a recent study, the impact of Chinese eye exercises on the development of myopia has been examined using a longitudinal design [70]. No association between eye exercises and myopia onset has been found [70]. However, due to the limited sample size, low level of intervention time, and performance qualities of the exercises in the study, the actual impact is still not conclusive and needs to be justified by further studies.

7.7 Future Prospects

It has been estimated that without any effective controls or interventions the proportion of myopes in the population will reach up to 50% and 10% for high myopes by 2050 [71]. Approaches that have produced a reduction of at least 50% in incidence, such as time outdoors, have the potential to make a significant difference on the impending myopia epidemic. But the level of impact of the full utility of available interventions needs to be evaluated by further studies.

Another critical issue is how to implement both education intensity and outdoor time interventions in East Asia. There needs to be a balance between educational achievement and interventions delivered, which don't exacerbate the prevalence of myopia in East Asia. This balance can be seen in Australia [72], with some of the highest educational ranks in the world (PISA, https://www.oecd.org/pisa/data/) but

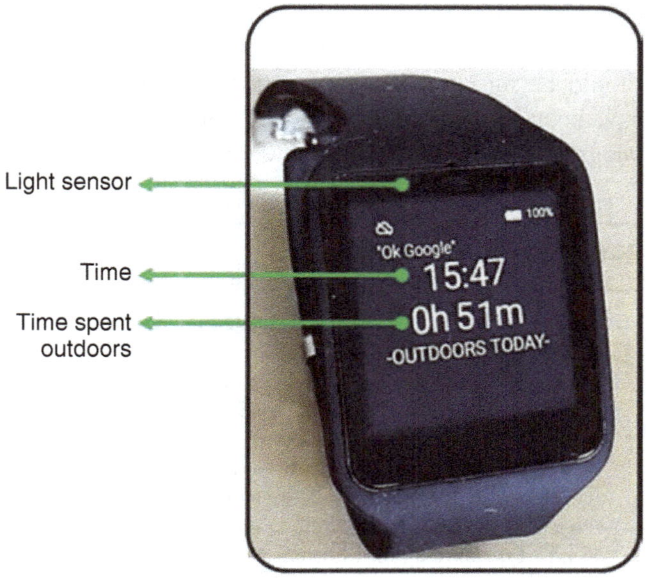

Fig. 7.11 FitSight fitness tracker to record time outdoors. ©Verkicharla et al. [73]

also high levels of outdoor activity and light intensity. Preventing the onset of myopia is certainly challenging in the East Asian population and requires a collaborative effort among clinics, schools, parents, and the entire society.

Nonetheless, maximizing the utility of time outdoors is still the priority in the prevention of myopia onset. The implementation of outdoor activities in school programs and daily life necessitates further propagation and feedback from parents and children. Novel devices combined with the internet and even social networks are a potential direction. An example is FitSight, which was developed by Saw et al. (Fig. 7.11) and comprises of a smartwatch with a light sensor and smartphone app that records time outdoors and sends feedback to parents and children [73]. This kind of devices needs to be proven to be useful by undertaking field study and determining wearability. Additionally, the price of the device should be considered in the design.

Another behavior control method focuses on limiting the screen time on computers, tablets, and smart phones. Though the role of screen time in myopia development is still ambiguous, the restriction may enable more time for children to go outdoors. Applications to provide screen distance and time monitoring, alerts to rest eyes, blue light filters, and remote locking capability for parents are available in some countries (plano, https://www.plano.co/). The effect of this technology on myopia prevention remains to be seen.

Other approaches to prevent myopia onset still require further investigations, such as imposed myopic defocus, low-dose atropine, or some novel pharmacological agents for non-myopes. They may help to prevent myopia in those who are rapidly progressing or have high-risk genetic forms. Thus, a question is raised: how do we identify children that have an increased risk of becoming myopic or highly myopic? Risk estimation is therefore critical to achieve personalized treatment for individuals. For children who are non-myopic but at an increased risk of developing high myopia in the future, additional outdoor activities and aggressive approaches should be introduced with frequent follow-up visits. Tools of myopia prediction have been developed as mentioned before, and we expect to see the outcomes of the integration of risk prediction and clinical practice in the near future.

References

1. Wu LJ, et al. Prevalence and associated factors of myopia in high-school students in Beijing. PLoS One. 2015;10:e0120764. https://doi.org/10.1371/journal.pone.0120764.
2. Wu JF, et al. Refractive error, visual acuity and causes of vision loss in children in Shandong, China. The Shandong Children Eye Study. PLoS One. 2013;8:e82763. https://doi.org/10.1371/journal.pone.0082763.
3. Goh WS, Lam CS. Changes in refractive trends and optical components of Hong Kong Chinese aged 19-39 years. Ophthalmic Physiol Opt. 1994;14:378–82.
4. Lin LL, et al. Epidemiologic study of the prevalence and severity of myopia among schoolchildren in Taiwan in 2000. J Formos Med Assoc. 2001;100:684–91.
5. Jung SK, Lee JH, Kakizaki H, Jee D. Prevalence of myopia and its association with body stature and educational level in 19-year-old male conscripts in Seoul, South Korea. Invest Ophthalmol Vis Sci. 2012;53:5579–83. https://doi.org/10.1167/iovs.12-10106.
6. Matsumura H, Hirai H. Prevalence of myopia and refractive changes in students from 3 to 17 years of age. Surv Ophthalmol. 1999;44(Suppl 1):S109–15.
7. Wu HM, et al. Does education explain ethnic differences in myopia prevalence? A population-based study of young adult males in Singapore. Optom Vis Sci. 2001;78:234–9.
8. Shah RL, Huang Y, Guggenheim JA, Williams C. Time outdoors at specific ages during early childhood and the risk of incident myopia. Invest Ophthalmol Vis Sci. 2017;58:1158–66. https://doi.org/10.1167/iovs.16-20894.
9. Ku P.-W. et al. The associations between near visual activity and incident myopia in children. Ophthalmology. https://doi.org/10.1016/j.ophtha.2018.05.010.
10. He M, et al. Effect of time spent outdoors at school on the development of myopia among children in China: a randomized clinical trial. JAMA. 2015;314:1142–8. https://doi.org/10.1001/jama.2015.10803.
11. Lin LL, Shih YF, Hsiao CK, Chen CJ. Prevalence of myopia in Taiwanese schoolchildren: 1983 to 2000. Ann Acad Med Singap. 2004;33:27–33.
12. Guo X, et al. Significant axial elongation with minimal change in refraction in 3- to 6-year-old Chinese preschoolers: The Shenzhen Kindergarten Eye Study. Ophthalmology. 2017;124:1826–38. https://doi.org/10.1016/j.ophtha.2017.05.030.
13. Giordano L, et al. Prevalence of refractive error among preschool children in an urban population: the Baltimore Pediatric Eye Disease Study. Ophthalmology. 2009;116:739–46. https://doi.org/10.1016/j.ophtha.2008.12.030.
14. Multi-Ethnic Pediatric Eye Disease Study Group. Prevalence of myopia and hyperopia in 6- to 72-month-old african american and Hispanic children: the multi-ethnic pediatric eye disease study. Ophthalmology. 2010;117:140–147.e143. https://doi.org/10.1016/j.ophtha.2009.06.009.
15. Dirani M, et al. Prevalence of refractive error in Singaporean Chinese children: the strabismus, amblyopia, and refractive error in young Singaporean Children (STARS) study. Invest Ophthalmol Vis Sci. 2010;51:1348–55. https://doi.org/10.1167/iovs.09-3587.
16. Zhao J, et al. The progression of refractive error in school-age children: Shunyi district, China. Am J Ophthalmol. 2002;134:735–43.
17. Xiang F, et al. Increases in the prevalence of reduced visual acuity and myopia in Chinese children in Guangzhou over the past 20 years. Eye. 2013;27:1353–8. https://doi.org/10.1038/eye.2013.194.

18. Wang SK, et al. Incidence of and factors associated with myopia and high myopia in Chinese children, based on refraction without cycloplegia. JAMA Ophthalmol. 2018;136:1017–24. https://doi.org/10.1001/jamaophthalmol.2018.2658.
19. Saw SM, et al. Incidence and progression of myopia in Singaporean school children. Invest Ophthalmol Vis Sci. 2005;46:51–7. https://doi.org/10.1167/iovs.04-0565.
20. Tsai DC, et al. Myopia development among young schoolchildren: The Myopia Investigation Study in Taipei. Invest Ophthalmol Vis Sci. 2016;57:6852–60. https://doi.org/10.1167/iovs.16-20288.
21. Xiang F, He M, Morgan IG. Annual changes in refractive errors and ocular components before and after the onset of myopia in Chinese children. Ophthalmology. 2012;119:1478–84. https://doi.org/10.1016/j.ophtha.2012.01.017.
22. Mutti DO, et al. Refractive error, axial length, and relative peripheral refractive error before and after the onset of myopia. Invest Ophthalmol Vis Sci. 2007;48:2510–9. https://doi.org/10.1167/iovs.06-0562.
23. COMET Group. Myopia stabilization and associated factors among participants in the Correction of Myopia Evaluation Trial (COMET). Invest Ophthalmol Vis Sci. 2013;54:7871–84. https://doi.org/10.1167/iovs.13-12403.
24. French AN, Morgan IG, Burlutsky G, Mitchell P, Rose KA. Prevalence and 5- to 6-year incidence and progression of myopia and hyperopia in Australian schoolchildren. Ophthalmology. 2013;120:1482–91. https://doi.org/10.1016/j.ophtha.2012.12.018.
25. Jones-Jordan LA, et al. Early childhood refractive error and parental history of myopia as predictors of myopia. Invest Ophthalmol Vis Sci. 2010;51:115–21. https://doi.org/10.1167/iovs.08-3210.
26. Jones LA, et al. Parental history of myopia, sports and outdoor activities, and future myopia. Invest Ophthalmol Vis Sci. 2007;48:3524–32. https://doi.org/10.1167/iovs.06-1118.
27. Williams C, Miller LL, Gazzard G, Saw SM. A comparison of measures of reading and intelligence as risk factors for the development of myopia in a UK cohort of children. Br J Ophthalmol. 2008;92:1117–21. https://doi.org/10.1136/bjo.2007.128256.
28. Huang HM, Chang DS, Wu PC. The association between near work activities and myopia in children-a systematic review and meta-analysis. PLoS One. 2015;10:e0140419. https://doi.org/10.1371/journal.pone.0140419.
29. Zadnik K, et al. Prediction of juvenile-onset myopia. JAMA Ophthalmol. 2015;133:683–9. https://doi.org/10.1001/jamaophthalmol.2015.0471.
30. Chen Y, Zhang J, Morgan IG, He M. Identifying children at risk of high myopia using population centile curves of refraction. PLoS One. 2016;11:e0167642. https://doi.org/10.1371/journal.pone.0167642.
31. Chua SY, et al. Age of onset of myopia predicts risk of high myopia in later childhood in myopic Singapore children. Ophthalmic Physiol Opt. 2016;36:388–94. https://doi.org/10.1111/opo.12305.
32. Sankaridurg PR, Holden BA. Practical applications to modify and control the development of ametropia. Eye. 2014;28:134–41. https://doi.org/10.1038/eye.2013.255.
33. Parssinen O, Lyyra AL. Myopia and myopic progression among school children: a three-year follow-up study. Invest Ophthalmol Vis Sci. 1993;34:2794–802.
34. Mutti DO, Mitchell GL, Moeschberger ML, Jones LA, Zadnik K. Parental myopia, near work, school achievement, and children's refractive error. Invest Ophthalmol Vis Sci. 2002;43:3633–40.
35. Rose KA, et al. Outdoor activity reduces the prevalence of myopia in children. Ophthalmology. 2008;115:1279–85. https://doi.org/10.1016/j.ophtha.2007.12.019.
36. Dirani M, et al. Outdoor activity and myopia in Singapore teenage children. Br J Ophthalmol. 2009;93:997.
37. Wu PC, Tsai CL, Wu HL, Yang YH, Kuo HK. Outdoor activity during class recess reduces myopia onset and progression in school children. Ophthalmology. 2013;120:1080–5. https://doi.org/10.1016/j.ophtha.2012.11.009.

38. Nina J, Hanne J, Ernst G. Does the level of physical activity in university students influence development and progression of myopia?--a 2-year prospective cohort study. Invest Ophthalmol Vis Sci. 2008;49:1322.
39. Feldkaemper M, Schaeffel F. An updated view on the role of dopamine in myopia. Exp Eye Res. 2013;114:106–19.
40. Prepas SB. Light, literacy and the absence of ultraviolet radiation in the development of myopia. Med Hypotheses. 2008;70:635–7.
41. Jeremy AG, et al. Does vitamin D mediate the protective effects of time outdoors on myopia? Findings from a prospective birth cohort. Invest Ophthalmol Vis Sci. 2015;55:8550–8.
42. Mutti DO, Marks AR. Blood levels of vitamin D in teens and young adults with myopia. Optom Vis Sci. 2011;88:377–82.
43. Tideman JWL, et al. Low serum vitamin D is associated with axial length and risk of myopia in young children. Eur J Epidemiol. 2016;31:491–9.
44. Hammond DS, Josh W, Wildsoet CF. Dynamics of active emmetropisation in young chicks--influence of sign and magnitude of imposed defocus. Ophthalmic Physiol Opt. 2013;33: 215–26.
45. Flitcroft DI. The complex interactions of retinal, optical and environmental factors in myopia aetiology. Prog Retin Eye Res. 2012;31:622–60.
46. Zhou Z, et al. Pilot study of a novel classroom designed to prevent myopia by increasing children's exposure to outdoor light. PLoS One. 2017;12:e0181772. https://doi.org/10.1371/journal.pone.0181772.
47. Cindy K, Regan Scott A. Correlation between light levels and the development of deprivation myopia. Invest Ophthalmol Vis Sci. 2015;56:299–309.
48. Lan W, Yang Z, Feldkaemper M, Schaeffel F. Changes in dopamine and ZENK during suppression of myopia in chicks by intense illuminance. Exp Eye Res. 2016;145:118–24.
49. Wu PC, et al. Myopia prevention and outdoor light intensity in a school-based cluster randomized trial. Ophthalmology. 2018;125(8):1239–50.
50. Mcknight CM, et al. Myopia in young adults is inversely related to an objective marker of ocular sun exposure: The Western Australian Raine Cohort Study. Am J Ophthalmol. 2014;158:1079–1085.e1072.
51. Lingham G, et al. Investigating the long-term impact of a childhood sun-exposure intervention, with a focus on eye health: protocol for the Kidskin-Young Adult Myopia Study. BMJ Open. 2018;8:e020868. https://doi.org/10.1136/bmjopen-2017-020868.
52. Li SM, et al. Near work related parameters and myopia in chinese children: the Anyang Childhood Eye Study. PLoS One. 2015;10:e0134514. https://doi.org/10.1371/journal.pone.0134514.
53. Ip JM, et al. Role of near work in myopia: findings in a sample of Australian school children. Invest Ophthalmol Vis Sci. 2008;49:2903–10. https://doi.org/10.1167/iovs.07-0804.
54. Charman WN. Myopia, posture and the visual environment. Ophthalmic Physiol Opt. 2011;31:494–501. https://doi.org/10.1111/j.1475-1313.2011.00825.x.
55. Vincent SJ, Collins MJ, Read SA, Carney LG, Yap MK. Corneal changes following near work in myopic anisometropia. Ophthalmic Physiol Opt. 2013;33:15–25. https://doi.org/10.1111/opo.12003.
56. Hua WJ, et al. Elevated light levels in schools have a protective effect on myopia. Ophthalmic Physiol Opt. 2015;35:252–62. https://doi.org/10.1111/opo.12207.
57. Leung TW, et al. A novel instrument for logging nearwork distance. Ophthalmic Physiol Opt. 2011;31:137–44. https://doi.org/10.1111/j.1475-1313.2010.00814.x.
58. Wen L, et al. A novel device to record the behavior related to myopia development— preliminary results in the lab. Invest Ophthalmol Vis Sci. 2016;57:2491.
59. Lan WZ, et al. The correlation between an objective index summarizing individual environmental risk factors and the change of refractive error. Invest Ophthalmol Vis Sci. 2018;41:59.
60. Winawer J, Wallman J. Temporal constraints on lens compensation in chicks. Vis Res. 2002;42:2651–68.

61. Zhu X, Winawer JA, Wallman J. Potency of myopic defocus in spectacle lens compensation. Invest Ophthalmol Vis Sci. 2003;44:2818–27.
62. Morgan I, Megaw P. Using natural STOP growth signals to prevent excessive axial elongation and the development of myopia. Ann Acad Med. 2004;33:16–20.
63. Tarutta E, Khodzhabekyan N, Filinova O, Milash S, Kruzhkova G. Long -term effects of optical defocus on eye growth and refractogenesis. Pomeranian J Life Sci. 2016;62:25–30.
64. Lin J. Observation of ocular haemodynamic change pre and post doing the eye exercises using color Doppler flood image. Chin J Ultrasound Diagn. 2004;5:446–7.
65. Li SM, et al. Efficacy of Chinese eye exercises on reducing accommodative lag in school-aged children: a randomized controlled trial. PLoS One. 2015;10:e0117552. https://doi.org/10.1371/journal.pone.0117552.
66. Changjun L, Wang J, Gou H, Jianzhou W. A survey on prevalence of myopia and its influential factors in middle school students. Mod Prev Med. 2010;37:3047–51.
67. Lin Z, et al. Eye exercises of acupoints: their impact on refractive error and visual symptoms in Chinese urban children. BMC Complement Altern Med. 2013;13:306. https://doi.org/10.1186/1472-6882-13-306.
68. Lin Z, et al. Eye exercises of acupoints: their impact on myopia and visual symptoms in Chinese rural children. BMC Complement Altern Med. 2016;16:349. https://doi.org/10.1186/s12906-016-1289-4.
69. Ping Z, Wang K, Chunhua Z, Bin Z. The epidemiological investigation of myopia in junior students. Prac J Med Pharm. 2004;21:543–5.
70. Kang MT, et al. Chinese eye exercises and myopia development in school age children: a Nested Case-Control Study. Sci Rep. 2016;6:28531. https://doi.org/10.1038/srep28531.
71. Holden BA, et al. Global prevalence of myopia and high myopia and temporal trends from 2000 through 2050. Ophthalmology. 2016;123:1036–42. https://doi.org/10.1016/j.ophtha.2016.01.006.
72. Morgan IG. New perspectives on the prevention of myopia. Eye Sci. 2011;26:3.
73. Verkicharla PK, et al. Development of the fitsight fitness tracker to increase time outdoors to prevent myopia. Transl Vis Sci Technol. 2017;6:20.

8

Myopia in Children: Clinical Treatment Strategies

Audrey Chia and Su Ann Tay

Key Points

- Our understanding of the pathogenesis and etiology of myopia continues to evolve, and with it, various interventions that prevent or slow the progression of myopia. These include the use of bifocal spectacles, peripheral defocus spectacles and contact lenses, orthokeratology contact lenses, atropine and environmental interventions.
- With various interventions available for myopia control, understanding the effectiveness, safety profile and cost of each intervention can aid the clinician in making collective decisions with patients and their families on the most appropriate intervention for each child.
- An atropine-based protocol for the treatment of myopia developed based on evidence from studies collected thus far is discussed. This includes assessment of risk factors for myopia progression, factors to consider when starting atropine, monitoring response to atropine treatment and factors to consider before cessation of treatment.
- It is important that there is continued assessment of the long-term effect and value of these treatments in preventing high myopia and its associated complications.

A. Chia (✉) · S. A. Tay
Singapore National Eye Centre, Singapore, Singapore

Singapore Eye Research Institute, Singapore, Singapore
e-mail: audrey.chia.w.l@singhealth.com.sg; tay.su.ann@singhealth.com.sg

8.1 Introduction

The understanding of the pathogenesis of myopia and various interventions has evolved over time. The belief of an association between myopia and near work in the 1980s [1–5] led to interventions targeting accommodation such as bifocal glasses [6–8] and topical atropine [9–12]. The discovery of the importance of the peripheral retina [13–15], and how peripheral hyperopic defocus may aggravate eye growth and myopia [16–19] resulted in the exploration of peripheral defocus glasses and contact lenses as potential interventions in the 2000s. Induced peripheral myopic defocus is now thought to be how orthokeratology contact lenses slow myopia [16]. Research has moved on to novel contact lens designs, which also induce peripheral or dual defocus. More recently, it is hoped that with greater understanding of gene and molecular processes involved in eye growth, novel genetic and pharmacological treatments may be developed over time to control myopia.

8.2 Near Activity and Accommodation

8.2.1 Bifocal and Progressive Addition Spectacles

Progressive and bifocal glasses were introduced in the 1990s to try and slow myopia. However, studies with progressive addition lenses (PALs) showed a small and clinically insignificant or no effect on myopia progression [20–23]. One meta-analysis noted small reductions in myopia progression (0.25 D, 95% CI 0.13–0.38; nine trials) and axial length (−0.12 mm, 95% CI −0.18 to −0.05; six trials) [24]. This effect may be greater for children with a higher myopia (<−3.0 D), accommodative lag, or near esophoria [24–28].

In contrast, randomized controlled trials (RCTs) showed that executive bifocal lenses slowed myopia progression by 39% and up to 51% with base-in prisms incorporated [29]. It is possible that the larger near segment made it more likely for children to use the near add during near work, and may also induce more peripheral myopic defocus. However, because of the lack of collaborating evidence, meta-analysis across trials found data to be limited and inconsistent [20].

8.2.2 Atropine

Atropine is a non-specific muscarinic acetylcholine receptor antagonist and was initially thought to work by blocking accommodation. This theory has since been disproved in animal studies [30]. Its exact mechanism is still unknown but it is thought to work through muscarinic or non-muscarinic pathways either in the retina or in the sclera [31, 32]. Atropine has a strong dose-dependent inhibitory effect of myopia progression [30]. The initial high doses of atropine (i.e., 0.5% or 1.0%) slowed myopia progression by more than 70% over 1–2 years [33–36]. However, lower doses (0.1% or less) can also slow myopia by 30–60%, and may be associated with fewer side effects (pupil dilation, glare or blur) [36, 37]. Huang et al. in a review of the data, found that high-dose and low-dose atropine slowed spherical equivalent by 0.68 D

[0.52–0.84] and 0.53 D [0.21–0.85] respectively, and axial length by −0.21 mm [−0.28 to −0.16] and−0.15 mm [−0.25 to −0.05] respectively over 1 year [38].

Washout data from the Atropine Treatment of Myopia (ATOM) studies, however, showed that there was a myopic rebound if atropine was stopped suddenly, especially at higher doses and in younger children [39, 40]. Up to 12% of children may exhibit a poor response (i.e., progress >1.0 D over 1 year) even on high-dose atropine. A poorer response was associated with younger children, a higher degree of myopia at baseline and myopic parents [41]. Similarly, in the ATOM2 study, 9.3%, 6.4%, and 4.3% of children in the 0.01%, 0.1%, and 0.5% group, respectively, progressed by 1.5 D or more in the first 2 years of treatment [42].

More recently, in the Low-Concentration Atropine for Myopia Progression (LAMP) study involving children aged 4–12 years, those treated with 0.01%, 0.02%, and 0.05% atropine showed a reduction of SE progression of 27%, 43%, and 67%, and axial length growth of 12%, 29%, and 51%, respectively [37]. Overall, the effect on spherical equivalent was larger than that of axial length.

8.3 Peripheral Defocus

From animal studies, it is known that eyeball growth (i.e., hyperopia or myopia) could be induced by using positive and negative lenses, respectively [43, 44]. These studies also showed that peripheral refraction could influence eye growth, independent of central vision. Excessive near work could induce hyperopic defocus in the peripheral retina and promote eye growth [25, 45–48]. The increased prolate growth of the myopic eyeball and use of spherical glasses correcting for central vision may aggravate this effect [46, 49–52]. Based on this theory, optical interventions that induce a myopic defocus in the periphery should slow myopia.

8.3.1 Peripheral Myopic Defocus Glasses

In 2010, Sankaridurg et al. published their results of three novel spectacle lenses. All lenses had a central clear aperture with varying amounts of plus defocus in the periphery. Unfortunately, there was no significant effect on myopic progression with all three designs compared to single vision lenses (SVLs). In a subgroup of younger children with parental myopia, however, the prototype where the central aperture extended into the horizontal and inferior meridians with a peripheral power of +1.9 D did result in less myopia progression [53]. However, in a recent RCT conducted in Japanese children involving this design, no difference in myopia reduction was found [54].

8.3.2 Bifocal or Dual-Focus Contact Lenses

Bifocal contact lens designs often include a central distance focus, and peripheral rings with near add, creating a peripheral myopic defocus. Studies exploring the effect of these bifocal soft contact lenses indicate slowing of myopia progression by

30–38% and axial length by 31–51% over a period of 24 months [55–57]. Different studies suggest that efficacy may improve with increase in wear time, in children with faster rates of progression [58], near esophoria [59], and with designs possessing a higher hyperopic power in the mid-periphery (up to 6 D) [60]. With the myriad of lens designs possible, the challenge now is to develop the most effective design with the least compromise to visual quality, comfort, and safety [61].

8.3.3 Orthokeratology

Orthokeratology (Ortho-k) lenses optically correct myopia by flattening the central cornea, resulting in a relative peripheral myopic defocus [62, 63]. Individual studies and meta-analyses have shown a 40–60% reduction in the rate of myopia progression with ortho-k lenses compared with controls using SVL spectacles [64–69]. In a meta-analysis by Sun et al., the combined results showed a mean AL reduction of 0.27 mm (95% CI: 0.22, 0.32) after 2 years, corresponding to a 45% reduction in myopic progression [69]. Younger children (aged 7–8 years) with faster myopic progression (>1.0 D/year) might benefit more [66], and benefits were noted even in partially corrected children with high myopia [68]. However, studies show that the efficacy may decrease over time, especially after 4–5 years [70–72], and a potential "rebound" after discontinuation, especially in children under 14 years [73]. There is also a potential non-response rate of 7–12% [74, 75]. The risk of infective keratitis remains [76–81]; a recent systemic review suggested an infection rate similar to overnight wear of soft contact lenses, which is estimated at 13.9 per 10,000 [82, 83].

8.4 Time Spent Outdoors

While initial strategies were targeted at minimizing near work, it became apparent that increasing time spent outdoors could be more important [84, 85]. In the Sydney Myopia Study, exposure to more than 2 h of outdoor activity per day decreased the odds of myopia and countered the effects of near work [86]. Interventions involving increasing time outdoors appeared to reduce the onset of myopia and also its progression in myopic children [87, 88]. A meta-analysis has suggested a 2% reduced odds of myopia per additional hour of time spent outdoors per week [89]. Another meta-analysis showed that time outdoors protected children against incident myopia with a risk ratio (RR) of 0.536–0.574 in clinical trials and longitudinal cohort studies, and an odds ratio of 0.964 in cross-sectional studies, but had less effect in slowing progression in children who were already myopic [90].

8.4.1 Environmental Interventions

Based on new evidence, the advice has shifted from spending at least 2 h/day outdoors in addition to avoiding excessive near work. This has changed health and school messaging in many East Asian countries [88].

8.4.2 Higher Light Intensities and Dopamine

Potential reasons why time outdoors may be protective include higher light intensities [91, 92], differences in chromatic composition [93–95], the reduction in dioptric accommodative focus and psychometric influences encountered outdoors [96]. Higher light intensities increase retina dopamine production, which is believed to retard axial length elongation [97]. In animal studies, higher light levels greatly retarded form-deprivation myopia [91, 92, 98], a reaction which is abolished by dopamine antagonists [97]. The role of chromaticity (red and blue) and ultraviolet (UV) light is still uncertain [99–102], while that of higher vitamin D levels has been debunked [103, 104].

8.5 Inheritance and Genetics of Myopia

Epidemiology studies suggest that the risk of myopia is doubled if children had one myopic parent, and 3–5 times if they had two [105], with a possible additive effect with subsequent generations [106]. In addition, monozygous twins have a 75–90% chance of having a similar refraction compared to 30% in dizygous twins [107–109].

From pedigree analysis, multiple inheritance patterns (i.e., autosomal dominant, autosomal recessive, and X-linked) have been identified. Genome-wide sequencing analyses have identified more than 20 myopia and high myopia loci and over 130 potential genes (MYP1-3, 5–19) in different populations [107, 110]. These loci have been linked to neuronal signaling, retinoic acid synthesis, ion transport, channel activity, and membrane potential [110], which may influence ocular development, differentiation, and growth [111]. It is hoped that by understanding the genetics of myopia, it may be possible to predict who may develop high myopia or complications of myopia early, how people may respond to various interventions, and uncover novel interventions.

8.6 Application to Clinical Practice

In deciding on treatment regimes, questions on which children would benefit most from treatment in terms of age, baseline myopia, rate of progression, and family history remain. In addition, the appropriate duration of treatment and the best time to start, stop, and restart treatment need to be further studied. With the various interventions available for myopia control, decisions need to be made in conjunction with patients and their families on the most appropriate one, taking into consideration the effectiveness, safety profile, and cost of the each intervention (Table 8.1).

The following is an atropine-based protocol which has been developed, based on evidence collected thus far (Table 8.2 and Fig. 8.1). On presentation, the risk of the child developing myopia and its potential complications are assessed. Low-risk children may be older children (aged >11 years), those with little or no myopia progression in the last 1 year, and relatively low myopia. High-risk children may be those who have a strong family history of high myopia or myopic complications, are younger (<9 years), and with documented rapid progression of myopia over the last year. Parental and child

Table 8.1 Summary of interventions for myopia control efficacy, safety, and accessibility

	Effectiveness	Safety	Accessibility
Time outdoors	Decrease onset of myopia by 30%; and progression of myopia by 18% [87, 88]	Safe. Requires sun protection of eyes and skin	Available to all. Limited by social factors (academic expectations), weather, and seasonal variations
Executive bifocal spectacles	Decrease myopia progression by 39%; 51% with base-in prisms incorporated [29]	Safe although may result in some visual distortion	Moderately expensive Readily available in most spectacle shops
PAL spectacles	Decrease myopia progression 0–20% [24]		
Peripheral myopic defocus spectacles	No significant difference from SVL [53, 54]		
Bifocal or dual focus soft contact lenses	Decrease myopia progression 30–38% over 24 months [57] Better effect with near esophoria [59]	Possible risk of infective keratitis, contact lens intolerance No data on discontinuation and rebound effect	Moderately expensive although likely readily available in most spectacle shops
Orthokeratology contact lenses	40–50% reduction in myopia progression over 1–2 years Effect may wane over time Rebound noted if stopped suddenly [69, 70]	Risk of infective keratitis similar to overnight soft CL wear: 13.9 per 10,000 [83] Ocular surface problems, corneal staining [82]	Can be expensive Require clinical expertise to ensure proper fit
Atropine	Dose-related response for myopia control with 70–80% reduction with high dose (0.5–1%) [33–36] and 30–60% with low dose (0.01–0.05%) [36, 37] Rebound noted if stopped suddenly (esp. in younger children and at higher doses) [39, 40]	Glare and near blur with higher doses Allergy 1–4% Systemic effects rare Effect on spherical equivalent greater than axial length	Can be cost-effective if manufactured in bulk Lower doses not readily available in all communities

sentiments are also assessed (e.g., overall anxiety, willingness to administer eye drops every day, possibly till the child is in his/her mid-teens). Various options are discussed, ensuring that parents have realistic expectations of the outcome. The possibility of a poor response and need for a higher dose of atropine or alternative treatments are also carefully explained. Options would then include starting atropine or waiting another 6–12 months to monitor the natural progression of refraction.

In this protocol, children are first started on a lower dose of atropine with a plan to increase the dose as necessary. However, an alternative would be to start initially

Table 8.2 An atropine-based protocol for myopia treatment

A. Starting atropine
- Assess child's risk of myopia
- High risk: family history of high myopia or myopic complications, younger age, documented rapid progression of myopia, poor life-style profile (outdoor–near work)
- Assess parents' and children's risk aversion to treatment, willingness to continue on treatment till at least teenage years
- Age 4–13 years of age with documented progression of myopia of at least >0.5 D in the last year

B1: Not keen on treatment: monitor over next 6–12 months
B2: Keen on treatment: commence atropine 0.01% daily for at least 2 years

C. Follow-up on treatment
- Review child every 6 months
- Monitor for compliance and side effects : near blur, glare, and allergy
- Cycloplegic refraction and axial length measurements at least once per year

D1: Good or acceptable response to treatment (<0.5 D/year)
Age <12 years old: consider continuing dose or slowly taper if no myopia progression noted in the past year
Age >12 years old: consider taper of medication if no/little progression noted in the past year

D2: Poor response to treatment (>0.5 D/year)
- Particularly in younger children (<9 years), with strong family history, with baseline high myopia and rapid progression prior to starting atropine
- Consider an increased dose (e.g., atropine 0.01% 2× per day, 0.1% daily or 1.0% 2–3× per week)
- Consider tinted glasses with near add if required
- Once stabilization of myopia is achieved, continue at that dose, and taper frequency of drops as child reaches teenage years

D3: Poor response despite maximum atropine dose
- Consider stopping and changing or adding different treatment options

E. Long-term follow-up
- Continue to monitor child for at least 1 year after stopping treatment

on a higher dose, with an aim to taper medication over time. Once medication is started, progression (refraction and/or axial length) is monitored every 6 months, with an initial aim to continue children on medication (i.e., atropine 0.01% daily) for at least 2 years. Children may respond to treatment in three ways: well (with little or no progression); adequately (with acceptable amount of progression, e.g., <0.5 D/year); or poorly (>0.5 D/year).

If a good response is obtained, the next question is how long treatment should continue for and when treatment should be stopped. From the ATOM 2 study, we know that stopping atropine 0.01% between 8 and 10 years resulted in a 60% risk of a rebound effect, compared to 30% at age 10–12 years and 8% after the age of 12 years. In addition, children who did not demonstrate rebound tended to show little or no myopic progression within the last year [67]. This suggests that in children younger than 12 years who showed no progression in the past year, atropine 0.01% may be slowly tapered (e.g., by reducing drop frequency by 1–2 days/week each year). However, if children are older than 12 years, then the frequency of eye drops could be tapered more quickly (e.g., by 1–2 days/week every 6 months). Using this regime, most children will be off medication by about 14–15 years of age.

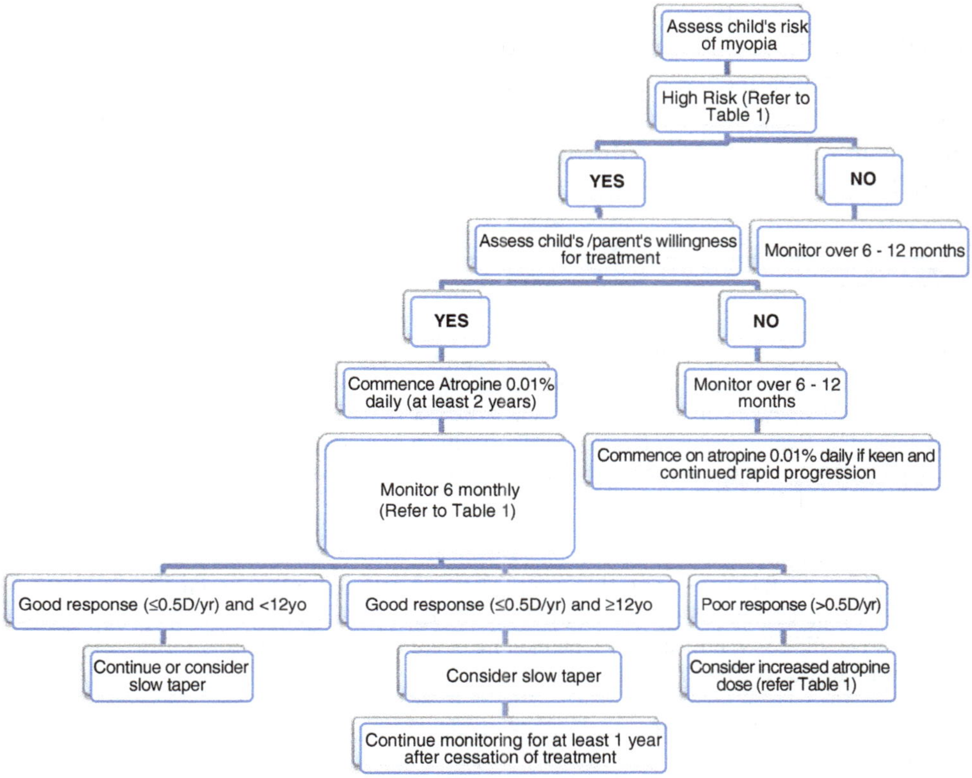

Fig. 8.1 Flow chart of atropine-based protocol for myopia treatment.

In children who progress on low-dose atropine, the frequency of application or dose could be increased (e.g., using atropine 0.01% twice a day; or using a higher concentration, e.g., 0.1% or 1%). Note that while using higher concentrations, a daily dose may not be necessary and children may require tinted glasses with near add to cope with any glare or near blur. Once an adequate control of myopia is achieved, medication can be continued till the child reaches teenage years and then tapered as required. There are some children (10%), however, who may progress rapidly even on higher doses of atropine [68]. If this occurs, then the possibility of stopping treatment or trying other treatment modalities should be discussed. Even after stopping treatment, it may be necessary to monitor children for a further 6–12 months to ensure that there is no further rebound.

Since our knowledge of how children respond to atropine and other interventions continues to increase over time, any protocol developed needs to be evaluated regularly, taking full advantage of our knowledge and accessibility to different treatment options.

8.7 Conclusion

Our management of myopia continues to evolve over time with a better understanding of the pathogenesis of myopia and its interventions. The challenge is to identify which individuals to treat, when to start treatment and which interventions one should use. There are differences in efficacy, safety, and cost which need to be balanced. More work is required to determine how to combine or time treatments to optimize outcome, and when treatments can be safely stopped. It is also important that there is continued assessment of the long-term effect and value of these treatments in preventing high myopia and its associated complications.

References

1. Parssinen O, Lyyra AL. Myopia and myopic progression among schoolchildren: a three-year follow-up study. Invest Ophthalmol Vis Sci. 1993;34:2794–802.
2. Goss DA. Nearwork and myopia. Lancet. 2000;356:1456–7.
3. Hepsen IF, Evereklioglu C, Bayramlar H. The effect of reading and near-work on the development of myopia in emmetropic boys: a prospective, controlled, three-year follow-up study. Vis Res. 2001;41:2511–20.
4. Saw SM, Chua WH, Hong CY, et al. Nearwork in early-onset myopia. Invest Ophthalmol Vis Sci. 2002;43:332–9.
5. Li SM, Li SY, Kang MT, et al. Near work related parameters and myopia in Chinese children: The Anyang Childhood Eye Study. PLoS One. 2015;10:e0134514.
6. Goss DA. Effect of bifocal lenses on the rate of childhood myopia progression. Am J Optom Physiol Optic. 1986;63:135–41.
7. Parssinen O, Hemminki E, Klemetti A. Effect of spectacle use and accommodation on myopic progression: final results of a three-year randomised clinical trial among schoolchildren. Br J Ophthalmol. 1989;73:547–51.
8. Grosvenor T, Perrigin DM, Perrigin J, Maslovitz B. Houston Myopia Control Study: a randomized clinical trial. Part II. Final report by the patient care team. Am J Optom Physiol Optic. 1987;64:482–98.
9. Bedrossian RH. The effect of atropine on myopia. Ann Ophthalmol. 1971;3:891–7.
10. Gimbel HV. The control of myopia with atropine. Can J Ophthalmol. 1973;8:527–32.
11. Bedrossian RH. The effect of atropine on myopia. Ophthalmology. 1979;86:713–9.
12. Brodstein RS, Brodstein DE, Olson RJ, et al. The treatment of myopia with atropine and bifocals. A long-term prospective study. Ophthalmology. 1984;91:1373–9.
13. Wallman J, Gottlieb MD, Rajaram V, et al. Local retinal regions control local eye growth and myopia. Science. 1987;237:73–8.
14. Diether S, Schaeffel F. Local changes in eye growth induced by imposed local refractive error despite active accommodation. Vis Res. 1997;37:659–68.
15. Miles FA, Wallman J. Local ocular compensation for imposed local refractive error. Vis Res. 1990;30:339–49.
16. Wallman J, Winawer J. Homeostasis of eye growth and the question of myopia. Neuron. 2004;43:447–68.
17. Smith EL III, Hung LF, Ramamirtham R, et al. Optically imposed hyperopic defocus in the periphery can produce central axial myopia in infant monkeys. Invest Ophthalmol Vis Sci. 2007;48(13):1533.
18. Smith EL, Hung LF, Huang J. Relative peripheral hyperopic defocus alters central refractive development in infant monkeys. Vis Res. 2009;49:2386–92.
19. Smith EL III, Hung LF, Huang J, et al. Effects of optical defocus on refractive development in monkeys: evidence for local, regionally selective mechanisms. Invest Ophthalmol Vis Sci. 2010;51:3864–73.
20. Walline JJ, Lindsley K, Vedula SS, et al. Interventions to slow progression of myopia in children. Cochrane Database Syst Rev. 2011;12:CD004916.
21. Gwiazda JE, Hyman L, Everett D, The COMET Group, et al. Five–year results from the correction of myopia evaluation trial (COMET). Invest Ophthalmol Vis Sci. 2006;47(13):1166.

22. Hasebe S, Ohtsuki H, Nonaka T, et al. Effect of progressive addition lenses on myopia progression in Japanese children: a prospective, randomized, double-masked, crossover trial. Invest Ophthalmol Vis Sci. 2008;49(7):2781–9.
23. Hasebe S, Jun J, Vamas SR, et al. Myopia control with positively aspherised progressive additional lenses: a 2 year, multicentre, randomized, controlled trial. Invest Ophthalmol Vi Sci. 2014;55(11):7177–88.
24. Li SM, Ji YZ, Wu SS, et al. Multifocal versus single vision lenses intervention to slow progression of myopia in school-age children: a meta-analysis. Surv Ophthalmol. 2011;56:451–60.
25. Gwiazda JE, Hyman L, Norton TT, COMET Group, et al. Accommodation and related risk factors associated with myopia progression and their interaction with treatment in COMET children. Invest Ophthalmol Vis Sci. 2004;45(7):2143–51.
26. Correction of Myopia Evaluation Trial 2 Study Group for the Pediatric Eye Disease Investigator Group. Progressive-addition lenses versus single-vision lenses for slowing progression of myopia in children with high accommodative lag and near esophoria. Invest Ophthalmol Vis Sci. 2011;52:2749–57.
27. Berntsen DA, Sinnott LT, Mutti DO, Zadnik K. A randomized trial using progressive addition lenses to evaluate theories of myopia progression in children with a high lag of accommodation. Invest Ophthalmol Vis Sci. 2012;53:640–9.
28. Yang Z, Lan W, Ge J, Liu W, Chen X, Chen L, Yu M. The effectiveness of progressive addition lenses on the progression of myopia in Chinese children. Ophthalmic Physiol Opt. 2009;29:41–8.
29. Cheng D, Woo GC, Drobe B, Schmid KL. Effect of bifocal and prismatic bifocal spectacles on myopia progression in children: three-year results of a randomized clinical trial. Ophthamology. 2014;132:258–64.
30. McBrien NA, Moghaddam HO, Reeder AP. Atropine reduces experimental myopia and eye enlargement via a nonaccommodative mechanism. Invest Ophthalmol Vis Sci. 1993;34:205–15.
31. McBrien NA, Stell WK, Carr B. How does atropine exert its anti-myopia effects? Ophthalmic Physiol Opt. 2013;33(3):373–8.
32. Lind GJ, Chew SJ, Marzani D, Wallman J. Muscarinic acetylcholine receptor antagonists inhibit chick scleral chondrocytes. Invest Ophthalmol Vis Sci. 1998;39:2217–31.
33. Yen MY, Liu JH, Kao SC, Shiao CH. Comparison of the effect of atropine and cyclopentolate on myopia. Ann Ophthalmol. 1989;21:180–2.
34. Shih YF, Chen CH, Chou AC, et al. Effects of different concentrations of atropine on controlling myopia in myopic children. J Ocul Pharmacol Ther. 1999;15:85–90.
35. Chua WH, Balakrishnan V, Chan YH, et al. Atropine for the treatment of childhood myopia. Ophthalmology. 2006;113(12):2285–91.
36. Chia A, Chua WH, Cheung YB, et al. Atropine for the treatment of childhood myopia: safety and efficacy of 0.5%, 0.1%, and 0.01% doses (Atropine for the Treatment of Myopia 2). Ophthalmology. 2012;119(2):347–54.
37. Yam JC, Jiang Y, Tang SM, et al. Low-concentration atropine for myopia progression (LAMP) study: a randomized, double-blinded, placebo-controlled trial of 0.05%, 0.025%, and 0.01% atropine eye drops in myopia control. Ophthalmology. 2019;126(1):113–24.
38. Huang J, Wen D, Wang Q, et al. Efficacy comparison of 16 interventions for myopia control in children: a network meta-analysis. Ophthalmology. 2016;123(4):697–708.
39. Tong L, Huang XL, Koh AL, et al. Atropine for the treatment of childhood myopia: effect on myopia progression after cessation of atropine. Ophthalmology. 2009;116:572–9.
40. Chia A, Chua WH, Wen L, et al. Atropine for the treatment of childhood myopia: changes after stopping atropine 0.01%, 0.1% and 0.5%. Am J Ophthalmol. 2014;157(2):451–457.e1.
41. Loh KL, Lu Q, Tan D, Chia A. Risk factors for progressive myopia in the atropine therapy for myopia study. Am J Ophthalmol. 2015;159:945–9.
42. Chia A, Lu QS, Tan D. Five-year clinical trial on atropine for the treatment of myopia 2: myopia control with atropine 0.01% eyedrops. Ophthalmology. 2016;123(2):391–9.
43. Troilo D, Wallman J. The regulation of eye growth and refractive state: an experimental study of emmetropization. Vis Res. 1991;31:1237–50.

44. Schaeffel F, Troilo D, Wallman J, Howland HC. Developing eyes that lack accommodation grow to compensate for imposed defocus. Vis Neurosci. 1990;4:177–83.
45. Seidemann A, Schaeffel F. An evaluation of the lag of accommodation using photorefraction. Vis Res. 2003;43:419–30.
46. Gwiazda J, Bauer J, Thorn F, et al. A dynamic relationship between myopia and blur-driven accommodation in school-aged children. Vis Res. 1995;35:1299–304.
47. Gwiazda J, Thorn F, Bauer J, et al. Myopic children show insufficient accommodative response to blur. Invest Ophthalmol Vis Sci. 1993;34:690–4.
48. Charman WN. Near vision, lags of accommodation and myopia. Ophthalmic Physiol Opt. 1999;19:126–33.
49. Mutti DO, Sinnott LT, Mitchell GL, CLEERE Study Group, et al. Relative peripheral refractive error and the risk of onset and progression of myopia in children. Invest Ophthalmol Vis Sci. 2011;52(1):199–205.
50. Atchison DA, Jones CE, Schmid KL, et al. Eye shape in emmetropia and myopia. Invest Ophthalmol Vis Sci. 2004;45(10):3380–6.
51. Schmid GF. Association between retinal steepness and central myopic shift in children. Optom Vis Sci. 2011;88(6):684–90.
52. Sng CCA, Lin XY, Gus G, et al. Change in peripheral refraction over time in Singapore Chinese children. Invest Ophthalmol Vis Sci. 2011;52(11):7880–7.
53. Sankaridurg P, Donovan L, Varnas S, et al. Spectacle lenses designed to reduce progression of myopia: 12-month results. Optom Vis Sci. 2010;87(9):631–41.
54. Kanda H, Oshika T, Hiraoka T, et al. Effect of spectacle lenses designed to reduce relative peripheral hyperopia on myopia progression in Japanese children: a 2-year multicenter randomized controlled trial. Jpn J Ophthalmol. 2018;62:537–43.
55. Benavente-Pérez A, Nour A, Troilo D. Axial eye growth and refractive error development can be modified by exposing the peripheral retina to relative myopic or hyperopic defocus. Invest Ophthalmol Vis Sci. 2014;55(10):6765–73.
56. Walline JJ. Myopia control: a review. Eye Contact Lens. 2016;42(1):3–8.
57. Li SM, Kang MT, Wu SS, et al. Studies using concentric ring bifocal and peripheral add multifocal contact lenses to slow myopia progression in school-aged children: a meta-analysis. Ophthalmic Physiol Opt. 2017;37(1):51–9.
58. Lam CSY, Tang WC, Tse DY-Y, Tang YY, To CH. Defocus incorporated soft contact (DISC) lens slows myopia progression in Hong Kong Chinese schoolchildren: a 2-year randomised clinical trial. Br J Ophthalmol. 2014;98:40–5.
59. Aller TA, Liu M, Wildsoet CF. Myopia control with bifocal contact lenses: a randomized clinical trial. Optom Vis Sci. 2016;93(4):344–52.
60. Paune J, Morales H, Armengol J, et al. Myopia control with a novel peripheral gradient soft lens and orthokeratology: a 2-year clinical trial. Biomed Res Int. 2015;2015:507572.
61. Anstice NS, Phillips JR. Effect of dual-focus soft contact lens wear on axial myopia progression in children. Ophthalmology. 2011;118:1152–61.
62. Charman WN, Mountford J, Atchison DA, et al. Peripheral refraction in orthokeratology patients. Optom Vis Sci. 2006;83:641–8.
63. Queirós A, González-Méijome JM, Jorge J, et al. Peripheral refraction in myopic patients after orthokeratology. Optom Vis Sci. 2010;87(5):323–9.
64. Wen D, Huang J, Chen H, et al. Efficacy and acceptability of orthokeratology for slowing myopic progression in children: a systematic review and meta-analysis. J Ophthalmol. 2015;2015:360806.
65. Si JK, Tang K, Bi HS, et al. Orthokeratology for myopia control: a meta-analysis. Optom Vis Sci. 2015;92:252–7.
66. Cho P, Cheung SW, Edwards M, et al. The longitudinal orthokeratology research in children (LORIC) in Hong Kong: a pilot study on refractive changes and myopic control. Curr Eye Res. 2005;30:71–80.
67. Santodomingo-Rubido J, Villa-Collar C, Gilmartin B, et al. Myopia control with orthokeratology contact lenses in Spain: refractive and biometric changes. Invest Ophthalmol Vis Sci. 2012;53:5060–5.

68. Charm J, Cho P. High myopia partial reduction ortho-k: a 2-year randomized study. Optom Vis Sci. 2013;90:530–9.
69. Sun Y, Xu F, Zhang T, Liu M, Wang D, Chen Y, Liu Q. Orthokeratology to control myopia progression: a meta-analysis. PLoS One. 2015;10(4):e0124535.
70. Hiraoka T, Kakita T, Okamoto F, et al. Long-term effect of overnight orthokeratology on axial length elongation in childhood myopia: a 5-year follow-up study. Invest Ophthalmol Vis Sci. 2012;53:3913–9.
71. Lee YC, Wang JH, Chiu CJ. Effect of Orthokeratology on myopia progression: twelve-year results of a retrospective cohort study. BMC Ophthalmol. 2017;17(1):243.
72. Santodomingo-Rubido J, Villa-Collar C, Gilmartin B, Gutiérrez-Ortega R, Sugimoto K. Long-term efficacy of orthokeratology contact lens wear in controlling the progression of childhood myopia. Curr Eye Res. 2017;42(5):713–20.
73. Cho P, Cheung SW. Discontinuation of orthokeratology on eyeball elongation (DOEE). Cont Lens Anterior Eye. 2017;40:82–7.
74. Cho P, Cheung SW. Retardation of myopia in orthokeratology (ROMIO) study: a 2-year randomized clinical trial. Invest Ophthalmol Vis Sci. 2012;53:7077–85.
75. Chen C, Cheung SW, Cho P. Myopia control using toric orthokeratology (TO-SEE Study). Invest Ophthalmol Vis Sci. 2013;54(10):6510–7.
76. Sun X, Zhao H, Deng S, et al. Infectious keratitis related to orthokeratology. Ophthalmic Physiol Opt. 2006;26:133–6.
77. Yepes N, Lee SB, Hill V, et al. Infectious keratitis after overnight orthokeratology in Canada. Cornea. 2005;24:857–60.
78. Tseng CH, Fong CF, Chen WL, et al. Overnight orthokeratology-associated microbial keratitis. Cornea. 2005;24:778–82.
79. Young AL, Leung AT, Cheng LL, et al. Orthokeratology lens–related corneal ulcers in children: a case series. Ophthalmology. 2004;111:590–5.
80. Xuguang S, Lin C, Yan Z, et al. Acanthamoeba keratitis as a complication of orthokeratology. Am J Ophthalmol. 2003;136:1159–61.
81. Chan TC, Li EY, Wong VW, Jhanji V. Orthokeratology-associated infectious keratitis in a tertiary care eye hospital in Hong Kong. Am J Ophthalmol. 2014;158:1130–5.
82. Liu YM, Xie P. The safety of orthokeratology—a systematic review. Eye Contact Lens. 2016;42:35–42.
83. Meter V, Woodford S, et al. Safety of overnight orthokeratology for myopia. Ophthalmology. 2008;115(12):2301–13.
84. Guggenheim JA, Northstone K, McMahon G, et al. Time outdoors and physical activity as predictors of incident myopia in childhood: a prospective cohort study. Invest Ophthalmol Vis Sci. 2012;53(6):2856–65.
85. Rose KA, Morgan IG, Smith W, Burlutsky G, Mitchell P, Saw SM. Myopia, lifestyle, and schooling in students of Chinese ethnicity in Singapore and Sydney. Arch Ophthalmol. 2008;126(4):527–30.
86. Rose KA, Morgan IG, Ip J, Kifley A, Huynh S, Smith W, Mitchell P. Outdoor activity reduces the prevalence of myopia in children. Ophthalmology. 2008;115(8):1279–85.
87. He M, Xiang F, Zeng Y, et al. Effect of time spent outdoors at school on the development of myopia among children in china a randomized clinical trial. JAMA. 2015;314(11):1142–8.
88. Wu PC, Chen CT, Lin KK, et al. Myopia prevention and outdoor light intensity in a school-based cluster randomized trial. Ophthalmology. 2018;125(8):1239–50.
89. Sherwin JC, Reacher MH, Keogh RH, et al. The association between time spent outdoors and myopia in children and adolescents: a systematic review and meta-analysis. Ophthalmology. 2012;119:2141–51.
90. Xiong S, Sankaridurg P, Naduvilath T, Zang J, Zou H, Zhu J, Lv M, He X, Xu X. Time spent in outdoor activities in relation to myopia prevention and control: a meta-analysis and systematic review. Acta Ophthalmol. 2017;95(6):551–66.
91. Ashby R, Ohlendorf A, Schaeffel F. The effect of ambient illuminance on the development of deprivation myopia in chicks. Invest Ophthalmol Vis Sci. 2009;50:5348–54.

92. Karouta C, Ashby RS. Correlation between light levels and the development of deprivation myopia. Invest Ophthalmol Vis Sci. 2015;56:299–309.
93. Rohrer B, Schaeffel F, Zrenner E. Longitudinal chromatic aberration and emmetropization: results from the chicken eye. J Physiol. 1992;449:363–76.
94. Seidemann A, Schaefel F. Effects of longitudinal chromatic aberration on accommodation and emmetropization. Vis Res. 2002;42:2409–17.
95. Rucker FJ, Wallman J. Chick eyes compensate for chromatic simulations of hyperopic and myopic defocus: evidence that the eye uses longitudinal chromatic aberration to guide eye growth. Vis Res. 2009;49:1775–83.
96. Flitcroft DI. The complex interactions of retinal, optical and environmental factors in myopia aetiology. Prog Retin Eye Res. 2012;31:622–60.
97. Feldkaemper M, Schaeffel F. An updated view on the role of dopamine in myopia. Exp Eye Res. 2013;114:106–19.
98. Smith EL 3rd, Hung LF, Huang J. Protective effects of high ambient lighting on the development of form-deprivation myopia in rhesus monkeys. Invest Ophthalmol Vis Sci. 2012;53:421–8.
99. Prepas SB. Light, literacy and the absence of ultraviolet radiation in the development of myopia. Med Hypotheses. 2008;70:635–7.
100. Foulds WS, Barathi VA, Luu CD. Progressive myopia or hyperopia can be induced in chicks and reversed by manipulation of the chromaticity of ambient light. Invest Ophthalmol Vis Sci. 2013;54(13):8004–12.
101. Smith EL, Hung LF, Arumugam B, et al. Effects of long-wavelength lighting on refractive development in infant rhesus monkeys. Invest Ophthalmol Vis Sci. 2015;56(11):6490–500.
102. Hung LF, Arumugam B, She Z, et al. Narrow-band, long-wavelength lighting promotes hyperopia and retards vision-induced myopia in infant rhesus monkeys. Exp Eye Res. 2018;4(176):147–60.
103. Guggenheim JA, Williams C, Northstone K, et al. Does vitamin D mediate the protective effects of time outdoors on myopia? Findings from a prospective birth cohort. Invest Ophthalmol Vis Sci. 2014;55:8550–8.
104. Cuellar-Partida G, Williams KM, Yazar S, et al. Genetically low vitamin D concentrations and myopic refractive error: a Mendelian randomization study. Int J Epidemiol. 2017;46:1882–90.
105. Wenbo L, Congxia B, Hui L. Genetic and environmental-genetic interaction rules for the myopia based on a family exposed to risk from a myopic environment. Gene. 2017;626:305–8.
106. Ahn H, Lyu IS, Rim TH. The influence of parental myopia on children's myopia in different generations of parent-offspring pairs in South Korea. Semin Ophthalmol. 2018;33(3):419–28.
107. Li J, Zhang Q. Insight into the molecular genetics of myopia. Mol Vis. 2017;23:1048–80.
108. Chen Y, Zhang J, Morgan IG, He M. Identifying children at risk of high myopia using population centile curves of refraction. PLoS One. 2016;11(12):e0167642.
109. Guggenheim JA, Ghorbani Mojarrad N, Williams C, et al. Genetic prediction of myopia: prospects and challenges. Ophthalmic Physiol Opt. 2017;37:549–56.
110. Rong SS, Chen LJ, Pang CP. Myopia Genetics-The Asia-Pacific Perspective. Asia Pac J Ophthalmol. 2016;5(4):236–44.
111. Flitcroft DI, Loughman J, Wildsoet CF, Williams C, Guggenheim JA, CREAM Consortium. Novel myopia genes and pathways identified from syndromic forms of myopia. Invest Ophthalmol Vis Sci. 2018;59(1):338–48.

9

Pathologic Myopia: A Comprehensive Overview

Kyoko Ohno-Matsui and Jost B. Jonas

Key Points

- Pathologic myopia is defined by the presence of posterior staphylomas and/or the presence of myopic chorioretinal atrophy equal to or more serious than diffuse atrophy.
- Myopic CNV is the most frequent cause of central vision loss.
- Ultra wide-field OCT is a useful tool to detect posterior staphylomas.
- Anti-VEGF therapies have greatly improved the prognosis of myopic CNV.
- Vitreoretinal surgeries for myopic macular retinoschisis are useful.

9.1 Introduction

Pathologic myopia (PM) is a major cause of blindness in the world, especially in East Asian countries [1–5]. The cause of blindness in patients with PM includes myopic maculopathy with or without posterior staphyloma, myopic macular retinoschisis, and glaucoma or glaucoma-like optic neuropathy. In this chapter, the lesions of myopic fundus complications including posterior staphylomas are described.

K. Ohno-Matsui (✉)
Department of Ophthalmology and Visual Science, Tokyo Medical and Dental University, Tokyo, Japan
e-mail: k.ohno.oph@tmd.ac.jp

J. B. Jonas
Department of Ophthalmology, University of Heidelberg, Heidelberg, Germany

9.2 Definition of Pathologic Myopia

The terms "pathologic myopia," "high myopia," and "axial myopia" have long been used in a parallel manner in the literature. According to recent discussions, the term "high myopia" simply describes the status of a "high degree of myopia" and should be defined by a cut-off value of myopic refractive error. The term "axial myopia" may be used to describe the situation with an axial elongation as cause for the myopic refractive error. It is in contrast to the term refractive myopia, which is used for eyes with an abnormally high refractive power of their optical media. The term "pathologic myopia" describes the situation of pathologic consequences of a myopic axial elongation. According to a recent consensus article by Ohno-Matsui et al. [6], pathologic myopia was defined by myopic chorioretinal atrophy equal to or more serious than diffuse atrophy (by META-PM study group classification [7]) and/or the presence of posterior staphylomas.

9.3 Posterior Staphyloma

Posterior staphyloma has been considered a hallmark lesion of pathologic myopia. While axial elongation may primarily start in the equatorial and retro-equatorial region with secondary changes taking place at the posterior fundus, posterior staphylomas occur in the posterior segment of the eye and can be associated with, or lead to, vision-threatening complications in the macula as part of a myopic maculopathy [7–11] and myopic optic neuropathy/glaucoma [12, 13].

9.3.1 Definition of Staphyloma by Spaide (Fig. 9.1)

A posterior staphyloma is an outpouching of a circumscribed area of the posterior fundus, where the radius of curvature is less than the curvature radius of the surrounding eye wall [14].

9.3.2 Detection of Posterior Staphyloma

Moriyama et al. recently applied three-dimensional magnetic resonance imaging (3D-MRI) to analyze the shape of the entire eye from the corneal surface to the posterior pole including even large posterior staphylomas (Fig. 9.2) [15–17]. The technique allowed visualizing a staphyloma from any angle. The advantage of 3D-MRI of visualizing the shape of the whole eye including the anterior ocular segment is combined with its disadvantage of not being feasible as a screening technique. Instead, a new prototype of a wide-field swept-source optical coherence tomographic (OCT) system has been developed, which uses not only one but multiple scan lines and which generates scan maps allowing a three-dimensional

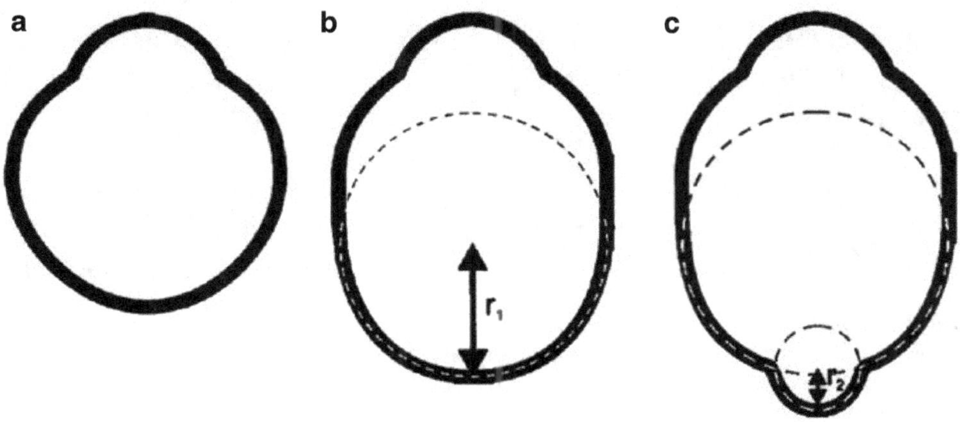

Fig. 9.1 Definition of posterior staphyloma (cited from the textbook *Pathologic Myopia* [14]). (**a**) Normal eye shape. (**b**) Axial expansion occurring in the equatorial region that does not induce any altered curvature in the posterior aspect of the eye. This eye would have axial myopia but no staphyloma. (**c**) Posterior staphyloma. A second curvature occurs in the posterior portion of the eye, and this second curvature has a small radius (r_2) than the surrounding eye wall (r_1). This secondary curve is a staphyloma. (This figure does not take into account changes in scleral thickness)

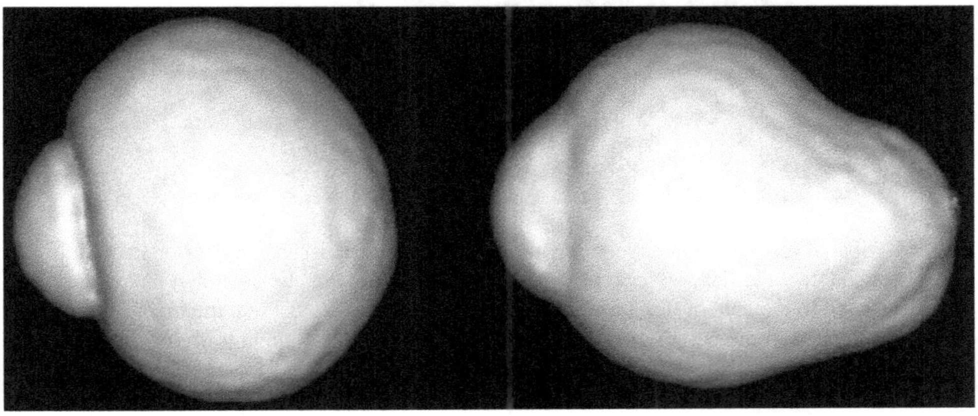

Fig. 9.2 Three-dimensional magnetic resonance images of eyes with emmetropia and posterior staphyloma. The shape of the emmetropic eye (left) is almost spherical and symmetrical, while the eye with a posterior staphyloma shows an outpouching of its posterior segment

reconstruction of posterior staphylomas in a region of interest of 23 × 20 mm with a depth of 5 mm. Applying a wide-field OCT (WF-OCT), Shinohara et al. [18] showed that WF-OCT could provide tomographic images of posterior staphylomas in a resolution and size unachievable up to that time, and that WF-OCT might replace 3D-MRI in examining posterior staphylomas. Upon WF-OCT, the edges of the staphylomas showed consistent features, consisting of a gradual thinning of the choroid from the periphery toward the staphyloma edge and a gradual re-thickening of the choroid from the staphyloma edge in direction to the posterior pole (Fig. 9.3).

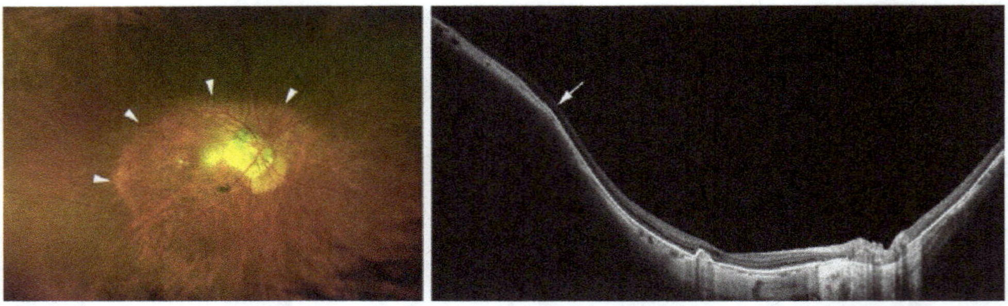

Fig. 9.3 Swept-source wide-field optical coherence tomographic (OCT) image of a posterior staphyloma. (Left) Right fundus shows a wide staphyloma (arrowheads). (Right) The wide-field OCT image shows the staphyloma edge (arrow) with a gradual thinning of the choroid from the periphery toward the staphyloma edge and a gradual re-thickening of the choroid toward the posterior pole. The white arrow indicates the change in the curvature radius of the sclera at the staphyloma edge

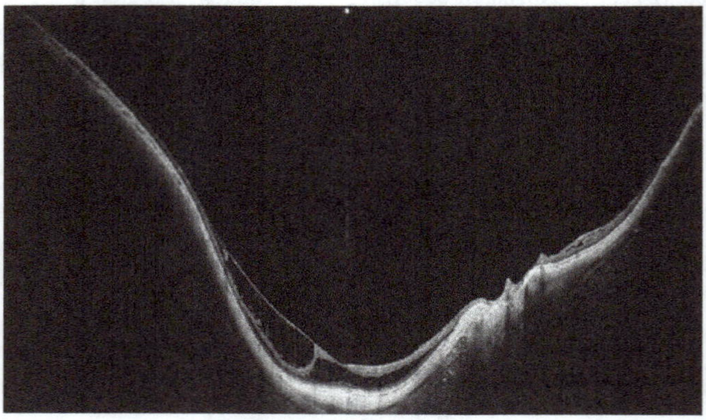

Fig. 9.4 Spatial relationship between myopic macular retinoschisis and posterior staphyloma. In this swept-source wide-field optical coherence tomographic image, the outer and inner retinoschisis is restricted to the area of the posterior staphyloma. It may suggest that the inner retinal structures as compared to the outer retinal structures were not flexible enough to follow the elongated circumference of Bruch's membrane and sclera

An additional advantage of the swept-source WF-OCT technology was the relatively large depth of focus so that structures from the posterior vitreous to the sclera could be imaged in the same image. It allowed the analysis of relationships between vitreoretinal abnormalities and other lesions in the inner retinal layers, such as myopic macular retinoschisis and posterior staphylomas as reported by Shinohara et al. [19] (Fig. 9.4).

9.3.3 Classification (Ohno-Matsui's Modified Classification, Fig. 9.3)

Based upon and modifying Curtin's [20] classical categorization of posterior staphylomas, with Types I–V as primary staphylomas and Types VI–X as compound staphylomas, Ohno-Matsui [17] used 3D-MRI and wide-field fundus

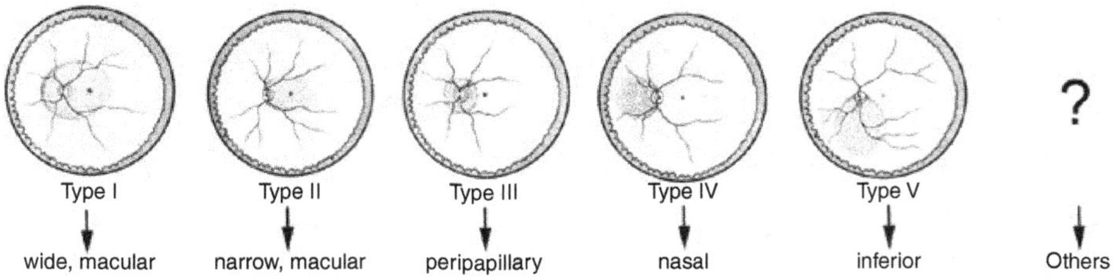

Fig. 9.5 Classification staphyloma (cited from [17] with permission). New classification of posterior staphyloma according to its location and extent. The staphyloma type is renamed according to its location and distribution. Type I → wide, macular staphyloma, Type II → narrow, macular staphyloma, Type III → peripapillary staphyloma, Type IV → nasal staphyloma, Type V → inferior staphyloma, others → staphylomas other than Types I–V

imaging to reclassify staphylomas into six types: the wide macular type, the narrow macular type, the peripapillary type, the nasal type, the inferior type, and others (Fig. 9.5).

9.4 Fundus Complications of Pathologic Myopia

9.4.1 Myopic Chorioretinal Atrophy (META-PM Study, Table 9.1)

In the META-PM classification [7], myopic maculopathy lesions have been categorized into five categories from "no myopic retinal lesions" (Category 0), "tessellated fundus only" (Category 1; Fig. 9.6a), "diffuse chorioretinal atrophy" (Category 2; Fig. 9.6b), "patchy chorioretinal atrophy" (Category 3; Fig. 9.6c), to "macular atrophy" (Category 4; Fig. 9.6d). These categories were defined based on long-term clinical observations that showed the progression patterns and associated factors of the development of myopic choroidal neovascularization (CNV) for each stage. Three additional features were added to these categories and were included as "plus signs": (1) lacquer cracks (Fig. 9.6e) and (2) myopic CNV (Fig. 9.6f) (Table 9.1). Since a Fuchs' spot represented a scarred form of myopic CNV, Fuchs' spots were categorized under the term of myopic CNV. The reason for separately listing the "plus signs" was that all three lesions have been shown to be strongly associated with central vision loss; however, they did not fit into any particular category and might develop from, or coexist, in eyes with any

Table 9.1 Myopic Chorioretinal Atrophy Classification (META-PM Study)

		Plus lesions
Category 0	Normal fundus	Myopic CNV lacquer cracks
Category 1	Tesselated fundus	
Category 2	Diffuse chorioretinal atrophy	
Category 3	Patchy chorioretinal atrophy	
Category 4	Macular atrophy	

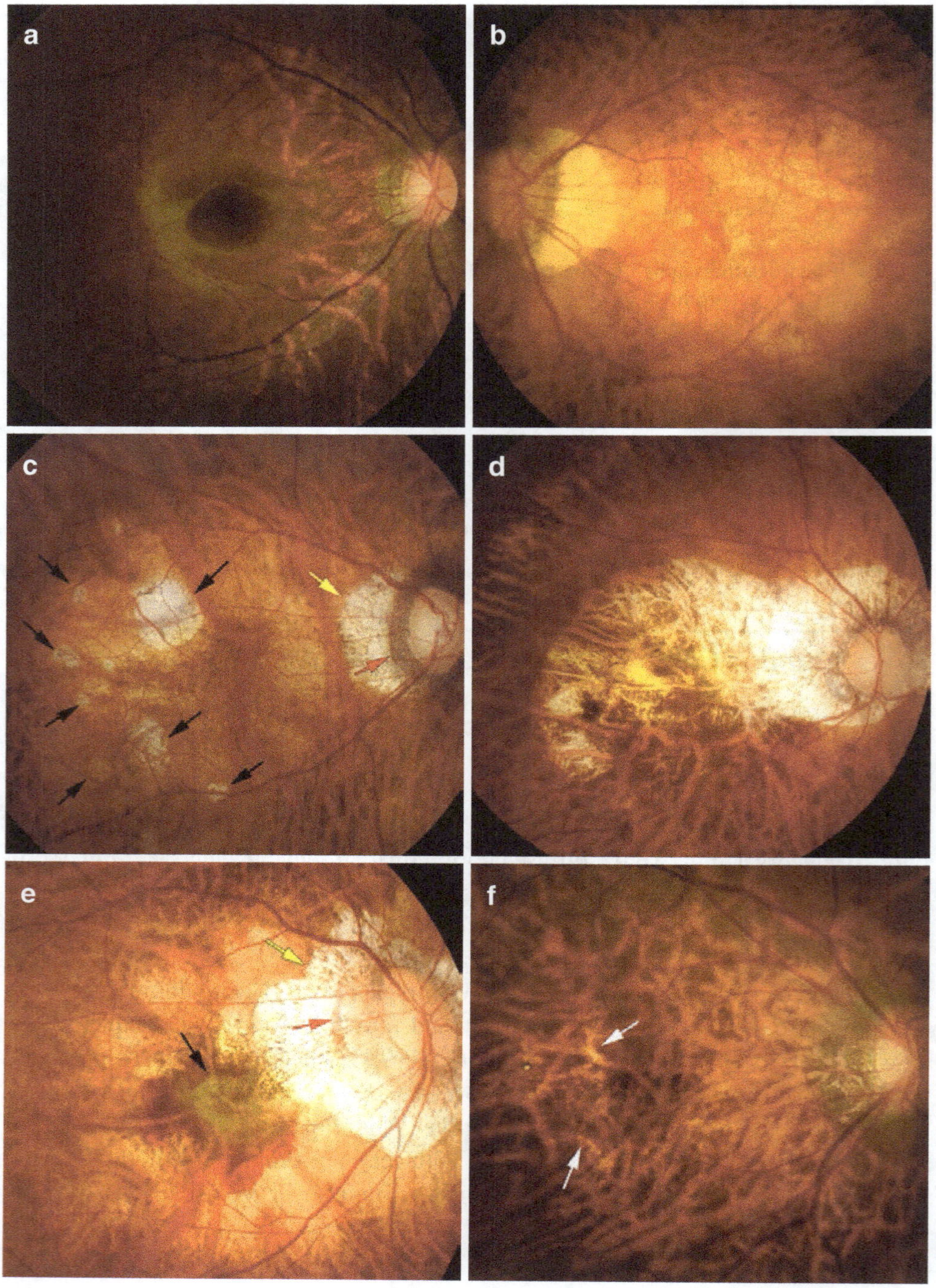

Fig. 9.6 Myopic maculopathy. (**a**) Fundus tessellation temporal to the optic disc. (**b**) Diffuse chorioretinal atrophy. Ill-defined, yellowish atrophy is seen in the posterior fundus. (**c**) Patchy chorioretinal atrophy. Within the area of diffuse atrophy, multiple areas of well-defined, whitish atrophic lesions are seen (arrows); yellow arrows: parapapillary gamma zone; red arrow: parapapillary delta zone. (**d**) Macular atrophy, several years after the formation of myopic choroidal neovascularization (CNV), a well-defined atrophic lesion is seen in the macular area. (**e**) Myopic CNV. Subretinal hemorrhage is seen around the CNV (arrow); yellow arrows: parapapillary gamma zone; red arrow: parapapillary delta zone. (**f**) Lacquer cracks. Multiple yellowish linear lesions are seen (arrows)

of the myopic maculopathy categories described above. Based on this classification, pathologic myopia has now been defined as myopic maculopathy Category 2 or above, or the presence of "plus" sign or posterior staphyloma [7, 21].

9.4.2 Diffuse Chorioretinal Atrophy (Category 2)

Diffuse chorioretinal atrophy is characterized by a yellowish white appearance of the posterior pole. The region of the diffuse atrophy may extend from a restricted area around the optic disc and a part of the macula to the entire posterior pole. The atrophy generally first appears around the optic disc, often increases with age, and finally covers the entire area within a staphyloma if a staphyloma is present. Both older age and longer axial length have been described as risk factors for the development of diffuse atrophy [9]. Marked thinning of the choroidal layer in the area of diffuse atrophy can be detected upon OCT, with occasional large choroidal vessels remaining.

9.4.3 Patchy Chorioretinal Atrophy (Category 3)

Patchy chorioretinal atrophy appears as well-defined, grayish white lesion(s) in the macular area or around the optic disc. Upon OCT, the area of patchy atrophy is characterized by the absence of the entire choroid and the RPE as well as of the outer retina. Hyper-transmission through the underlying sclera can be seen upon OCT. Using swept-source OCT, Ohno-Matsui et al. [22] showed that patchy atrophy was not simply a chorioretinal atrophy but was combined with a defect in Bruch's membrane (BM).

9.4.4 Lacquer Cracks (Plus Sign)

Lacquer cracks appear as yellowish linear lesions in the macula. Lacquer cracks have been considered to represent breaks in BM [9, 23–25]. Progression patterns of lacquer cracks include an increased number, elongation, and progression to patchy atrophy [8, 26].

Detection of lacquer cracks can sometimes be difficult especially in eyes with diffuse atrophy. Assessments of hyper-fluorescence by fluorescein angiography and hypo-fluorescence upon indocyanine green angiography have been useful for the diagnosis. Other linear lesions due to pathologic myopia with a similar hypo-fluorescence upon by indocyanine green angiography, such as myopic stretch lines, have to be differentiated [27].

Due to their small width, linear defects in BM as the base of lacquer cracks are difficult to be directly detected. Instead, hyper-reflective lines of the choroidal and scleral tissue layers on the OCT images indirectly indicate the linear BM defect by an optical window effect (Fig. 9.7). The recently developed imaging technique of OCT angiography may be useful for detecting a rupture of the choriocapillaris in

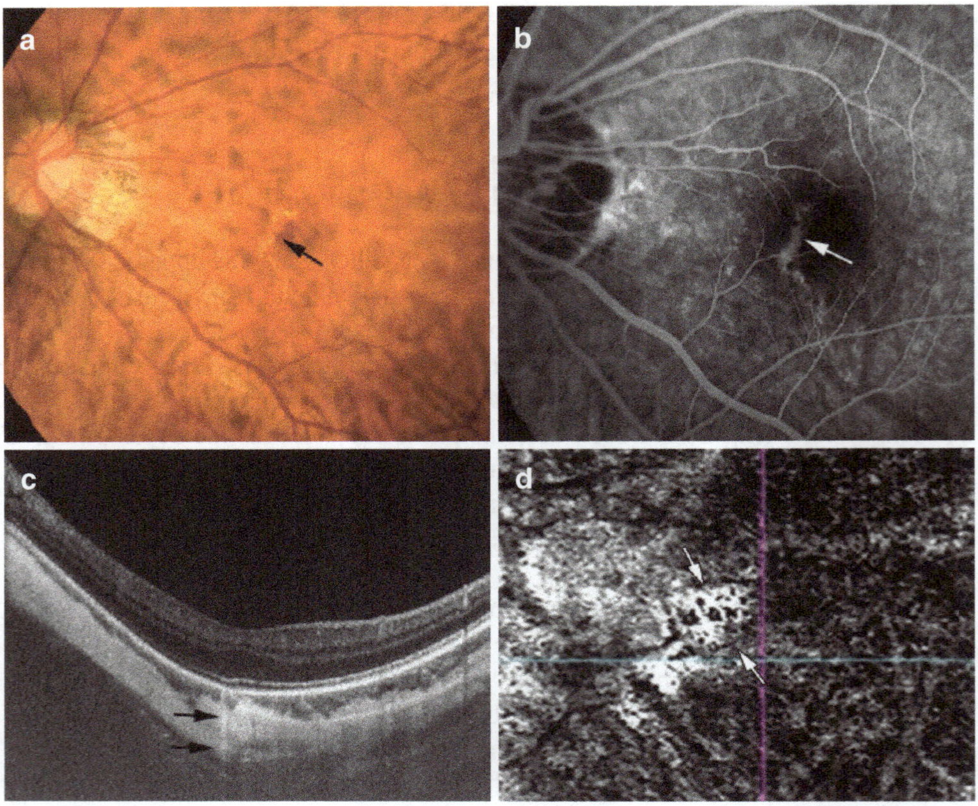

Fig. 9.7 Multimodal imaging of lacquer cracks. (**a**) Left fundus shows lacquer crack as yellowish linear lesion (arrow). (**b**) Fluorescein angiogram shows linear hyper-fluorescence at the site of lacquer crack (arrow). (**c**) Optical coherent tomographic image shows deep penetration of light (arrows) at the site of lacquer cracks. (**d**) OCT angiography shows a defect of choriocapillaris (arrows)

the area of lacquer cracks, again indirectly indicating a defect in BM [28]. Since a subretinal bleeding can often be observed at the onset of the development of lacquer cracks [29–31] (Fig. 9.8), it is important to exclude the presence of a myopic CNV in cases of subretinal bleeding in the region of lacquer cracks.

9.4.5 Myopic CNV and CNV-Related Macular Atrophy

Myopic CNV is a major sight threatening complication of pathologic myopia. It is the most common cause of CNV in individuals younger than 50 years, and it is the second most common cause of CNV overall [25, 32]. Myopic CNV is a Type II CNV and shows a clear hyper-fluorescence by fluorescein angiography. Anti-VEGF therapy is the first-line treatment for myopic CNV, as shown by the RADIANCE study [33] and the MYRROR study [34].

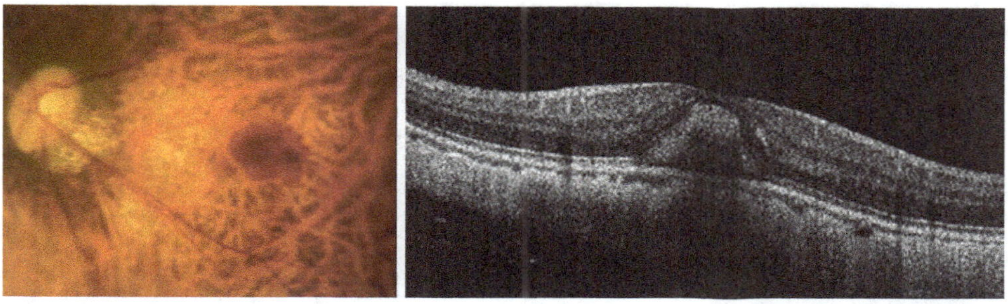

Fig. 9.8 Subretinal bleeding due to new lacquer crack formation. Left fundus shows subretinal bleeding. There are some projections along the temporal border of the hemorrhage. Optical coherent tomographic image shows subretinal hemorrhage. Serous retinal detachment or macular edema is not seen

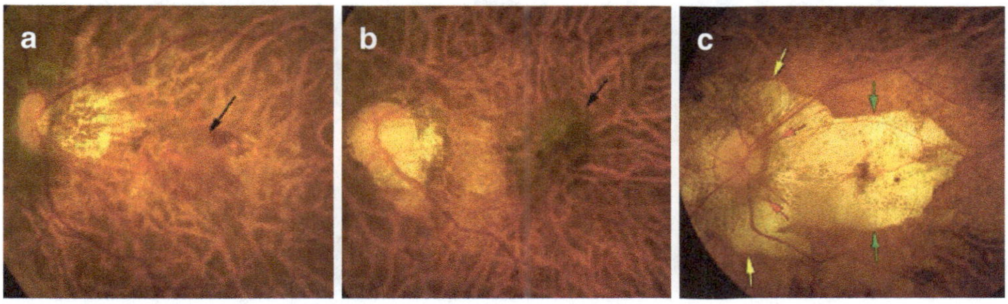

Fig. 9.9 Fundus photographs showing various phases of myopic CNV in different eyes. (**a**) Active phase. Subretinal bleeding is observed around the grayish CNV (black arrow). (**b**) Scar phase with pigmented scarred CNV (black arrow). (**c**) Atrophic phase at about 10 years after the first occurrence of a CNV; a well-defined macular atrophy (green arrows) appears as a macular Bruch's membrane defect, merging with a large parapapillary gamma zone (yellow arrows) around a parapapillary delta zone (red arrows)

In the long-term, both in treated eyes and in eyes exposed to the natural course of the disorder, macular atrophy develops around the scarred CNV and impairs central vision (Fig. 9.9). Swept-source OCT showed that CNV-related macular atrophy was not simply a chorioretinal atrophy but was BM hole [35], like patchy chorioretinal atrophy.

As shown upon OCT-angiography, the CNV maintains its blood flow even when the CNV transforms into the scar phase, including the area of CNV-related macular atrophy (Fig. 9.10). Louzada et al. [36] and Giuffre et al. [37] reported that blood vessels originating from the sclera were found at the site of myopic CNVs. Recently Ishida et al. [38] reported that the blood vessels of myopic CNVs were continuous to scleral branches of short posterior ciliary arteries (Fig. 9.11).

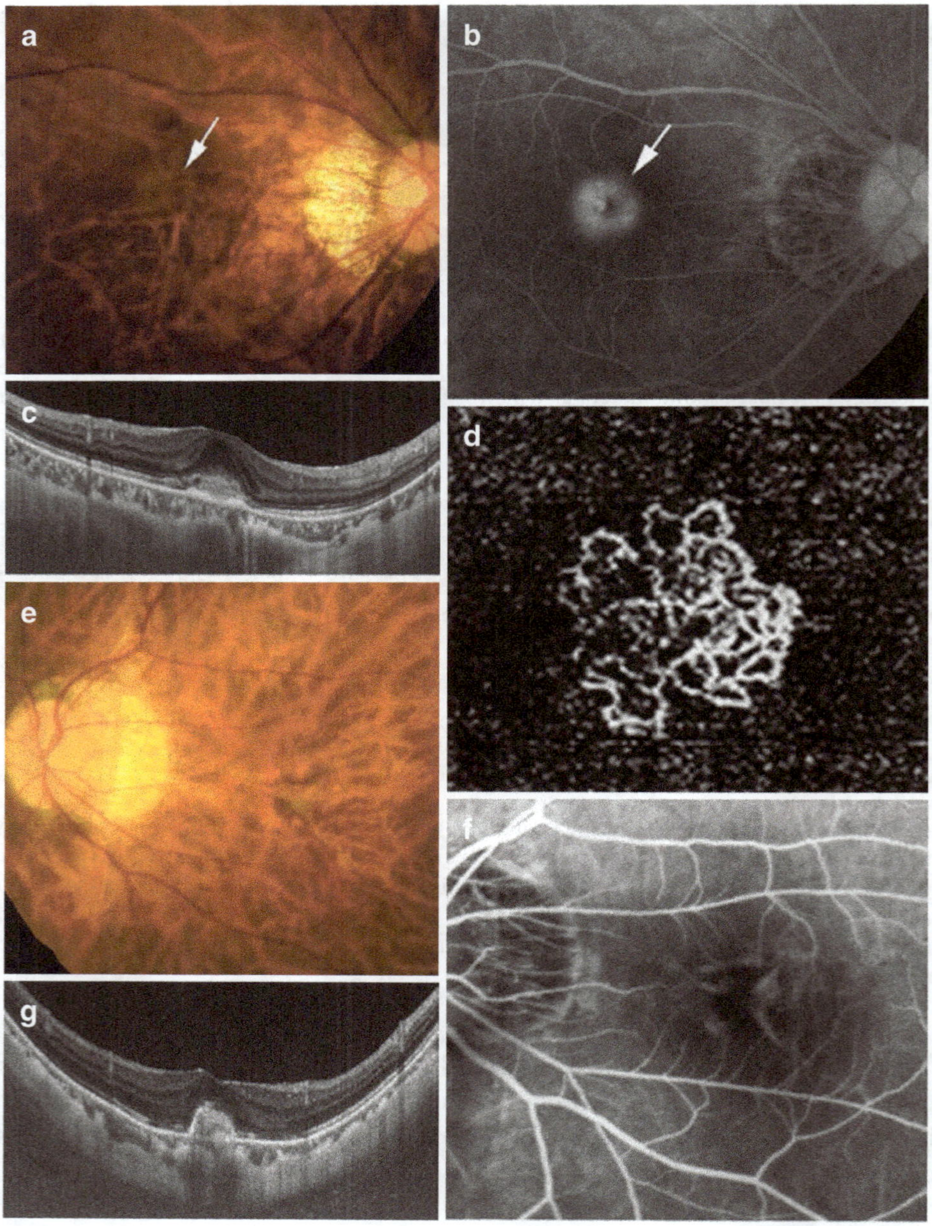

Fig. 9.10 Detection of choroidal neovascularization (CNV) with blood flow in all of the three phases of myopic CNV by optical coherent tomographic angiography (OCTA) [38]. (**a–d**) Active phase. Right fundus shows a grayish CNV (arrow in **a**). Fluorescein angiography (FA) shows hyper-fluorescence at the CNV (arrow in **b**). (**c**) Type II CNV is observed as subretinal tissue with fuzzy border by OCT. (**d**) OCTA shows newly formed vessels. (**e–h**) Scar phase. (**e**) Left fundus shows irregular shape of CNV. (**f**) FA shows tissue staining of irregular shape of CNV. (**g**) OCT shows subretinal CNV with sharp margins. (**h**) OCTA shows spiky shaped CNV. (**i–l**) Atrophic phase. CNV-related macular atrophy (margined by arrowheads) is seen around the remnants of a CNV (arrow in **i**). Fundus autofluorescence shows clear hypo-fluorescence in the area of the macular atrophy around the CNV (arrow in **j**). OCT shows subretinal CNV (arrow in **k**) surrounded by a large defect of Bruch's membrane. The inner retina directly sits on the sclera in the area of macular atrophy. The choroid is barely seen in the area of the macular atrophy. (**l**) OCTA shows CNV with blood flow. Large blood vessels appear to be connected to the CNV

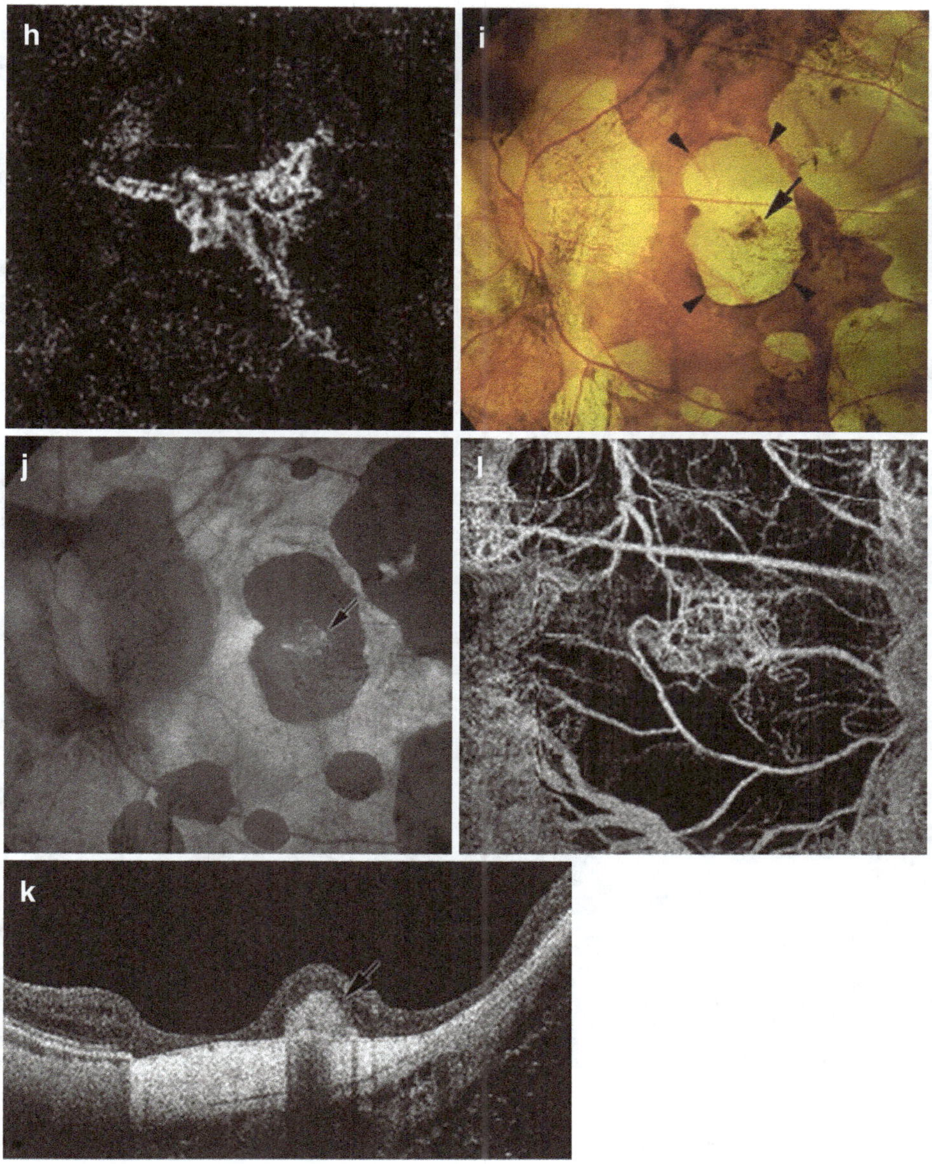

Fig. 9.10 (continued)

9.5 Myopic Macular Retinoschisis

Using optical coherence tomography, Takano and Kishi first demonstrated a foveal retinal detachment and retinoschisis in severely myopic eyes with posterior staphylomas [39]. Panozzo and Mercanti proposed the term "myopic traction maculopathy (MTM)" to encompass various findings characterized by a traction as visualized by OCT in highly myopic eyes [40]. Myopic traction maculopathy,

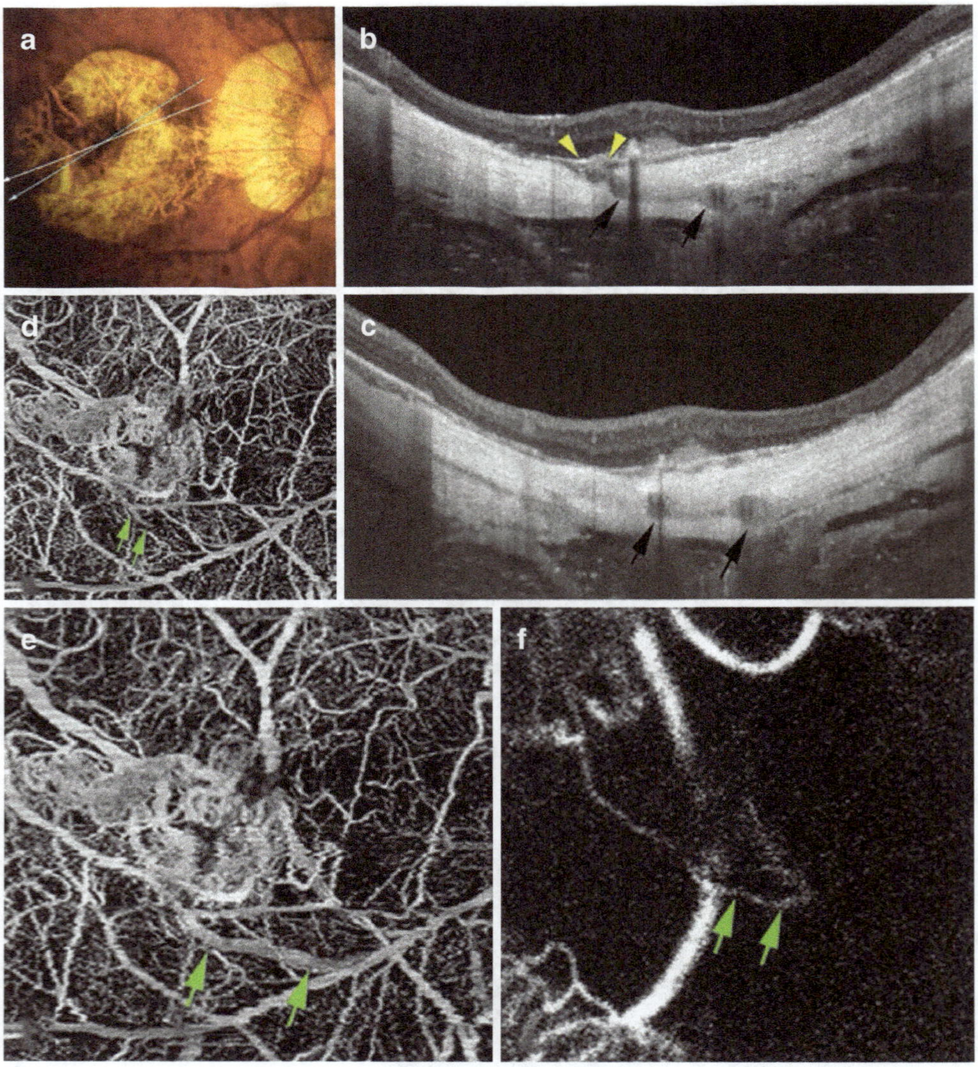

Fig. 9.11 Continuity between scleral perforating vessels and myopic choroidal neovascularization (CNV) in the atrophic phase [38]. (**a**) Fundus photograph of the right eye shows a sharp-margined macular atrophy around a CNV (arrow). Arrows indicate scanned line by OCT. (**b**, **c**) Swept-source OCT images show subretinal CNV. Cross sections of blood vessels coursing within the sclera can be seen (arrows in **c**) in a section scanned by swept-source OCT (blue arrow in **a**). In a serial OCT section (**b**, in a section scanned at white arrow in **a**), this vessel (arrows) is observed to be continuous with the CNV through a defect of Bruch's membrane (between arrowheads). (**d**, **e**) OCT angiogram shows the intrascleral vessel in Fig. 9.4b begins to be seen at the depth just posterior to the CNV (arrows, **d**). At a deeper slab **e**, the longer course of this vessel is seen (arrow, **e**). (**f**, **g**) Arterial phase of ICG angiogram (6 s after dye injection in **f**, and 8 s after dye injection in **g**) shows that the intrascleral vessel shown in OCT angiogram and OCT **b** scans was already filled with dye in the arterial phase (arrows). (**h**) Arterial phase of fluorescein angiogram (10 s after dye injection) shows that the intrascleral vessel observed in **f** and **g** is fairly seen (arrows)

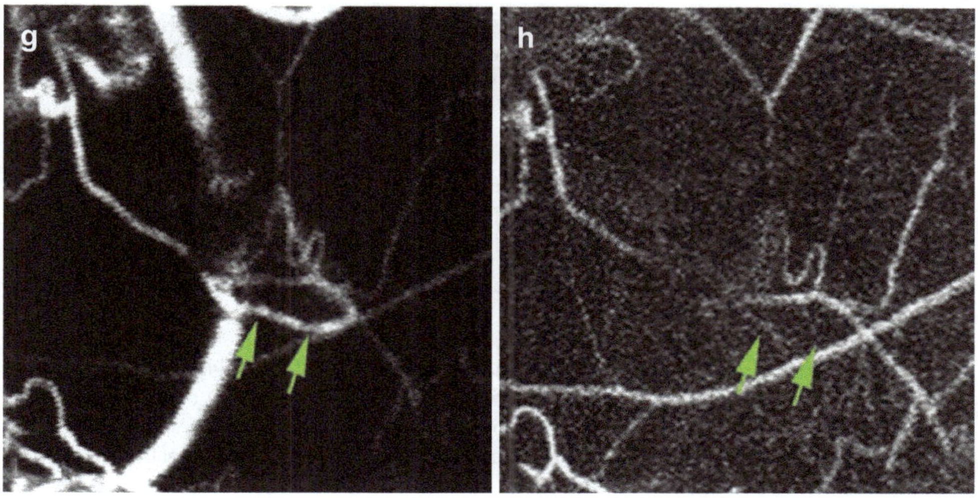

Fig. 9.11 (continued)

also called foveal retinoschisis [39], macular retinoschisis [41], or myopic foveoschisis [42], includes the features of schisis-like inner retinal fluid, schisis-like outer retina fluid, foveal detachment, lamellar or full-thickness macular hole, and/or macular detachment [43]. These features can best be detected by OCT as an indispensable tool to diagnose MTM. Additional examination techniques are a retro-mode imaging which uses an infrared laser in the confocal scanning laser ophthalmoscope and which can produce a pseudo-three-dimensional image showing the details of deep retinal structures (Fig. 9.12). Applying retro-mode imaging, a characteristic fingerprint and firework pattern at the corresponding area of a macular retinoschisis have been detected in the region of a macula retinoschisis [44, 45].

Shimada et al. have classified myopic traction maculopathy according to its location and extent from S0 through S4: S0: no retinoschisis; S1: extrafoveal; S2: foveal; S3: both foveal and extrafoveal but not the entire macula; and S4: entire macula [46].

9.6 Dome-Shaped Macula (DSM)

A dome-shaped macula (DSM) is an inward protrusion of the macula as visualized by OCT (Fig. 9.13) [47–49]. Imamura et al. reported that a DSM was associated with, and caused by, a local thickening of the subfoveal sclera [50]. It was postulated that the local thickening of the subfoveal sclera was an adaptive or

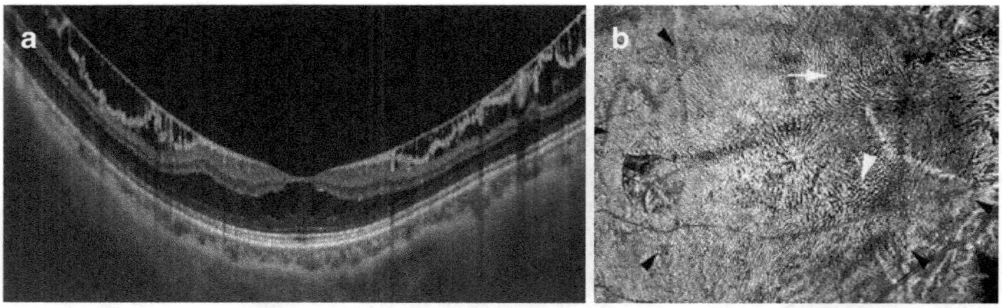

Fig. 9.12 Myopic macular retinoschisis. (**a**) OCT image shows outer and inner retinoschisis. (**b**) Columnar structures are seen within the area of outer retinoschisis (cited from [44]). Retro-mode image by F10 (Nidek, Aichi, Japan) showing a fingerprint pattern (black arrowheads) consisting of central radiating retinal striae and surrounding multiple dots (arrowhead) and lines (arrow). Many lines appear in parallel or in a whorled pattern. The inner lamellar hole appears as a circular defect at the central fovea

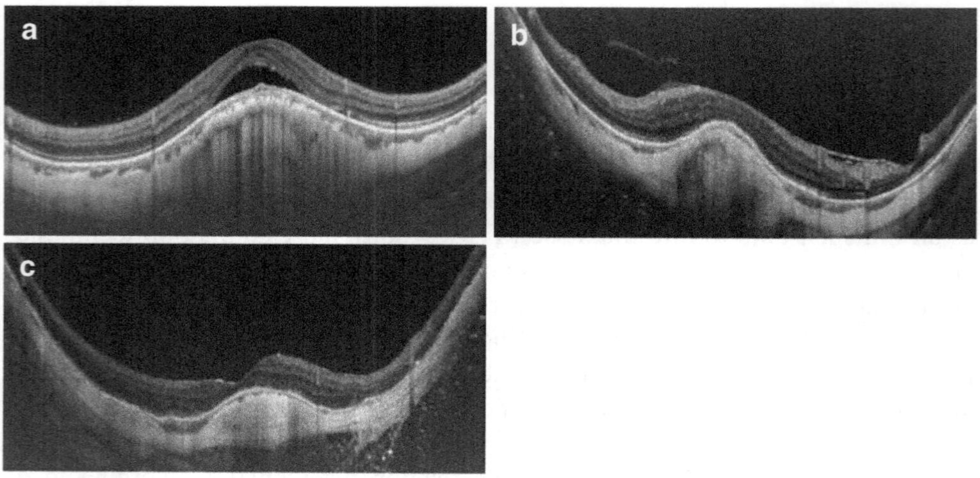

Fig. 9.13 Various types of Dome-shaped macula (DSM). (**a**) Serous retinal detachment is seen on the top of the dome. The sclera is too thick to allow the visualization of its outer surface. (**b**) The subfoveal sclera is thick; however, the scleral outer surface is visible in the surrounding area. (**c**) The subfoveal sclera is thick; however, the scleral outer surface is visible in all regions

compensatory response to the defocus of the image on the fovea in highly myopic eyes. Fang et al. [51] found the high prevalence of macular BM defects around the dome (Figs. 9.14 and 9.15). Ohno-Matsui et al. reported a similar finding [52] as peri-dome choroidal deepening. The morphology of the DSM in association with macular BM defects may be associated with a focal relaxation of the posterior sclera, no longer pushed outward by an expanding BM but allowed to partially bulge inward, leading to the formation of a DSM.

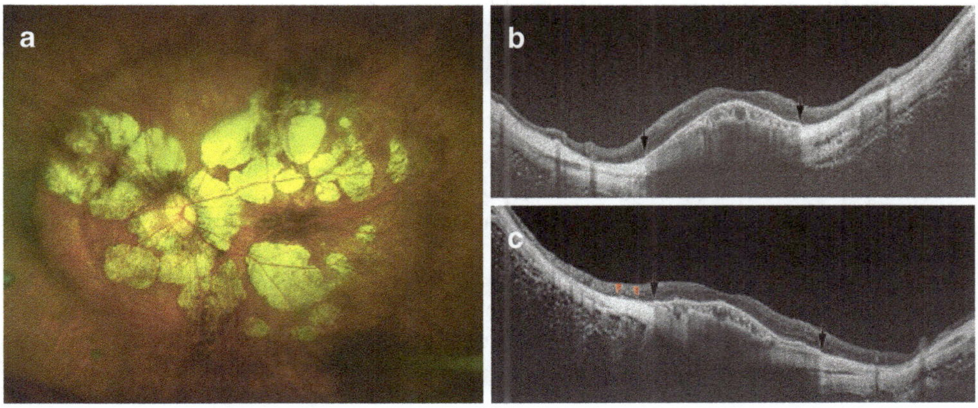

Fig. 9.14 Dome-shaped macula (DSM) coexisting with the macular Bruch's membrane defects (MBMD) associated with patchy atrophy [51]. (**a**) Left fundus of a 65-year-old woman with an axial length of 33.2 mm shows multiple patches of whitish, well-defined patchy atrophy in the regions superior and inferior to the fovea. Two long arrows show scanned lines examined by optical coherence tomography (OCT) in the images (**b**) and (**c**), respectively. (**b**) Oblique OCT section across the fovea demonstrates an inward protrusion due to DSM. Bruch's membrane is present at the center of the macula, but is interrupted abruptly (arrow) on both sides of the dome. (**c**) Oblique OCT section across the fovea shows the inward protrusion of macula due to DSM. Bruch's membrane is present at the center of macula, but is abruptly interrupted (arrow) on both sides of the dome. The remnants of Bruch's membrane are seen near the edge of the macular Bruch's membrane defect (arrowheads)

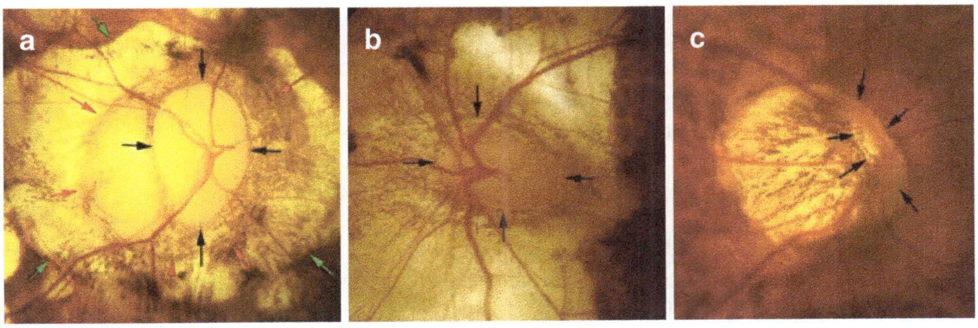

Fig. 9.15 Severe deformity of the optic disc due to pathologic myopia. (**a**) Acquired megalodisc. The optic disc shows irregular shape. (**b**) Horizontally stretched optic disc. (**c**) Extreme tilting of the optic disc. Black arrows: peripapillary rim; red arrows: parapapillary delta zone; green arrows: parapapillary gamma zone

References

1. Iwase A, Araie M, Tomidokoro A, et al. Prevalence and causes of low vision and blindness in a Japanese adult population: the Tajimi Study. Ophthalmology. 2006;113:1354–62.
2. Xu L, Wang Y, Li Y, et al. Causes of blindness and visual impairment in urban and rural areas in Beijing: the Beijing Eye Study. Ophthalmology. 2006;113:1134.e1.

3. You QS, Xu L, Yang H, et al. Five-year incidence of visual impairment and blindness in adult Chinese the Beijing Eye Study. Ophthalmology. 2011;118:1069–75.
4. Yamada M, Hiratsuka Y, Roberts CB, et al. Prevalence of visual impairment in the adult Japanese population by cause and severity and future projections. Ophthalmic Epidemiol. 2010;17:50–7.
5. Hsu WM, Cheng CY, Liu JH, et al. Prevalence and causes of visual impairment in an elderly Chinese population in Taiwan: the Shihpai Eye Study. Ophthalmology. 2004;111:62–9.
6. Ohno-Matsui K, Lai TYY, Cheung CMG, Lai CC. Updates of pathologic myopia. Prog Retin Eye Res. 2016;52:156–87.
7. Ohno-Matsui K, Kawasaki R, Jonas JB, et al. International photographic classification and grading system for myopic maculopathy. Am J Ophthalmol. 2015;159:877–83.
8. Fang Y, Yokoi T, Nagaoka N, et al. Progression of myopic maculopathy during 18-year follow-up. Ophthalmology. 2018;125(6):863–77.
9. Hayashi K, Ohno-Matsui K, Shimada N, et al. Long-term pattern of progression of myopic maculopathy: a natural history study. Ophthalmology. 2010;117:1595–611.
10. Yan YN, Wang YX, Yang Y, et al. Ten-year progression of myopic maculopathy: The Beijing Eye Study 2001-2011. Ophthalmology. 2018;125(8):1253–63.
11. Vongphanit J, Mitchell P, Wang JJ. Prevalence and progression of myopic retinopathy in an older population. Ophthalmology. 2002;109:704–11.
12. Xu L, Wang Y, Wang S, Jonas JB. High myopia and glaucoma susceptibility the Beijing Eye Study. Ophthalmology. 2007;114:216–20.
13. Nagaoka N, Jonas JB, Morohoshi K, et al. Glaucomatous-type optic discs in high myopia. PLoS One. 2015;10:e0138825.
14. Spaide RF. Staphyloma: part 1. New York: Springer; 2014. p. 167–76.
15. Moriyama M, Ohno-Matsui K, Hayashi K, et al. Topographical analyses of shape of eyes with pathologic myopia by high-resolution three dimensional magnetic resonance imaging. Ophthalmology. 2011;118:1626–37.
16. Moriyama M, Ohno-Matsui K, Modegi T, et al. Quantitative analyses of high-resolution 3D MR images of highly myopic eyes to determine their shapes. Invest Ophthalmol Vis Sci. 2012;53:4510–8.
17. Ohno-Matsui K. Proposed classification of posterior staphylomas based on analyses of eye shape by three-dimensional magnetic resonance imaging. Ophthalmology. 2014;121:1798–809.
18. Shinohara K, Shimada N, Moriyama M, et al. Posterior staphylomas in pathologic myopia imaged by widefield optical coherence tomography. Invest Ophthalmol Vis Sci. 2017;58: 3750–8.
19. Shinohara K, Tanaka N, Jonas JB, et al. Ultra-widefield optical coherence tomography to investigate relationships between myopic macular retinoschisis and posterior staphyloma. Ophthalmology. 2018;125(10):1575–86.
20. Curtin BJ. The posterior staphyloma of pathologic myopia. Trans Am Ophthalmol Soc. 1977;75:67–86.
21. Verkicharla PK, Ohno-Matsui K, Saw SM. Current and predicted demographics of high myopia and an update of its associated pathological changes. Ophthalmic Physiol Opt. 2015;35:465–75.
22. Ohno-Matsui K, Jonas JB, Spaide RF. Macular Bruch membrane holes in highly myopic patchy chorioretinal atrophy. Am J Ophthalmol. 2016;166:22–8.
23. Gao LQ, Liu W, Liang YB, et al. Prevalence and characteristics of myopic retinopathy in a rural Chinese adult population: the Handan Eye Study. Arch Ophthalmol. 2011;129:1199–204.
24. Zheng Y, Lavanya R, Wu R, et al. Prevalence and causes of visual impairment and blindness in an urban Indian population: the Singapore Indian Eye Study. Ophthalmology. 2011;118:1798–804.
25. Neelam K, Cheung CM, Ohno-Matsui K, et al. Choroidal neovascularization in pathological myopia. Prog Retin Eye Res. 2012;31:495–525.

26. Xu X, Fang Y, Uramoto K, et al. Clinical features of lacquer cracks in eyes with pathologic myopia. Retina. 2018. https://doi.org/10.1097/IAE.0000000000002168.
27. Shinohara K, Moriyama M, Shimada N, et al. Myopic stretch lines: linear lesions in fundus of eyes with pathologic myopia that differ from lacquer cracks. Retina. 2014;34:461–9.
28. Sayanagi K, Ikuno Y, Uematsu S, Nishida K. Features of the choriocapillaris in myopic maculopathy identified by optical coherence tomography angiography. Br J Ophthalmol. 2017;101:1524–9.
29. Ohno-Matsui K, Ito M, Tokoro T. Subretinal bleeding without choroidal neovascularization in pathologic myopia. A sign of new lacquer crack formation. Retina. 1996;16:196–202.
30. Shapiro M, Chandra SR. Evolution of lacquer cracks in high myopia. Ann Ophthalmol. 1985;17:231–5.
31. Klein RM, Green S. The development of lacquer cracks in pathologic myopia. Am J Ophthalmol. 1988;106:282–5.
32. Ohno-Matsui K, Yoshida T, Futagami S, et al. Patchy atrophy and lacquer cracks predispose to the development of choroidal neovascularisation in pathological myopia. Br J Ophthalmol. 2003;87:570–3.
33. Wolf S, Balciuniene VJ, Laganovska G, et al. RADIANCE: a randomized controlled study of ranibizumab in patients with choroidal neovascularization secondary to pathologic myopia. Ophthalmology. 2014;121:682–92.
34. Ikuno Y, Ohno-Matsui K, Wong TY, et al. Intravitreal aflibercept injection in patients with myopic choroidal neovascularization: The MYRROR Study. Ophthalmology. 2015;122:1220–7.
35. Ohno-Matsui K, Jonas JB, Spaide RF. Macular Bruch's membrane holes in choroidal neovascularization-related myopic macular atrophy by swept-source optical coherence tomography. Am J Ophthalmol. 2015;162:133–9.
36. Louzada RN, Ferrara D, Novais EA, et al. Analysis of scleral feeder vessel in myopic choroidal neovascularization using optical coherence tomography angiography. Ophthalmic Surg Lasers Imaging Retina. 2016;47:960–4.
37. Giuffre C, Querques L, Carnevali A, et al. Choroidal neovascularization and coincident perforating scleral vessels in pathologic myopia. Eur J Ophthalmol. 2017;27:e39–45.
38. Ishida T, Watanabe T, Yokoi T, et al. Possible connection of short posterior ciliary arteries to choroidal neovascularisations in eyes with pathologic myopia. Br J Ophthalmol. 2018;103(4):457–62.
39. Takano M, Kishi S. Foveal retinoschisis and retinal detachment in severely myopic eyes with posterior staphyloma. Am J Ophthalmol. 1999;128:472–6.
40. Panozzo G, Mercanti A. Optical coherence tomography findings in myopic traction maculopathy. Arch Ophthalmol. 2004;122:1455–60.
41. Benhamou N, Massin P, Haouchine B, et al. Macular retinoschisis in highly myopic eyes. Am J Ophthalmol. 2002;133:794–800.
42. Ikuno Y, Sayanagi K, Ohji M, et al. Vitrectomy and internal limiting membrane peeling for myopic foveoschisis. Am J Ophthalmol. 2004;137:719–24.
43. Johnson MW. Myopic traction maculopathy: pathogenic mechanisms and surgical treatment. Retina. 2012;32(Suppl 2):S205–10.
44. Tanaka Y, Shimada N, Ohno-Matsui K, et al. Retromode retinal imaging of macular retinoschisis in highly myopic eyes. Am J Ophthalmol. 2010;149:635–40.e1.
45. Su Y, Zhang X, Wu K, et al. The noninvasive retro-mode imaging of confocal scanning laser ophthalmoscopy in myopic maculopathy: a prospective observational study. Eye. 2014;28:998–1003.
46. Shimada N, Tanaka Y, Tokoro T, Ohno-Matsui K. Natural course of myopic traction maculopathy and factors associated with progression or resolution. Am J Ophthalmol. 2013;156:948–57.
47. Gaucher D, Erginay A, Lecleire-Collet A, et al. Dome-shaped macula in eyes with myopic posterior staphyloma. Am J Ophthalmol. 2008;145:909–14.
48. Caillaux V, Gaucher D, Gualino V, et al. Morphologic characterization of dome-shaped macula in myopic eyes with serous macular detachment. Am J Ophthalmol. 2013;156:958–67.

49. Ellabban AA, Tsujikawa A, Matsumoto A, et al. Three-dimensional tomographic features of dome-shaped macula by swept-source optical coherence tomography. Am J Ophthalmol. 2012;3:578.
50. Imamura Y, Iida T, Maruko I, et al. Enhanced depth imaging optical coherence tomography of the sclera in dome-shaped macula. Am J Ophthalmol. 2011;151:297–302.
51. Fang Y, Jonas JB, Yokoi T, et al. Macular Bruch's membrane defect and dome-shaped macula in high myopia. PLoS One. 2017;12:e0178998.
52. Ohno-Matsui K, Fang Y, Uramoto K, et al. Peri-dome choroidal deepening in highly myopic eyes with dome-shaped maculas. Am J Ophthalmol. 2017;183:134–40.

10

Myopia Evaluation and the Role of Imaging

Quan V. Hoang, Jacqueline Chua, Marcus Ang, and Leopold Schmetterer

Q. V. Hoang
Singapore Eye Research Institute, Singapore, Singapore

Singapore National Eye Centre, Singapore, Singapore

Eye Academic Clinical Program, Duke-NUS Medical School, Singapore, Singapore

Department of Ophthalmology, Harkness Eye Institute, Columbia University Medical Center, New York, NY, USA

J. Chua
Singapore Eye Research Institute, Singapore, Singapore

Singapore National Eye Centre, Singapore, Singapore

Eye Academic Clinical Program, Duke-NUS Medical School, Singapore, Singapore

M. Ang
Singapore Eye Research Institute, Singapore, Singapore

Singapore National Eye Centre, Singapore, Singapore

Eye Academic Clinical Program, Duke-NUS Medical School, Singapore, Singapore

Myopia Centre, Cornea and Refractive Service, Singapore National Eye Centre, Singapore, Singapore

L. Schmetterer (✉)
Singapore Eye Research Institute, Singapore, Singapore

Singapore National Eye Centre, Singapore, Singapore

Eye Academic Clinical Program, Duke-NUS Medical School, Singapore, Singapore

Department of Ophthalmology, Lee Kong Chian School of Medicine, Nanyang Technological University, Singapore, Singapore

School of Chemical and Biomedical Engineering, Nanyang Technological University, Singapore, Singapore

Department of Clinical Pharmacology, Medical University of Vienna, Vienna, Austria

Center for Medical Physics and Biomedical Engineering, Medical University of Vienna, Vienna, Austria
e-mail: leopold.schmetterer@seri.com.sg

Key Points

- Advances in ocular imaging devices including optical coherence tomography, ultrasound, and magnetic resonance imaging have enabled the visualization of pathologic changes due to myopia, identifying microscopic changes ranging from the posterior segment (sclera, choroid, retina, and/or the optic nerve) to the anterior segment.
- Imaging-derived measures (imaging biomarkers) are potentially useful in assessing degenerative changes occurring in the myopic fundus, in evaluating the early changes preceding myopic macular degeneration, and in providing objective measures of ocular structures to aid in detecting staphyloma formation and progression, myopic macular degeneration-tilted disc syndrome, and glaucoma in highly myopic eyes.
- Imaging the highly myopic eye is not straightforward and is associated with challenges such as optics-related aberrations, focusing ability of current devices, and morphological alterations of the myopic fundus and optic nerve.
- An understanding of the imaging of microstructural changes associated with pathological myopia, challenges associated with imaging devices, and potential usefulness and limitations of imaging devices will better inform clinicians of its future potential in the diagnosis and management of vision-threatening complications associated with pathological myopia.

10.1 Introduction

In evaluating the myopic eye, imaging has been proven vital in assessing disease complications [1] and prognostication for future management. Early identification of these changes would help predict the development of future complications, which include retinal tears and retinal detachments [2]. Additionally, the possibility of identifying subtle changes in the macula (such as macular schisis or early macular holes; Fig. 10.1) via high-resolution images of the macula could perchance aid clinicians in predicting the development of complications such as macular holes and retinal detachments [3].

Furthermore, imaging may help detect, prognosticate, and guide management of other myopia-related eye diseases. This includes the early detection of atrophy and defects in the basement membrane, located between retinal pigment epithelium (RPE) and Bruch's membrane (BM), which would help predict the risk of developing choroidal neovascularization (CNV) [4]—a leading cause of low vision and blindness in 5–17% of eyes in patients with pathological myopia (PM) [5]. In addition, imaging is vital for monitoring progression of posterior staphylomas and geographic atrophy, both of which can cause visual impairment in older age groups of patients [6].

Optic disc imaging can also be used to predict the development of glaucoma, where visualization of myopic tilting of the optic disc with peripapillary atrophy and pitting of the optic disc [7], is a possible predisposing factor [8, 9]. Serial imaging investigative measures can therefore be utilized for monitoring the development

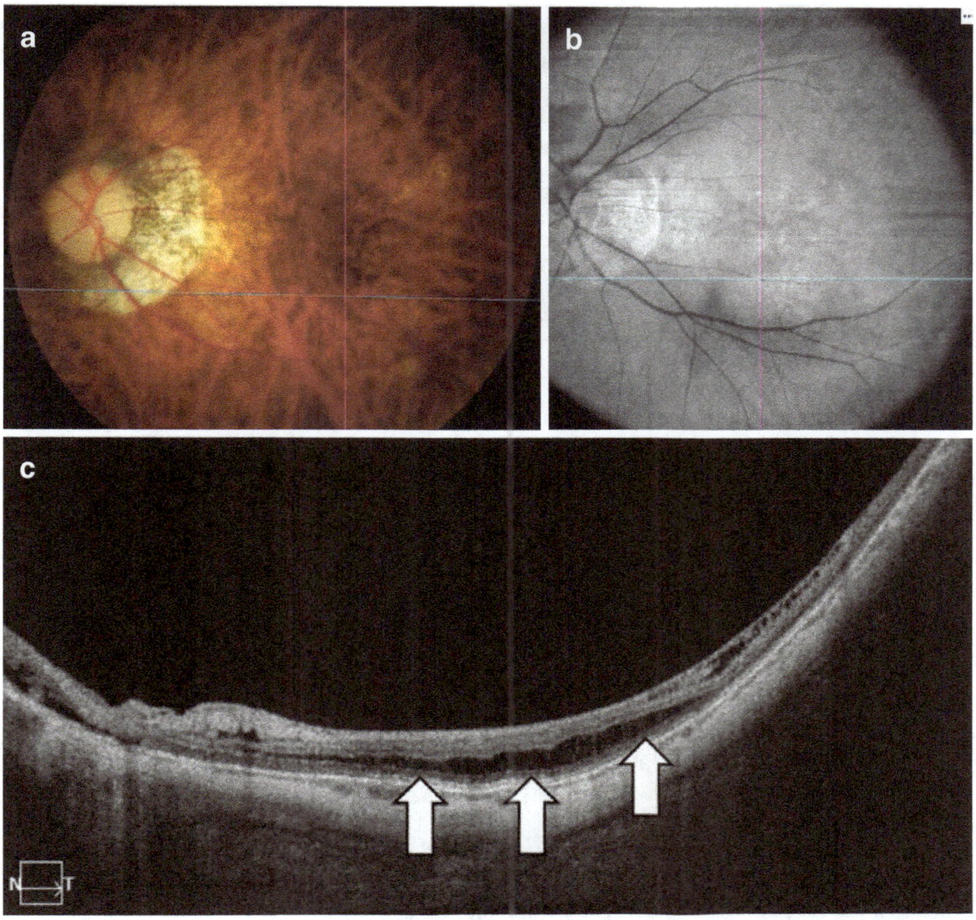

Fig. 10.1 Optical coherence tomography (OCT) imaging findings of a patient with myopic macular degeneration, showing the benefits of using the OCT over color fundus photograph in detecting retinoschisis. (**a**) Color fundus photograph showing tilted disc with large temporal peripapillary atrophy. (**b**, 12 × 12 mm; PLEX Elite, Zeiss) OCT of the fundus showing slight elevation of the retina where the crosshair is positioned. (**c**) OCT B-scan showing distinct retinoschisis (white arrows)

of open-angle, normal-tension glaucoma [10]. With the hope of exploring novel developments and prospective future clinical applications in the field of imaging in myopia, this chapter thus outlines the significance and challenges of imaging myopic eyes (from the anterior and posterior segments and optic nerve).

10.2 Disease Characteristics of Myopia

To best understand how one should approach imaging eyes with myopia, one needs to gear imaging modalities based on the pathophysiology of the disease, which has already been outlined in previous chapters. For example, not only does the sclera of these extremely elongated eyes show marked scleral thinning [12, 13], some eyes thin to the extent that local outpouchings or staphylomas form (Figs. 10.2 and 10.3). Staphylomas are often recognized as the harbinger of PM, reported in up to 90% of

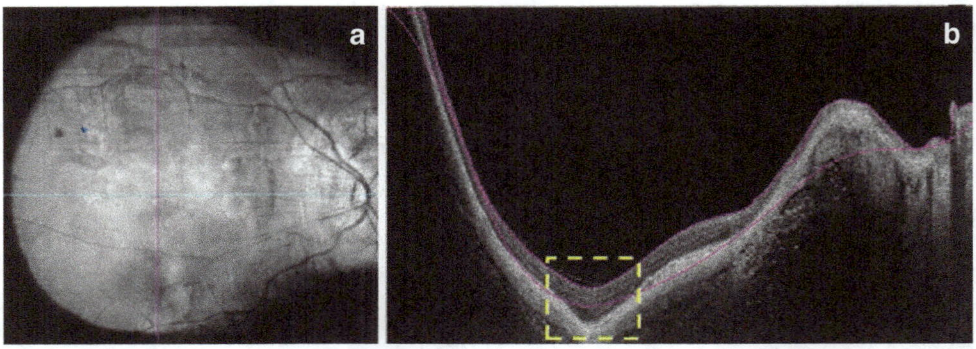

Fig. 10.2 Optical coherence tomography (OCT) imaging findings of a highly myopic patient, showing the benefits of using the OCT over fundus photograph to detect posterior staphyloma. (**a**, 12 × 12 mm; PLEX Elite, Zeiss) OCT fundus photograph showing tilted disc with large temporal peripapillary atrophy. (**b**) OCT B-scan showing distinct posterior staphyloma (yellow dotted box)

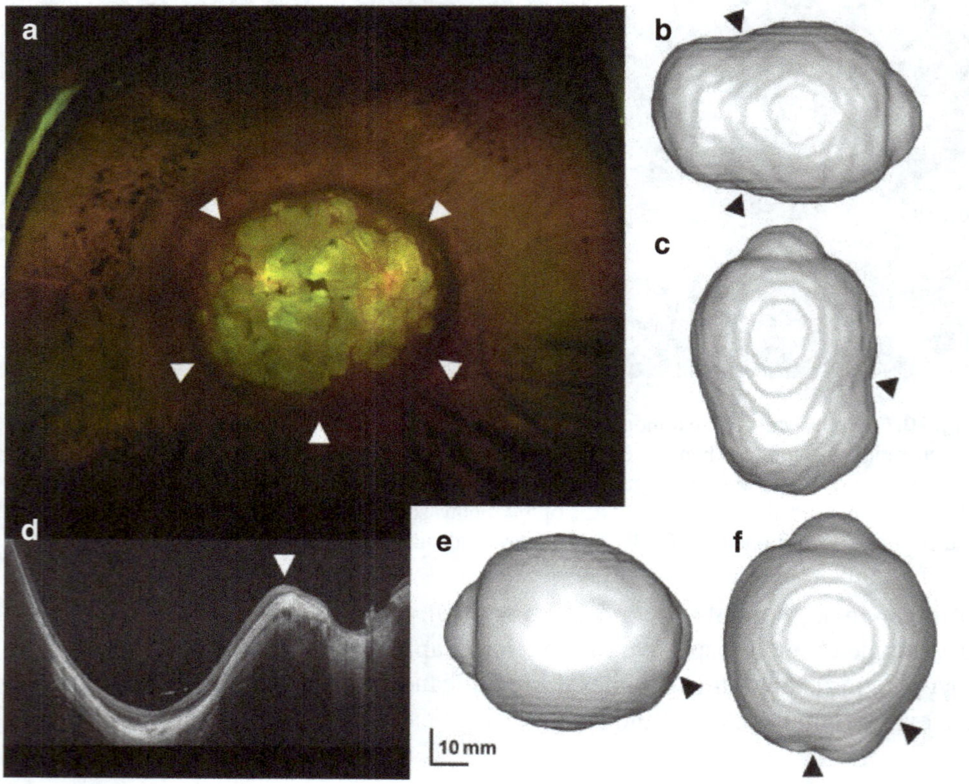

Fig. 10.3 Fundus photography, swept source optical coherence tomography (SSOCT), and 3-dimensional magnetic resonance imaging (MRI) of patients with posterior staphyloma. Patient 1 (**a**, **b**, **c**) was a 58-year-old woman with an axial length of 35.4 mm in the right eye (OD). The right fundus shows a deep, circular-shaped posterior staphyloma, with an abrupt change in scleral curvature (arrowheads) apparent on fundus photography (A) and OD MRI volume renderings (B- temporal view, C- inferior view). Patient 2 (**d**, **e**, **f**) was a 61-year-old woman with an OD axial length of 33.8 mm. A posterior staphyloma was present, with an abrupt change in scleral curvature (arrowheads) apparent on OD SSOCT (D) and OD MRI volume renderings (E- nasal view, F- superior view)

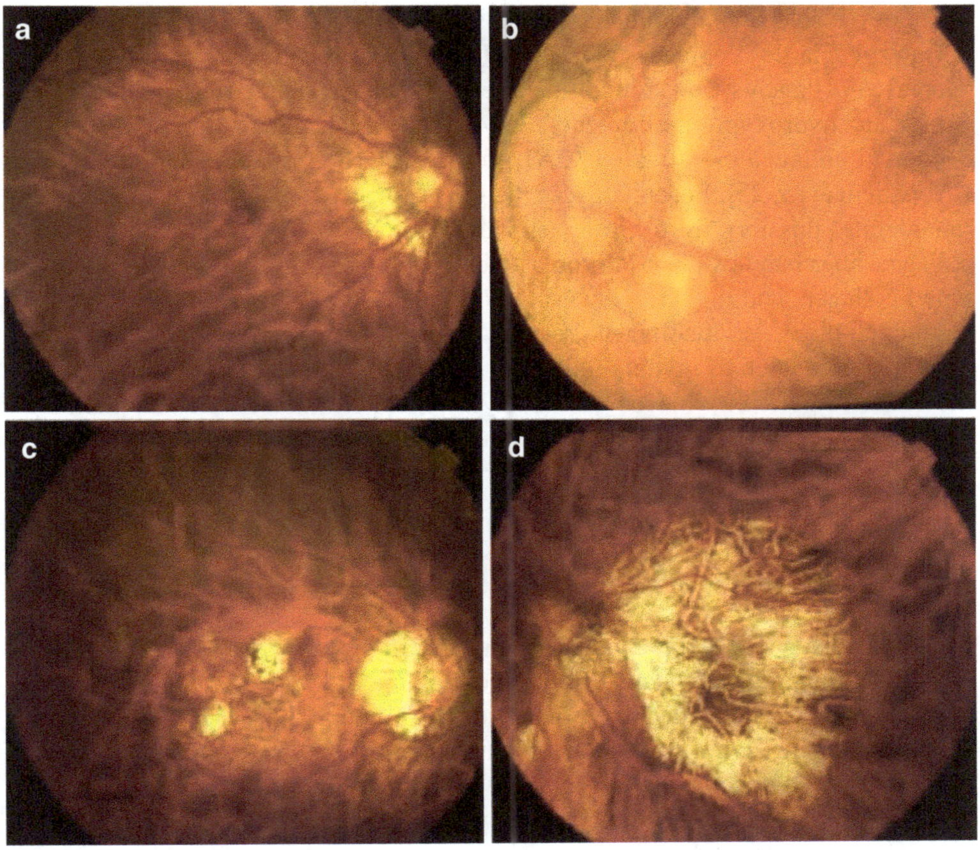

Fig. 10.4 Color fundus photographs showing the worsening levels of myopic macular degeneration; (**a**) Category 1, (**b**) Category 2, (**c**) Category 3 (**c**), and (**d**) Category 4

high myopia (HM) patients [14, 15]. More recent reports noted a severe grade of staphyloma being associated with further eye elongation [16] and more severe and progressive myopic macular degeneration (MMD; Fig. 10.4) [14, 17, 18]. Given that MMD is the leading cause of blindness in Japan [19], and the second leading cause in Chinese adults [20], it highlights the importance of closely monitoring patients with a severe grade of staphyloma. Risk of vision loss from myopic maculopathy (e.g., from splitting of retinal layers (foveoschisis), hole formation, atrophy, and CNV) may correlate with the specific location and conformation [11] of staphylomas [21].

10.3 Key Structures Altered in Myopia and Pathological Myopia

10.3.1 Sclera and Collagen

Changes in sclera and collagen structures may underlie axial elongation and staphyloma formation and progression. The anatomical changes underlying global eye elongation and local staphyloma formation likely occur in the component collagen fibers of the sclera. In mammalian models, there is scleral thinning and tissue loss during myopia development [11, 22] with a net decrease in scleral collagen (with decreased collagen synthesis and increased degradation) evidenced by reduced dry weight and hydroxyproline content [23, 24]. Decreased collagen fiber diameter and decreased collagen crosslinking (CXL) are seen in both mammalian models and HM patients [13, 25]. Specifically, in the guinea pig myopia model, there is scleral remodeling, possibly from greater slippage [26] between collagen fibrils and/or collagen fiber bundles due to fibroblast deactivation, with decreased expression of type I collagen, and α_2 and α_1 integrin [27, 28]. In the tree shrew mammalian myopia model, blockage of collagen crosslinking with β-aminopropionitrile resulted in an increased degree of myopia-induced vitreous elongation and scleral thinning at the posterior pole [29]. Moreover, the development of high myopia and pathologic myopia may be driven by genes such as the scleral remodeling gene LAMA2, leading to scleral thinning and staphyloma formation [30].

10.3.2 Choroidal Changes

Choroidal changes in myopia may contribute to atrophy and myopic macular degeneration. Morphological change such as the thinning of the choroidal vascular layer is closely associated with increasing levels of myopia and MMD (either immediately preceding, concurrent with or immediately following the development of MMD) [31–33]. Specifically, Wei et al. reported that subfoveal choroidal thickness in their Beijing-based cohort decreased by 15 μm per diopter of increased myopia [31]. There are various lesions comprising myopic maculopathy [3, 11, 18, 34, 35] that all involve the choroid, namely, diffuse chorioretinal atrophy, patchy chorioretinal atrophy, macular atrophy (bare sclera), lacquer cracks, and myopic choroidal neovascularization. Diffuse atrophy is a yellowish, ill-defined lesion [34], and is characterized by a marked thinning of the choroid as seen on optical coherence tomography (OCT), but with relatively preserved outer retina and retinal pigment epithelium, allowing for relatively good vision. Patchy chorioretinal atrophy is whitish, well-defined atrophy [34] with complete localized loss of the choroid with only the large choroidal vessels sporadically remaining within the atrophic area. Loss of the choroid is soon followed by loss of outer retina and retinal pigment epithelium. Macular atrophy is similar to patchy atrophy but tends to be centered at the fovea.

10.3.3 Bruch's Membrane and Retinal Pigment Epithelium Changes

The hallmark anatomical changes that occur alongside the development and progression of MMD are changes in BM and RPE as reflected in increasing degrees of atrophy [36]. Moreover, BM changes have been postulated to be the main driver of axial elongation overall [37]. Recently, Ohno-Matsui et al. reported the use of swept-source OCT (SS-OCT) to demonstrate that patchy atrophy was not simply chorioretinal atrophy, but also included a hole in Bruch's membrane [38]. Angiographically observed vessels within the area of patchy atrophy may include large choroidal vessels, intrascleral vessels, and retrobulbar vessels. Lacquer cracks are observed as yellowish linear lesions [34, 39, 40], and represent the mechanical rupture of BM [41]. Jonas et al. have reported an increase in disc–fovea distance due to an increase in the peripapillary gamma zone. Since BM thickness was found to be independent of axial length [42], even in the much larger surface area in an axially elongated eye in a human histomorphometric study, Jonas et al. inferred that the volume of BM increased with longer axial length and BM is actively produced during axial length elongation [37]. They postulated that BM was a primary driver of axial elongation that led to choroidal thinning through "compression." If this was indeed the mechanism, then the RPE is an ideal target for medical intervention in both eyes that are already severely elongated, as well as those undergoing progression, but still only minimally elongated.

10.4 Existing Imaging Modalities to Evaluate the Myopic Eye

10.4.1 Optical Coherence Tomography

Ophthalmic OCT systems can image the anterior segment as well as the posterior segment of the eye such as the retina, BM, RPE, and choroid. Spectral-domain OCT (SD-OCT, Spectralis, Heidelberg Eng., Carlsbad, CA) provides an axial resolution of 4 μm and a lateral resolution of 14 μm, but only about 1 mm of penetration into the retina. The extremely fine resolution of OCT allows better assessment of retinal layers such as photoreceptors, the ganglion cells, plexiform, and nuclear layers [43] and vitreous membranes in proximity to the retina. In contrast to the SD-OCT, SS-OCT uses a tunable laser with a longer wavelength of 1050 nm, which achieves greater penetration of tissue with less signal roll-off, allowing better visualization of choroidal anatomy [38, 44, 45] and has specifically been employed to correlate defects in BM with the atrophy of MMD [38]. In addition to utilizing choroidal thickness as biomarker for myopia progression [31–33], recent developments provide further insight into the function of the choroid, including the calculation of choroidal vascular index (CVI, the vessel-area-to-stromal-area ratio using a validated automated algorithm) [46] and OCTA using the SS-OCT (SS-OCTA, a noninvasive method of imaging choroidal vasculature, and specifically the foveal avascular zone (FAZ) without the administration of intravenous dye) [47, 48]. Newer UWF-OCT systems allow for even wider (100°) scans. Wider scans are likely crucial to accurately depicting staphyloma shape [49].

10.4.2 Ultrasound

Ophthalmic ultrasound can image the entire eye dynamically. Since their introduction in 1958, mechanically scanned, single element 10 MHz transducers have largely been the norm for imaging of the eye [50]. UBM systems (Escalon-Sonomed, Quantel, Ophthalmic Technologies, among others) have been used for diagnostic imaging and biometric characterization [51, 52]. Systems operating at 20 MHz were introduced (Quantel Medical, Bozeman, MT) for examination of the posterior segment of the eye and the vitreoretinal interface [51, 53]. With an axial resolution of about 75 μm, these systems provide superior resolution compared to conventional 10 MHz systems as well as the ability to image the retina. They also provide far deeper penetration than optical modalities (10 mm vs. 1 mm for OCT). Commercial single-element systems are designed such that during a contact examination, the geometric focus of the transducer falls just anterior to the retina. However, the anterior vitreous and anterior-segment structures (cornea, iris, ciliary body, and lens) are poorly visualized because they fall within the unfocused near field of the transducer which makes current ophthalmic systems unsuitable for imaging the entire vitreous. Recent advancements in annular-array imaging technology overcome these technical limits [54].

10.4.3 Magnetic Resonance Imaging

MRI allows for imaging of the whole eye (Fig. 10.3). The standard ophthalmology imaging modalities of ultrasound and optical coherence tomography are limited by a relatively narrow field of view. MRI does allow for imaging of the entire eye globe, but visualizing eye wall distortions at standard MR resolutions minimizes effect sizes and induces aliasing artifacts that obfuscate distortions. Super-resolution is an established MR approach that provides a means of detecting extremely small distortions by increasing signal to noise (with isotropic resolutions down to 50–100 μm), reducing scan time (which would allow patients to more readily maintain fixation, thereby reducing eye movement artifacts), and minimizing aliasing artifacts that can bias estimates [55, 56].

10.5 Challenges in Imaging of the Myopic Eye

10.5.1 Interaction Between Low- and High-Order Aberrations

Given the presence of two positive lenses (the cornea and the crystalline lens) in the eye, any imaging of intraocular structures is contingent on their properties. This makes direct visualization and imaging structures in the posterior segment, secondary to optical imperfections through the cornea and lens, the main challenge in imaging a myopic eye. Examples of such would include light diffraction in the pupil, intraocular scattering, and optical aberrations. As a result of these imperfections, imaging of patients with high myopia using any modality (such as fundus photography) would have a poorer image quality due to an imbalance of low- and high-order aberrations [57, 58]. Other causes to consider include the limitations of focusing lenses used by the imaging device. For example, the device may not be able to compensate (diopter compensation) sufficiently in patients with very high myopia (more than −12.0 D). Pathological myopia is also associated with varying structural changes within the eye (due to the abnormal eye elongation, scleral and corneal curvature irregularities, cataracts leading to poor clarity, or retinal thinning causing abnormal projections of the final image [58, 59]). Such structural changes are demonstrated in altered optic nerve head morphology.

Taking into considerations the challenges faced when imaging the myopic eye, current standards of practice for investigations include fundus photography, dye-based angiography, ultrasound (including biomicroscopy), and magnetic resonance imaging (MRI). The OCT has also become an often-used tool for the characterization of ocular tissue structural changes arising from myopia [60]. Swept source (SS)-OCT has a higher wavelength of 1050 nm and is hence able to penetrate into deeper layers. It is also capable of wide-angle scans, given its speed of capture and software engineering. More recently, OCT angiography (OCTA) has enabled visualization of the vasculature of the eye [61–63]. Nonetheless, there still exists room for improvement and various constraints. In the case of wide-field OCT (WF-OCT), problems with segmentation in the periphery may arise due to inadequate depth range to image the complete anterior–posterior extent of the posterior pole. Further considerations arise regarding the normative databases of OCT systems, where reference and patient cohorts should ideally be derived from the same population to reflect similar comorbidities [64]. Stratifications normally employed for covariates that affect measurements (such as age, ethnicity, and refractive error) are challenging to derive in myopic eyes—a result of large regional variation in refractive error prevalence [65]. In regions with a high prevalence of myopia and pathological myopia, this results in normative databases being poor representations of the existing patient population.

10.5.2 Challenges in Imaging the Anterior Segment

In high myopia, while most refractive errors in myopic eyes arise from an axial length, alterations in the anterior segment lead to significant optical and high-order aberrations [66]. Furthermore, the association between myopia and biomechanical changes in the cornea has implications in the assessment of intraocular pressure and may have a role in the pathogenesis of myopia [67]. Indeed, existing studies report inconsistent results—attributable to different imaging and measurement techniques, and the technological limitations in measuring biomechanical changes in the cornea associated with increasing myopia [68]. Preoperative clinical evaluation of patients with high myopia still necessitates imaging of the cornea and anterior segment, given their increasing risk of developing ectasia proportionate to the amount of corneal tissue removed in laser refractive surgeries [69]. Furthermore, as high myopes are more likely to require phakic lens implantation [70], accurate anterior segment imaging is necessary to ensure adequate safety measures prior to implantation and accurate intraocular lens (IOL) implantation. Especially in high myopes, accurate formulae, anterior segment imaging, and corneal topography are all necessary to prevent refractive surprises [71] and complications postoperatively. Significant improvements in IOL calculations and refractive prediction in high myopes [71] have fortunately been accomplished with new developments in biometry incorporating anterior segment OCT technology [72], coupled with next-generation formulae.

10.5.3 Challenges in Imaging the Retina

Prior to the discovery of modern imaging techniques, there were three main challenges faced in retinal imaging. First, the diagnosis of myopic foveoschisis was challenging based on clinical examination and fundus photography due to the lack of contrast between the retinal tissues and underlying choroid. Second, posterior staphylomas, a hallmark of pathological myopia [73], could not be identified from standalone two-dimensional fundus photography with ease. Finally, it is also challenging to capture lattice degeneration and retinal breaks in the peripheries on traditional 50° fundus photographs.

With the OCT, the way clinicians diagnosed and managed retinal complications of pathological myopia was transformed—with the ability to examine retinal layers *in vivo* and at high resolution. The ability to view distinct retinal layers has enhanced visualization of myopic traction maculopathy (MTM), for which splitting of the retinal layers can be well visualized on cross-sectional OCT scans of the retina. This can be taken a step further using retromode fundus imaging [74]. Examples of features that can be seen include inner or outer retinal schisis, foveal detachment, lamellar, or full thickness macular hole and/or macular detachment [75, 76].

Another aspect in which OCT has advanced the diagnosis and management of myopia-related eye diseases is in the characterization of posterior staphylomas, which are one of the hallmarks of pathological myopia. Nonstereoscopic fundus photographs are inadequate for detailed studies of posterior staphylomas as the change in contour at the staphyloma edge is not always discernible. The OCT overcomes this limitation because of its excellent depth resolution [21, 77]. Comparing their capability in visualizing posterior staphylomas, Shinohara et al. showed no significant differences between using WF-OCT and three-dimensional (3D) MRI imaging. It is noted, however, that ultrawide-field OCT (UWF-OCT) had the advantage in visualizing the spatial relationship of the staphylomas with the optic nerve and macula [78, 79].

Comparing the use of conventional fundus photography to UWF retinal imaging, the former has been shown capable of imaging up to 50° of the retina, while the latter covers a wider field of the retina at 200°. Given the high prevalence of lattice degeneration and retinal breaks in the peripheral retina in patients with highly myopic eyes, the advantages of UWF retinal imaging can be appreciated.

A potentially blinding complication of high myopia, myopic choroidal neovascularization (mCNV) is not easily diagnosed and monitored solely with clinical examinations. Multimodal imaging thus has a pertinent place in assessing mCNV. Verifying the diagnosis of mCNV requires the use of a fundus fluorescein angiography (FFA)—where leakage is seen as increasing size and intensity of hyperfluorescence with time [80]. A feature of pathological myopia, retinal avascularity in the 360° of the periphery, can also be revealed using wide-field FFA [81]. Distinguishing the myriad causes of subretinal exudation in high myopes (i.e., simple lacquer crack hemorrhage, inflammatory lesions, and mCNV [82, 83]) can be achieved with OCTA, which has the ability to identify neovascular membranes noninvasively. However, FFA remains the gold standard for mCNV diagnosis, given OCTA's comparatively lower sensitivity [84]. Furthermore, FFA is still necessary for monitoring disease activity, as OCTA lacks the ability to discern disease activity—where the flow signal may persist in an inactive mCNA [83–85]. Still, OCTA can assist with distinguishing the stages of mCNV via identification of signs of activity. These include ill-defined margins [86], disruption of the external limiting membrane [87], and variable amounts of intraretinal and subretinal fluids. These hyper-reflective lesions coalesce and develop a distinct border with appropriate treatment. Previous studies using the OCTA have suggested that rupture of the Bruch's membranes may be the cause of macular atrophy developing after mCNV [88]. However, the combination of OCTA and SS-OCT in multimodal imaging has given promising results—suggesting that mCNV is directly supplied by the short posterior ciliary artery instead of the choroidal vasculature as previously postulated [89].

10.5.4 Challenges in Imaging the Choroid and Sclera

Lying between the sclera and the RPE, the choroid's anatomical location makes imaging a challenge without the use of methods such as indocyanine green (ICG) angiography, ultrasonography (US), and OCT. Moreover, the choroid in pathological myopia is often extremely thin and thus difficult to measure. The addition of other, varied factors that interfere with choroid imaging in the myopic eye further complicate the process.

Typical fluorescein angiography has limited use in choroidal visualization since melanin impedes most of the spectra emitted from the agent. Imaging is also made near impossible with light absorption and scattering produced by the RPE pigment and choroidal blood. On the other hand, angiography via ICG has better use for the evaluation of various choroidal vasculopathy and inflammatory diseases [90]. This can be attributed to ICG's emitted spectrum being within the near-infrared wavelength—which is not disrupted by the RPE pigment or choroidal blood [91]. Nonetheless, other modalities such as OCT and autofluorescence imaging are still more feasible in the clinical setting and are thus still more often used than ICG angiography. Other modes of imaging include OCTA for assessing choroidal vasculature and its structures [46–48], as well as B-scan ultrasound to image the choroid with better penetration. However, B-scan images provide poorer resolution than those of OCTA—which is subsequently worsened by the thinning of the choroid in PM [53]. Yet, despite its flaws, the ultrasound remains useful in detecting staphylomas and globe contours.

With regard to OCT, we find that spectral domain OCT (SD-OCT) instruments with enhanced depth imaging can visualize the choroid more readily [92]. Inadequacies still exist in OCT images of the choroid, where deeper tissues imaged result in poorer sensitivity. The signals obtained in the choroid are also usually weak due to the high attenuation coefficient of the RPE. Nonetheless, ironically due to thinner choroids and relative depigmentation, full thickness imaging of the choroid is still attainable in high myopes. Yet, OCT image quality may still be compromised by distortions caused by the likely presence of staphylomas and abnormal eyewall contours in these same patients with high myopia. On the other hand, the extent of decreased sensitivities with increased tissue depth is comparatively lower in SS-OCT [93]. Clearly, notwithstanding the technique used, many challenges and limitations still exist in OCT imaging of high myopia—arising from the extreme axial length of highly myopic eyes, curvature deformity exaggeration on OCT, and the production of imaging artifacts [49].

The inability of OCT to readily distinguish the posterior scleral boundary makes scleral imaging a greater challenge than choroid imaging—where the choroid itself (unless extremely thin) reduces scleral image quality by disrupting signals. With the use of "Reflectivity" software, scleral boundaries may be augmented via adaptive compensation based on direct application of pixel intensity exponentiation. This would improve the precision of scleral thickness assessment [94, 95]. In retrospect, we conclude that the use of 3D MRI and ultrasound have more favorable results in visualizing scleral contours and characterizing staphylomas. Using animal experimentations on guinea pigs *ex vivo* and humans *in vivo*, we were able to demonstrate that quantitative ultrasound and super-resolution 3D MRI can be used to localize areas of scleral weakness and elasticity. These modalities could potentially detect scleral weakness preceding staphyloma formation; thereby discerning and even predicting which highly myopic eye is destined to develop staphylomas and MMD. This is critical in research studies targeted toward scleral reinforcement—such as macular buckling [96] or scleral collagen crosslinking [97, 98].

10.5.5 Challenges in Imaging the Optic Nerve

Features such as optic disc tilt (Fig. 10.5), peripapillary atrophy (PPA), and abnormally large or small optic discs are the earliest known structural alterations that potentially predict the development of pathological myopia, and can be observed even in young highly myopic adults. Unfortunately, these features (some also with associations to glaucoma) also interfere with the visualization of optic disc margins [99, 100], and are also not easy to discern in highly myopic eyes [101]. There is also added difficulty in eyes with myopic maculopathy, where visual field defects result in further interference [102]. As such, the answer to these challenges may lie in imaging deep optic nerve head structures (such as parapapillary sclera, scleral wall, and lamina cribrosa) [103] in highly myopic eyes for more precise diagnoses of glaucoma.

Glaucomatous optic nerve damage may be worsened by obstructed axoplasmic flow within the optic nerve head—possibly caused by a disrupted lamina cribrosa (LC) arising from optic disc tilt [104]. Imaging performed to evaluate the integrity of the lamina cribrosa may, therefore, aid in prognosticating risk for eventual glaucoma development. Indeed, Sawada et al. have shown via enhanced depth OCT imaging that LC defects in myopic eyes (with and without primary open-angle glaucoma) are associated with optic disc tilt angle, which can also explain the location and severity of glaucomatous visual field defects [104].

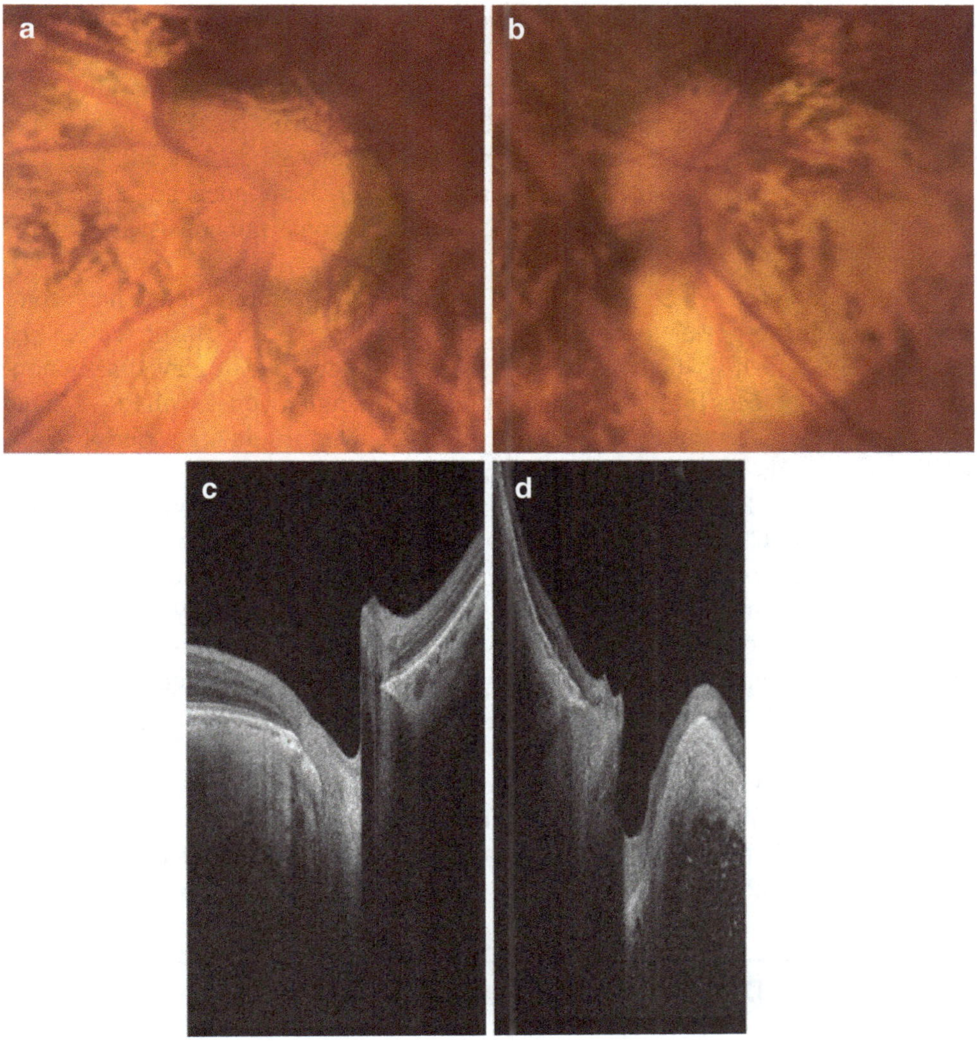

Fig. 10.5 Color photographs (top panels) and optical coherence tomography (bottom panels) of myopic tilted optic nerve discs showing moderately-tilted discs (left panels) and a severely tilted discs (right panels)

The optic nerve exits the eye at the Bruch's membrane opening (BMO), which can be easily discerned on OCT imaging. Using conventional disc margin-based measurements as a standard for comparison, Malik et al. investigated the utility of the BMO as a possible landmark for neuroretinal rim measurements, and has shown the BMO minimum rim width (BMO-MRW) to be markedly more sensitive (71% against 30%) than disc margin rim area (DM-RA) in diagnosing glaucoma [105].

Meanwhile, Enders et al. further demonstrated that a two-dimensional neuroretinal rim parameter based on BMO—namely, the BMO minimum rim area (BMO-MRA), outclassed all other measures (such as BMO-RMW, retinal nerve fiber layer thickness, and DM-RA) in diagnosing glaucoma [106]. Unfortunately, the diagnostic performance of this parameter has yet to be validated in myopic eyes.

Another deep optic nerve head structure that can be imaged on the enhanced depth OCT is the border tissue of Elschnig—a cuff of collagenous tissue arising from the sclera and joining the Bruch's membrane at the optic disc margin [104]. Having reviewed the externally oblique border tissue length (EOBT), optic nerve head tilt angle and optic canal obliqueness, Han et al. have concluded that temporally located maximal values for these parameters were both independently associated with the presence of myopic normal tension glaucoma and consistent with the location of retinal nerve fiber layer defects [103].

Macular ganglion cell complex (GCC) thickness has been reported to have comparable diagnostic power to circumpapillary retinal nerve fiber layer (cp-RNFL) thickness [107–110]—which on its own is strongly suggestive of glaucoma in non-myopic eyes, but faces limitations in interpretation in high myopes with PPA. Zhang et al. have indeed demonstrated that macular GCC parameters are superior to cp-RNFL parameters in diagnosing high myopes with glaucoma—with focal loss volume (FLV) on RTVue-OCT and minimum ganglion cell-inner plexiform layer (GCIPL) on the Cirrus HD OCT having the best diagnostic power among these macular parameters [111]. Yet, two obstacles persist in limiting the use of macular GCC measurements for the diagnosis of glaucoma in high myopes. Namely, these are the lack of a normative database in highly myopic eyes, as well as inaccurate measurements attributable to choroidal atrophy in myopic maculopathy. New developments regarding the use of OCTA on the optic nerve have suggested that it is a prospective adjunctive tool for evaluating the myopic disc for glaucomatous changes. Suwan et al. measured the perfused capillary density (PCD) via a 4.5 × 4.5 mm OCTA scan centered on the optic nerve head and has showed that eyes with myopia and open angle glaucoma had the lowest PCD compared to eyes with glaucoma alone and control eyes [112].

10.6 Future Developments

The primary aim of imaging in myopia would be to study the tissues involved with the pathological elongation of the eye, namely, the sclera as well as the choroid that is the regulator of scleral extracellular matrix remodeling [113], and its biomechanical properties [114]. As the RPE is highly scattering, it makes imaging of the myopic eye highly challenging. To make matters worse, the choroid is highly vascularized and perfused with a high concentration of red blood cells, this also causes a significant amount of light scattering making imaging more complicated [115]. One way to circumvent this problem would be to use OCT systems with wavelengths around 1060 nm to image the choroid [116]; however, the results obtained from this mode are less than satisfactory due to its relatively poor resolution capacity and inability to visualize the microvasculature and cellular structure of the choroid. Due to the complexity of this issue, there is no sensible nomenclature available to classify choroidal layers and boundaries, nor a definition of the choroidal–scleral interface [116]. As such, to facilitate comparisons and meta-analysis of existing data, there is a desperate need for a standardization for choroidal segmentation and OCT-based definition of the choroidal layers.

The OCT itself has its shortcomings: the sclera cannot be visualized using the OCT, higher wavelengths (around 1300 nm range) used for anterior segment OCT would not be able to be used to image the posterior pole either due to the high absorption coefficient of water contained in the vitreous [72]. These limitations also extend to the use of OCTA. There is currently no standard protocol for segmentation, the outcome parameters for OCTA have not been clearly defined either. Although some authors have tried to use analysis of flow voids or signal voids in the choriocapillaris to quantify the area taken up by the microvasculature [117, 118], the data pertaining to myopic patients are but insufficient [119]. Moreover, different authors have used different image analysis methods to quantify signal voids, as such, there is no clear common protocol in place to address the underlying issue. Looking into the future, there is however incipient research suggesting that the comprehension of blood supply and changes in vasculature from the anterior to the posterior segment of the myopic eye is crucial to the understanding of the disease [120–123].

Photoacoustic imaging has shown promise recently to fill the gaps between OCT and ultrasound in terms of penetration depth. Ultrasound biomicroscopy (higher ultrasound frequencies used) of the anterior segment simply does not have enough penetrative depth to image the posterior pole of the eye [124]. Photoacoustic imaging detects the waves generated by the absorption of pulsed laser light in tissues [125]; meanwhile, other modalities use contrast solely based on absorption. This modality has been used before to image the posterior pole of the eye in vitro and in animal models *in vivo*. This can also be used in concurrence with angiography, measuring oxygen saturation and pigment imaging [126]. However, there are some limitation pertaining to this modality notwithstanding moderate depth resolution, pure optical absorption sensing, need for contact detection with ultrasound sensor, and a relatively long acquisition time. In view of these limitations, we have yet to receive tangible results from photoacoustic imaging for posterior pole imaging in humans.

Recently, there has been a shift to elastography approaches to study the biochemical properties of ocular tissues with either OCT [127] or with ultrasound [128], the visualization of biochemical properties of the eye coats *in vivo* would otherwise be incredibly challenging This perspective is propelled by several studies proposing the measurement of ocular rigidity using noninvasive measures instead [129, 130]. However, none of these studies have addressed or included patients with myopia. The crux of this technique pertains to using an internal or external force to induce movement of tissue that is subsequently picked up using imaging devices, most *in vivo* work would be aimed at biochemical properties of the cornea [131, 132]. *In vivo* imaging using an ocular pulse with an internal excitation source is not yet able to produce results of biochemical parameters [133, 134]. Meanwhile, some *in vivo* work has been pursued involving the use of acoustic radiation force optical coherence elastography [135].

References

1. Chen L, et al. Rhegmatogenous retinal detachment due to paravascular linear retinal breaks over patchy chorioretinal atrophy in pathologic myopia. Arch Ophthalmol. 2010;128(12):1551–4.
2. Mitry D, et al. The epidemiology of rhegmatogenous retinal detachment: geographical variation and clinical associations. Br J Ophthalmol. 2010;94(6):678–84.
3. Hayashi K, et al. Long-term pattern of progression of myopic maculopathy: a natural history study. Ophthalmology. 2010;117(8):1595–611.
4. Yoshida T, et al. Myopic choroidal neovascularization: a 10-year follow-up. Ophthalmology. 2003;110(7):1297–305.
5. Ikuno Y, et al. Ocular risk factors for choroidal neovascularization in pathologic myopia. Invest Ophthalmol Vis Sci. 2010;51(7):3721–5.
6. Ohno-Matsui K, et al. Intrachoroidal cavitation in macular area of eyes with pathologic myopia. Am J Ophthalmol. 2012;154(2):382–93.
7. Samarawickrama C, et al. Myopia-related optic disc and retinal changes in adolescent children from singapore. Ophthalmology. 2011;118(10):2050–7.
8. Jonas JB, et al. Histology of the parapapillary region in high myopia. Am J Ophthalmol. 2011;152(6):1021–9.
9. Park HY, Lee K, Park CK. Optic disc torsion direction predicts the location of glaucomatous damage in normal-tension glaucoma patients with myopia. Ophthalmology. 2012;119(9):1844–51.
10. Marcus MW, et al. Myopia as a risk factor for open-angle glaucoma: a systematic review and meta-analysis. Ophthalmology. 2011;118(10):1989–1994.e2.
11. Curtin BJ. The myopias: basic science and clinical management. Philadelphia: Harper and Row; 1985.
12. Curtin BJ, Teng CC. Scleral changes in pathological myopia. Trans Am Acad Ophthalmol Otolaryngol. 1958;62(6):777–88.
13. Avetisov ES, et al. A study of biochemical and biomechanical qualities of normal and myopic eye sclera in humans of different age groups. Metab Pediatr Syst Ophthalmol. 1983;7(4):183–8.
14. Hsiang HW, et al. Clinical characteristics of posterior staphyloma in eyes with pathologic myopia. Am J Ophthalmol. 2008;146(1):102–10.
15. Curtin BJ, Karlin DB. Axial length measurements and fundus changes of the myopic eye. I. The posterior fundus. Trans Am Ophthalmol Soc. 1970;68:312–34.
16. Saka N, et al. Changes of axial length measured by IOL master during 2 years in eyes of adults with pathologic myopia. Graefes Arch Clin Exp Ophthalmol. 2013;251(2):495–9.
17. Lin LL, et al. Epidemiologic study of the prevalence and severity of myopia among schoolchildren in Taiwan in 2000. J Formos Med Assoc. 2001;100(10):684–91.
18. Steidl SM, Pruett RC. Macular complications associated with posterior staphyloma. Am J Ophthalmol. 1997;123(2):181–7.
19. Iwase A, et al. Prevalence and causes of low vision and blindness in a Japanese adult population: the Tajimi Study. Ophthalmology. 2006;113(8):1354–62.
20. Saka N, et al. Long-term changes in axial length in adult eyes with pathologic myopia. Am J Ophthalmol. 2010;150(4):562–568.e1.
21. Ohno-Matsui K, et al. Association between shape of sclera and myopic retinochoroidal lesions in patients with pathologic myopia. Invest Ophthalmol Vis Sci. 2012;53(10):6046–61.
22. McBrien NA, Cornell LM, Gentle A. Structural and ultrastructural changes to the sclera in a mammalian model of high myopia. Invest Ophthalmol Vis Sci. 2001;42(10):2179–87.
23. McBrien NA, Lawlor P, Gentle A. Scleral remodeling during the development of and recovery from axial myopia in the tree shrew. Invest Ophthalmol Vis Sci. 2000;41(12):3713–9.
24. Norton TT, Rada JA. Reduced extracellular matrix in mammalian sclera with induced myopia. Vis Res. 1995;35(9):1271–81.
25. Wollensak G, Iomdina E. Crosslinking of scleral collagen in the rabbit using glyceraldehyde. J Cataract Refract Surg. 2008;34(4):651–6.

26. McBrien NA, Jobling AI, Gentle A. Biomechanics of the sclera in myopia: extracellular and cellular factors. Optom Vis Sci. 2009;86(1):E23–30.
27. Wang Q, et al. Form-deprivation myopia induces decreased expression of bone morphogenetic protein-2, 5 in guinea pig sclera. Int J Ophthalmol. 2015;8(1):39–45.
28. Tian XD, et al. Expressions of type I collagen, alpha2 integrin and beta1 integrin in sclera of guinea pig with defocus myopia and inhibitory effects of bFGF on the formation of myopia. Int J Ophthalmol. 2013;6(1):54–8.
29. McBrien NA, Norton TT. Prevention of collagen crosslinking increases form-deprivation myopia in tree shrew. Exp Eye Res. 1994;59(4):475–86.
30. Li YT, Xie MK, Wu J. Association between Ocular axial length-related genes and high myopia in a Han Chinese population. Ophthalmologica. 2016;235(1):57–60.
31. Wei WB, et al. Subfoveal choroidal thickness: the Beijing Eye Study. Ophthalmology. 2013;120(1):175–80.
32. Wang NK, et al. Choroidal thickness and biometric markers for the screening of lacquer cracks in patients with high myopia. PLoS One. 2013;8(1):e53660.
33. Wang S, et al. Choroidal thickness and high myopia: a cross-sectional study and meta-analysis. BMC Ophthalmol. 2015;15:70.
34. Tokoro T. Types of fundus changes in the posterior pole. In: Atlas of posterior fundus changes in pathologic myopia. Tokyo: Springer; 1998. p. 5–22.
35. Ohno-Matsui K. Myopic chorioretinal atrophy. In: Spaide RF, Ohno-Matsui K, Yannuzzi LA, editors. Pathologic myopia. New York: Springer; 2014. p. 187–209.
36. Ohno-Matsui K, et al. International photographic classification and grading system for myopic maculopathy. Am J Ophthalmol. 2015;159(5):877–83.e7.
37. Jonas JB, et al. Bruch membrane and the mechanism of myopization: a new theory. Retina. 2017;37(8):1428–40.
38. Ohno-Matsui K, Jonas JB, Spaide RF. Macular bruch membrane holes in highly myopic patchy chorioretinal atrophy. Am J Ophthalmol. 2016;166:22–8.
39. Ohno-Matsui K, Tokoro T. The progression of lacquer cracks in pathologic myopia. Retina. 1996;16(1):29–37.
40. Pruett RC, Weiter JJ, Goldstein RB. Myopic cracks, angioid streaks, and traumatic tears in Bruch's membrane. Am J Ophthalmol. 1987;103(4):537–43.
41. Grossniklaus HE, Green WR. Pathologic findings in pathologic myopia. Retina. 1992;12(2):127–33.
42. Bai HX, et al. Bruch's membrane thickness in relationship to axial length. PLoS One. 2017;12(8):e0182080.
43. Puliafito CA, et al. Imaging of macular diseases with optical coherence tomography. Ophthalmology. 1995;102(2):217–29.
44. Tan CS, Ngo WK, Cheong KX. Comparison of choroidal thicknesses using swept source and spectral domain optical coherence tomography in diseased and normal eyes. Br J Ophthalmol. 2015;99(3):354–8.
45. Tan CS, et al. Comparison of retinal thicknesses measured using swept-source and spectral-domain optical coherence tomography devices. Ophthalmic Surg Lasers Imaging Retina. 2015;46(2):172–9.
46. Alshareef RA, et al. Subfoveal choroidal vascularity in myopia: evidence from spectral-domain optical coherence tomography. Ophthalmic Surg Lasers Imaging Retina. 2017;48(3):202–7.
47. Takase N, et al. Enlargement of foveal avascular zone in diabetic eyes evaluated by en face optical coherence tomography angiography. Retina. 2015;35(11):2377–83.
48. Tan CS, et al. Optical coherence tomography angiography evaluation of the parafoveal vasculature and its relationship with ocular factors. Invest Ophthalmol Vis Sci. 2016;57(9):224–34.
49. Shinohara K, et al. Ultrawide-field OCT to investigate relationships between myopic macular retinoschisis and posterior staphyloma. Ophthalmology. 2018;125:1575–86.
50. Baum G, Greenwood I. The application of ultrasonic locating techniques to ophthalmology. II. Ultrasonic slit lamp in the ultrasonic visualization of soft tissues. AMA Arch Ophthalmol. 1958;60(2):263–79.

51. Coleman DJ, et al. High-resolution ultrasonic imaging of the posterior segment. Ophthalmology. 2004;111(7):1344–51.
52. Reinstein DZ, Silverman RH, Coleman DJ. High-frequency ultrasound measurement of the thickness of the corneal epithelium. Refract Corneal Surg. 1993;9(5):385–7.
53. Hewick SA, et al. A comparison of 10 MHz and 20 MHz ultrasound probes in imaging the eye and orbit. Br J Ophthalmol. 2004;88(4):551–5.
54. Silverman RH, et al. Pulse-encoded ultrasound imaging of the vitreous with an annular array. Ophthalmic Surg Lasers Imaging. 2012;43(1):82–6.
55. Van Reeth E, et al. Isotropic reconstruction of a 4-D MRI thoracic sequence using super-resolution. Magn Reson Med. 2015;73(2):784–93.
56. Milanfar P. Super-resolution imaging. Boca Raton: CRC Press; 2010.
57. Collins MJ, Buehren T, Iskander DR. Retinal image quality, reading and myopia. Vis Res. 2006;46(1-2):196–215.
58. Pope JM, et al. Three-dimensional MRI study of the relationship between eye dimensions, retinal shape and myopia. Biomed Opt Express. 2017;8(5):2386–95.
59. Kuo AN, et al. Posterior eye shape measurement with retinal OCT compared to MRI. Invest Ophthalmol Vis Sci. 2016;57(9):196–203.
60. Ng DS, et al. Advances of optical coherence tomography in myopia and pathologic myopia. Eye. 2016;30(7):901–16.
61. Ang M, et al. Optical coherence tomography angiography: a review of current and future clinical applications. Graefes Arch Clin Exp Ophthalmol. 2018;256(2):237–45.
62. Tan ACS, et al. An overview of the clinical applications of optical coherence tomography angiography. Eye. 2018;32(2):262–86.
63. Ang M, et al. Optical coherence tomography angiography and indocyanine green angiography for corneal vascularisation. Br J Ophthalmol. 2016;100(11):1557–63.
64. Realini T, et al. Normative databases for imaging instrumentation. J Glaucoma. 2015;24(6):480–3.
65. Hashemi H, et al. Global and regional estimates of prevalence of refractive errors: systematic review and meta-analysis. J Curr Ophthalmol. 2018;30(1):3–22.
66. Kasahara K, et al. Characteristics of higher-order aberrations and anterior segment tomography in patients with pathologic myopia. Int Ophthalmol. 2017;37(6):1279–88.
67. Chansangpetch S, et al. Impact of myopia on corneal biomechanics in glaucoma and nonglaucoma patients. Invest Ophthalmol Vis Sci. 2017;58(12):4990–6.
68. Schehlein EM, Novack G, Robin AL. New pharmacotherapy for the treatment of glaucoma. Expert Opin Pharmacother. 2017;18(18):1939–46.
69. Chan C, et al. Validation of an objective scoring system for forme fruste keratoconus detection and post-LASIK Ectasia Risk Assessment in Asian eyes. Cornea. 2015;34(9):996–1004.
70. Lu Y, et al. Four-year follow-up of the changes in anterior segment after phakic collamer lens implantation. Am J Ophthalmol. 2017;178:140–9.
71. Chong EW, Mehta JS. High myopia and cataract surgery. Curr Opin Ophthalmol. 2016;27(1):45–50.
72. Ang M, et al. Anterior segment optical coherence tomography. Prog Retin Eye Res. 2018;66(9):132–56.
73. Ohno-Matsui K. What is the fundamental nature of pathologic myopia? Retina. 2017;37(6):1043–8.
74. Tanaka Y, et al. Retromode retinal imaging of macular retinoschisis in highly myopic eyes. Am J Ophthalmol. 2010;149(4):635–640.e1.
75. Johnson MW. Myopic traction maculopathy: pathogenic mechanisms and surgical treatment. Retina. 2012;32(Suppl 2):S205–10.
76. Wong CW, et al. Is choroidal or scleral thickness related to myopic macular degeneration? Invest Ophthalmol Vis Sci. 2017;58(2):907–13.
77. Shinohara K, et al. Characteristics of peripapillary staphylomas associated with high myopia determined by swept-source optical coherence tomography. Am J Ophthalmol. 2016;169:138–44.

78. Shinohara K, et al. Posterior staphylomas in pathologic myopia imaged by widefield optical coherence tomography. Invest Ophthalmol Vis Sci. 2017;58(9):3750–8.
79. Ohno-Matsui K, et al. Features of posterior staphylomas analyzed in wide-field fundus images in patients with unilateral and bilateral pathologic myopia. Retina. 2017;37(3):477–86.
80. Iacono P, et al. Fluorescein angiography and spectral-domain optical coherence tomography for monitoring anti-VEGF therapy in myopic choroidal neovascularization. Ophthalmic Res. 2014;52(1):25–31.
81. Kaneko Y, et al. Areas of nonperfusion in peripheral retina of eyes with pathologic myopia detected by ultra-widefield fluorescein angiography. Invest Ophthalmol Vis Sci. 2014;55(3):1432–9.
82. Miyata M, et al. Detection of myopic choroidal neovascularization using optical coherence tomography angiography. Am J Ophthalmol. 2016;165:108–14.
83. Bruyere E, et al. Neovascularization secondary to high myopia imaged by optical coherence tomography angiography. Retina. 2017;37(11):2095–101.
84. Querques G, et al. Optical coherence tomography angiography of choroidal neovascularization secondary to pathologic myopia. Dev Ophthalmol. 2016;56:101–6.
85. Querques L, et al. Optical coherence tomography angiography of myopic choroidal neovascularisation. Br J Ophthalmol. 2017;101(5):609–15.
86. Ohno-Matsui K, et al. Updates of pathologic myopia. Prog Retin Eye Res. 2016;52:156–87.
87. Battaglia Parodi M, Iacono P, Bandello F. Correspondence of leakage on fluorescein angiography and optical coherence tomography parameters in diagnosis and monitoring of myopic choroidal neovascularization treated with bevacizumab. Retina. 2016;36(1):104–9.
88. Ohno-Matsui K, Jonas JB, Spaide RF. Macular bruch membrane holes in choroidal neovascularization-related myopic macular atrophy by swept-source optical coherence tomography. Am J Ophthalmol. 2016;162:133–139.e1.
89. Ishida T, et al. Possible connection of short posterior ciliary arteries to choroidal neovascularisations in eyes with pathologic myopia. Br J Ophthalmol. 2018;103(4):457–62.
90. Hayashi K, et al. Value of indocyanine green angiography in the diagnosis of occult choroidal neovascular membrane. Jpn J Ophthalmol. 1988;42:827–9.
91. Geeraets WJ, Berry ER. Ocular spectral characteristics as related to hazards from lasers and other light sources. Am J Ophthalmol. 1968;66(1):15–20.
92. Spaide RF, Koizumi H, Pozonni MC. Enhanced depth imaging spectral-domain optical coherence tomography. Am J Ophthalmol. 2008;146(4):496–500.
93. Choma MA, et al. Sensitivity advantage of swept source and Fourier domain optical coherence tomography. Opt Express. 2003;11(18):2183–9.
94. Chung CW, et al. Enhancement of corneal visibility in optical coherence tomography images with corneal opacification. Transl Vis Sci Technol. 2016;5(5):3.
95. Girard MJ, et al. Enhancement of corneal visibility in optical coherence tomography images using corneal adaptive compensation. Transl Vis Sci Technol. 2015;4(3):3.
96. Alkabes M, Mateo C. Macular buckle technique in myopic traction maculopathy: a 16-year review of the literature and a comparison with vitreous surgery. Graefes Arch Clin Exp Ophthalmol. 2018;256(5):863–77.
97. Wollensak G, Iomdina E. Long-term biomechanical properties of rabbit sclera after collagen crosslinking using riboflavin and ultraviolet A (UVA). Acta Ophthalmol. 2009;87(2):193–8.
98. Kim M, et al. Pharmacologic alternatives to riboflavin photochemical corneal cross-linking: a comparison study of cell toxicity thresholds. Invest Ophthalmol Vis Sci. 2014;55(5):3247–57.
99. Chang RT, Singh K. Myopia and glaucoma: diagnostic and therapeutic challenges. Curr Opin Ophthalmol. 2013;24(2):96–101.
100. Jonas JB, Gusek GC, Naumann GO. Optic disk morphometry in high myopia. Graefes Arch Clin Exp Ophthalmol. 1988;226(6):587–90.
101. Jonas JB, et al. Intraocular pressure and glaucomatous optic neuropathy in high myopia. Invest Ophthalmol Vis Sci. 2017;58(13):5897–906.
102. Ohno-Matsui K, et al. Long-term development of significant visual field defects in highly myopic eyes. Am J Ophthalmol. 2011;152(2):256–265.e1.

103. Han JC, et al. The characteristics of deep optic nerve head morphology in myopic normal tension glaucoma. Invest Ophthalmol Vis Sci. 2017;58(5):2695–704.
104. Sawada Y, et al. Multiple temporal lamina cribrosa defects in myopic eyes with glaucoma and their association with visual field defects. Ophthalmology. 2017;124(11):1600–11.
105. Malik R, et al. Diagnostic accuracy of optical coherence tomography and scanning laser tomography for identifying glaucoma in myopic eyes. Ophthalmology. 2016;123(6):1181–9.
106. Enders P, et al. Novel Bruch's membrane opening minimum rim area equalizes disc size dependency and offers high diagnostic power for glaucoma. Invest Ophthalmol Vis Sci. 2016;57(15):6596–603.
107. Nakanishi H, et al. Sensitivity and specificity for detecting early glaucoma in eyes with high myopia from normative database of macular ganglion cell complex thickness obtained from normal non-myopic or highly myopic Asian eyes. Graefes Arch Clin Exp Ophthalmol. 2015;253(7):1143–52.
108. Hung KC, et al. Macular diagnostic ability in OCT for assessing glaucoma in high myopia. Optom Vis Sci. 2016;93(2):126–35.
109. Akashi A, et al. The ability of macular parameters and circumpapillary retinal nerve fiber layer by three SD-OCT instruments to diagnose highly myopic glaucoma. Invest Ophthalmol Vis Sci. 2013;54(9):6025–32.
110. Mwanza JC, et al. Diagnostic performance of optical coherence tomography ganglion cell--inner plexiform layer thickness measurements in early glaucoma. Ophthalmology. 2014;121(4):849–54.
111. Zhang Y, Wen W, Sun X. Comparison of several parameters in two optical coherence tomography systems for detecting glaucomatous defects in high myopia. Invest Ophthalmol Vis Sci. 2016;57(11):4910–5.
112. Suwan Y, et al. Association of myopia with peripapillary perfused capillary density in patients with glaucoma: an optical coherence tomography angiography study. JAMA Ophthalmol. 2018;136(5):507–13.
113. Summers JA. The choroid as a sclera growth regulator. Exp Eye Res. 2013;114:120–7.
114. Campbell IC, Coudrillier B, Ross Ethier C. Biomechanics of the posterior eye: a critical role in health and disease. J Biomech Eng. 2014;136(2):021005.
115. Kiss B, et al. Ocular hemodynamics during isometric exercise. Microvasc Res. 2001;61(1):1–13.
116. Ferrara D, Waheed NK, Duker JS. Investigating the choriocapillaris and choroidal vasculature with new optical coherence tomography technologies. Prog Retin Eye Res. 2016;52:130–55.
117. Spaide RF. Choriocapillaris flow features follow a power law distribution: implications for characterization and mechanisms of disease progression. Am J Ophthalmol. 2016;170:58–67.
118. Zhang Q, et al. A novel strategy for quantifying choriocapillaris flow voids using swept-source OCT angiography. Invest Ophthalmol Vis Sci. 2018;59(1):203–11.
119. Al-Sheikh M, et al. Quantitative OCT angiography of the retinal microvasculature and the choriocapillaris in myopic eyes. Invest Ophthalmol Vis Sci. 2017;58(4):2063–9.
120. Ang M, et al. Comparison of anterior segment optical coherence tomography angiography systems for corneal vascularisation. Br J Ophthalmol. 2018;102(7):873–7.
121. Cai Y, et al. Serial optical coherence tomography angiography for corneal vascularization. Graefes Arch Clin Exp Ophthalmol. 2017;255(1):135–9.
122. Ang M, et al. En face optical coherence tomography angiography for corneal neovascularisation. Br J Ophthalmol. 2016;100(5):616–21.
123. Grudzi E, et al. Modern diagnostic techniques for the assessment of ocular blood flow in myopia: current state of knowledge. J Ophthalmol. 2018;2018:8.
124. Silverman RH, et al. 75 MHz ultrasound biomicroscopy of anterior segment of eye. Ultrason Imaging. 2006;28(3):179–88.
125. Liu W, Zhang HF. Photoacoustic imaging of the eye: a mini review. Photoacoustics. 2016;4(3):112–23.
126. Xie D, et al. In vivo blind-deconvolution photoacoustic ophthalmoscopy with total variation regularization. J Biophotonics. 2018;11(9):e201700360.

127. Larin KV, Sampson DD. Optical coherence elastography - OCT at work in tissue biomechanics. Biomed Opt Express. 2017;8(2):1172–202.
128. Li G-Y, Cao Y. Mechanics of ultrasound elastography. Proc Math Phys Eng Sci. 2017;473(2199):20160841.
129. Karyotakis NG, et al. Manometric measurement of the outflow facility in the living human eye and its dependence on intraocular pressure. Acta Ophthalmol. 2015;93(5):e343–8.
130. Beaton L, et al. Non-invasive measurement of choroidal volume change and ocular rigidity through automated segmentation of high-speed OCT imaging. Biomed Opt Express. 2015;6(5):1694–706.
131. Sit AJ, et al. In vivo noninvasive measurement of young's modulus of elasticity in human eyes: a feasibility study. J Glaucoma. 2017;26(11):967–73.
132. Zaitsev VY, et al. Optical coherence elastography for strain dynamics measurements in laser correction of cornea shape. J Biophotonics. 2017;10(11):1450–63.
133. O'Hara KE, et al. Measuring pulse-induced natural relative motions within human ocular tissue in vivo using phase-sensitive optical coherence tomography. J Biomed Opt. 2013;18(12):121506.
134. Dragostinoff N, et al. Time course and topographic distribution of ocular fundus pulsation measured by low-coherence tissue interferometry. J Biomed Opt. 2013;18(12):121502.
135. Qu Y, et al. In vivo elasticity mapping of posterior ocular layers using acoustic radiation force optical coherence elastography. Invest Ophthalmol Vis Sci. 2018;59(1):455–61.

11

Interconnections between High Myopia and Glaucoma

Jost B. Jonas, Songhomitra Panda-Jonas, and Kyoko Ohno-Matsui

Key Points

- In all highly myopic eyes, glaucomatous optic neuropathy may specifically be ruled out, in attempt not to miss the diagnosis
- High axial myopia is a major risk factor for glaucomatous or glaucoma-like optic neuropathy, even at a normal intraocular pressure.
- Morphological risk factors for glaucoma in high myopia may be an enlarged optic disc and enlarged parapapillary delta zone.
- Histological hallmarks of the highly myopic optic nerve head are an elongated and thinned lamina cribrosa, steepened trans-lamina cribrosa pressure gradient, enlarged optic disc, elongated peripapillary scleral flange (as equivalent of parapapillary delta zone), and a shallowing of the physiological optic cup.

11.1 Introduction

Axial myopization leads to marked changes in the morphology of the posterior ocular segment including the anatomy of the optic nerve head. The changes of the optic nerve head include an enlargement of all three layers of the optic disc (i.e., optic disc Bruch's membrane opening, optic disc choroidal opening, and optic disc scleral

J. B. Jonas (✉) · S. Panda-Jonas
Department of Ophthalmology, Medical Faculty Mannheim, Ruprecht-Karls-University Heidelberg, Mannheim, Germany
e-mail: jost.jonas@medma.uni-heidelberg.de

K. Ohno-Matsui
Department of Ophthalmology and Visual Science, Tokyo Medical and Dental University, Tokyo, Japan

opening) with the development of a secondary macrodisc, and an enlargement and shallowing of the cup. Further morphological changes are an elongation and thinning of the lamina cribrosa with a secondary reduction in the distance between the intraocular space with the intraocular pressure (IOP) and the retro-lamina compartment with the orbital cerebrospinal fluid pressure, and a direct exposure of the peripheral posterior lamina cribrosa surface to the orbital cerebrospinal fluid space. In the parapapillary region, an elongation and thinning of the peripapillary scleral flange with development and enlargement of the parapapillary gamma zone (defined as the parapapillary Bruch's membrane free region) and delta zone (defined as the region between the optic disc border and the merging line of the optic nerve dura mater with the posterior sclera) occurs, in addition to an elongation and thinning of the peripapillary border tissue of the choroid (Jacoby). The optic rotates around the vertical axis, and less often and to a minor degree around the horizontal axis und the sagittal axis. These changes make it more difficult to differentiate between myopic changes and (additional) glaucoma-associated changes such as a loss of neuroretinal rim and thinning of the retinal nerve fiber layer, and these changes may make the optic nerve head more vulnerable potentially explaining the increased prevalence of glaucomatous optic neuropathy in highly myopic eyes.

11.2 Anatomy of the Optic Nerve Head in High Myopia

The anatomy of the optic nerve head in primary high myopia is markedly influenced by the axial elongation. This process of sagittal enlargement of the myopic globe takes place predominantly in the posterior hemisphere of the eye, and the changes are more pronounced the closer to the posterior pole [1–5]. Histological studies have shown that with longer axial length, the axial elongation-associated thinning of the sclera was most pronounced close to the posterior pole, while the scleral thickness in the pars plana region did not vary significantly between eyes of various axial length. In a similar manner, the thinning of the choroid was more marked the closer to the macula [6].

It has been postulated that the main driver for the scleral and choroidal thinning in the process of axial elongation may be a new production and elongation of Bruch's membrane in the equatorial and retroequatorial region of the eye [7]. Findings leading to this hypothesis were the following:

- the volume of the scleral and choroid did not markedly increase after the end of the second year of life and that both parameters were independent of axial length [3, 5];
- the thickness of Bruch's membrane was not associated with axial length so that its volume increased in the process of axial myopization [8];
- the main determinant of the process of emmetropization (and myopization) is the length of the optical axis which ends at the photoreceptor outer segments and not at the scleral posterior surface;
- the structure with a minimum of biomechanical strength and being located closest to the photoreceptor outer segments is Bruch's membrane;
- a biomechanical study revealed that the stiffness of Bruch's membrane was comparable or higher than those of other ocular tissues and that it could sustain a relatively high pressure of 80 mmHg or higher before rupture [9];

- the density of the retinal pigment epithelium cells and the retinal thickness decreased in the midperiphery with increasing axial length, while both parameters, measured in the macular region, were independent of axial length [10, 11]; and
- the optic disc-fovea distance increased with longer axial length by the development and enlargement of parapapillary gamma zone while the length of Bruch's membrane in the macular region was independent of axial length [12–14].

These anatomical findings and the postulated mechanism of Bruch's membrane enlargement in the midperiphery as the driver for the cylindrical-like sagittal enlargement of the globe are associated with typical myopic changes in the anatomy of the optic nerve head. These include the following: an enlargement of the optic nerve head with the development of a secondary or acquired macrodisc [15, 16]; enlargement and shallowing of the optic cup, so that the spatial contrast between the height of the neuroretinal rim and the depth of the optic cup is decreased; elongation and thinning of the lamina cribrosa [17, 18]; development and enlargement of parapapillary gamma zone and delta zone [19, 20]; and rotation of the optic disc mostly around the vertical axis [21, 22].

The enlargement of the optic disc (as defined by the peripapillary ring) affects all three optic disc layers: Bruch's membrane opening; the choroidal opening, in which the choroid is separated from the intrapapillary compartment by the peripapillary border tissue of the choroid (Jacoby); and the scleral opening which is spanned by the lamina cribrosa. The (passive) enlargement of all three optic disc layers may be due to the finding that the myopic axial elongation additionally includes a widening of the eye in the horizontal and vertical directions [23]. For each millimeter increase in axial length, both the horizontal globe diameter and the vertical globe diameter increase by approximately 0.2 mm [23]. Since the primary and active enlargement of Bruch's membrane may occur in the equatorial region, an increased tension within Bruch's membrane and within the choroid and the sclera may develop at the posterior pole. It would lead to a stretching of the openings of all three optic disc layers. It has been discussed that if the increased tension within Bruch's membrane is not sufficiently released by the enlargement of the physiological Bruch's membrane opening in the optic disc, secondary defects in Bruch's membrane may develop starting with the formation of lacquer cracks and ending the formation of macular Bruch's membrane defects [24–27]. If the enlargement of the optic disc Bruch's membrane opening is more marked than the enlargement of the optic disc choroidal opening, a part of the parapapillary region will no longer be covered by Bruch's membrane, so that parapapillary gamma zone as Bruch's membrane-free region develops [19, 20]. The uneven enlargement of the opening of the various layers of the optic disc may thus be one of the reasons for the development of parapapillary gamma zone.

The enlargement of the optic disc in axially elongating eyes leads secondarily to an enlargement of the optic cup, while the shape of the neuroretinal rim may still follow the so-called ISNT (inferior–superior–nasal–temporal) rule, with the small rim part being located usually in the temporal horizontal disc region [28]. Due to the stretching and enlargement of the optic disc and cup, the spatial contrast between the height of the neuroretinal rim and the depth of the optic cup appears to diminish, so that it becomes clinically more difficult to delineate the optic cup form the neuroretinal rim.

The enlargement of the opening in the scleral layer of the optic disc is associated with a stretching and thinning of the lamina cribrosa [17, 18]. Since the diameter of the retrobulbar optic nerve is not directly affected by the process of axial elongation, the myopic enlargement of the posterior surface of the lamina cribrosa has as consequence that a peripheral annular-like region of the lamina is no longer covered or buffered by the solid optic nerve but is directly facing the orbital cerebrospinal fluid space.

Outside of the optic disc border, parapapillary gamma zone and delta zone develop during axial elongation (Fig. 11.1) [19–21, 24, 29–35]. Gamma zone has been defined as the Bruch's membrane-free zone at the optic disc border. It is usually larger on the temporal side than on the nasal side. Prevalence and size of gamma zone is strongly associated with myopic axial elongation and the amount of the optic disc rotation around the vertical axis [21]. Two mechanisms may lead to the development of gamma zone. As pointed out above, gamma zone may develop if the enlargement of the optic disc Burch's membrane opening is more marked than the enlargement of the optic disc choroidal opening. A second mechanism may be connected with a shift of the three optic disc layers during axial elongation. One may assume that at birth all three optic disc layers are aligned to each other. If in the process of axial elongation Bruch's membrane is newly formed and enlarged in the equatorial region, the optic disc Bruch's membrane opening may shift in direction to the macula. If this movement is less marked for the optic disc choroidal layer and scleral layer than it is for the Bruch's membrane opening, a misalignment of the layers will occur, with the Bruch's membrane opening being located most to the macular side and the scleral opening being located most to the nasal side. This

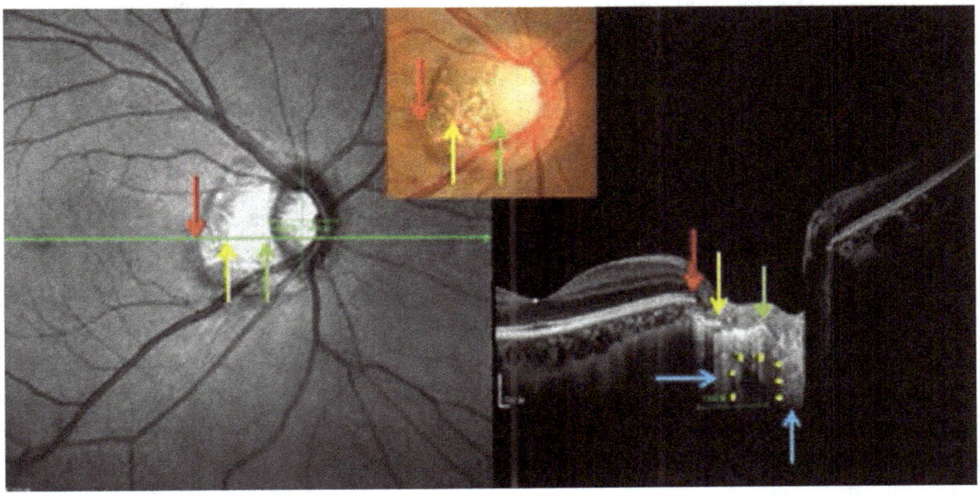

Fig. 11.1 Optical coherence tomographic image of the optic nerve head, showing parapapillary gamma zone (between red arrow and yellow arrow) with Bruch's membrane being absent, and parapapillary delta zone (between yellow arrow and green arrow (optic disc border)) showing an elongated peripapillary scleral flange as anterior border of the orbital cerebrospinal fluid space (yellow stars) between the optic nerve dura mater (horizontal blue arrow) and the optic nerve with its surrounding pia mater (vertical blue arrow)

phenomenon would explain the overhanging of Bruch's membrane on the nasal side of the optic disc in moderately myopic eyes, and it could be a second mechanism for the development of parapapillary gamma zone [36]. It would also explain the paradoxical course of the optic nerve through the optic nerve head channel with the optic nerve entering the canal from nasal anteriorly and reaching the vitreous compartment temporal posteriorly, although the optic nerve arrives at the eye globe coming from the posterior part of the orbit.

Parapapillary delta zone is located at the optic disc border within gamma zone and has been defined as the region of the elongated and thinned peripapillary scleral flange [19, 20]. The peripapillary scleral flange is the continuation of the inner half of the posterior sclera and continues into the lamina cribrosa, separated from the latter by the peripapillary scleral border tissue of Elschnig [37, 38]. It forms the anterior end of the orbital cerebrospinal fluid space. In axially elongated eyes, in particular beyond an axial length of 26.5 mm, the peripapillary scleral flange gets markedly elongated and thinned [37, 39]. It may change its dimensions from a normal thickness and length of about 0.5 mm to a length of 5 mm and a thickness of less than 100 μm. The ophthalmoscopical delineation between gamma zone and delta zone can be facilitated by searching for the peripapillary arterial circle of Zinn-Haller which is usually located at the merging line of the optic nerve dura mater with the sclera, i.e., at the peripheral end of delta zone [40, 41].

The optic disc shape as perceived upon ophthalmoscopy is normally slightly oval [42, 43]. It has to be taken into account that the ophthalmoscopically determined optic disc shape is different from the true optic disc shape, since the location of the optic disc close to the nasal side leads to perspective distortion, usually resulting in a perspective shortening of the horizontal disc diameter [44]. In addition, the optic disc undergoes rotational changes in the process of myopic axial elongation [22]. These are mainly an optic disc rotation around the vertical axis, and to a minor degree a rotation around the horizontal axis and the sagittal axis. A rotation round the vertical axis leads to a perspective shortening of the horizontal disc diameter, a rotation round the horizontal axis leads to a perspective shortening of the vertical disc diameter, a rotation round the sagittal axis does not change the perspective appearance of the disc diameters [44]. The rotation around the vertical axis is associated with the development and enlargement of gamma zone at the temporal side, and a rotation around the horizontal axis is associated with the development and enlargement of gamma zone at the inferior border of the optic disc. These optic disc rotations explain the ophthalmoscopical appearance of the markedly vertically oval shape of optic discs in highly myopic eyes [15, 16]. The difference between the two-dimensional ophthalmoscopical optic disc shape and the optic disc shape as determined three-dimensionally by optical coherence tomography increases with longer axial length, due to the progressing disc rotation around the vertical axis [44]. It has remained elusive which forces lead to the disc rotation around the vertical axis in progressive axial myopia. One reason could be, as outlined above, the increasing misalignment of the three optic disc openings, with the Bruch's membrane opening moving in temporally and the scleral opening staying partially behind. The resulting overhanging of Bruch's membrane into the nasal part of the optic disc channel leads to a shortening of the effective horizontal disc diameter. A second mechanism could be a backward strain or pull of the optic nerve dura mater on the peripapillary region [45, 46]. In a recent study, Demer and colleagues proposed that the backward pull of the optic nerve on the optic nerve head in markedly axially elongated eyes could lead to a novel mechanical load on the globe at the optic nerve head in ocular adduction [45]. Since the optic nerve originates in the nasal superior region of the orbit and inserts in the posterior nasal region of the eye, adduction of the globe would lead in axially elongated eyes to a backward pull of the optic nerve on the temporal and temporal inferior side of the optic nerve head. Such a mechanism could explain the marked rotation of the optic nerve head mainly around its vertical axis (and a slight rotation around its horizontal axis with a backward movement of the inferior optic disc pole) in highly elongated eyes. Since the optic nerve dura mater as compared to the pia mater or the neural tissue of the optic nerve may be biomechanically the strongest element, one may assume that the traction is forwarded by the optic nerve dura mater to its insertion on the globe, i.e., the merging line of the dura mater with the posterior sclera or the peripheral end of the peripapillary scleral flange. Traction on the merging line could also lead to an elongation of the peripapillary scleral flange and indirectly to the development and enlargement of parapapillary gamma zone. The study by Demer has been confirmed and extended by investigations conducted by Wang and colleagues who found that that the optic nerve head strains due to the pull by the optic nerve dura mater on the peripapillary sclera during a lateral eye movement of 13° were as high as, or higher than, those resulting from an IOP of 50 mmHg [46]. Fitting with the notion of a biomechanical role the optic nerve may play for the anatomy and physiology of the optic nerve head is the finding of peripapillary suprachoroidal cavitations which are located mostly in the inferior peripapillary region in about 17% of highly myopic eyes [47–50]. Their development may also be explained by a backward pull of the optic nerve dura mater on the temporal and inferior peripapillary sclera. Correspondingly, peripapillary suprachoroidal cavitations are associated with an optic disc rotation around the vertical disc axis and high axial myopia [50].

The cutoff for the differentiation between moderate myopia and high myopia at which the axial elongation associated enlargement of the optic nerve head starts has not concisely been assessed so far. According to hospital-based investigations and population-based studies, the optic disc and parapapillary gamma zone start to increase at about a value of approximately −8.00 diopters or an axial length of about 26.5 mm [51, 52]. At the same cutoff values, the prevalence of myopic retinopathy increases [53–55].

11.3 Increased Prevalence of Glaucoma in High Myopia and Associated Factors

Population-based investigations and hospital-based studies have shown that the prevalence of glaucomatous optic neuropathy (GON) was higher in highly myopic eyes than in emmetropic eyes [53, 56–69]. To cite an example, in the Beijing

Eye Study the prevalence of GON was significantly higher in eyes with a myopic refractive error exceeding −6 diopters than in the remaining eyes, while between the hyperopic eyes, the emmetropic eyes and the eyes with low to moderate myopia (myopic refractive up to −6 diopters or less), the frequency of glaucoma did not vary significantly [53]. Since the IOP pressure did not differ significantly between the highly myopic eyes and the remaining eyes, it suggested a higher glaucoma susceptibility in the highly myopic eyes. In the Blue Mountains Eye Study, the glaucoma prevalence was higher in moderate to high myopes (4.4%) than in emmetropes (1.5%) [63]. In the Barbados Eye Study, myopia increased the odds of having glaucoma while hyperopia reduced it [61]. In the Malmö eye survey on more than 30,000 individuals, the glaucoma prevalence increased with increasing myopia, and the association between myopia and glaucoma was strong at lower IOP levels, and weakened gradually with increasing IOP [64, 67]. The reason for a discrepancy between studies on an association between myopia and glaucoma may be that not all studies differentiated between moderate myopia, which may not be associated with an increased glaucoma prevalence, and high myopia with an increased frequency of GON [65]. Accordingly, in the Beijing Eye Study the low to moderate myopic group, the emmetropic group and the hyperopic group did not vary significantly in the prevalence of glaucoma in the present study [53]. By the same token, in non-highly myopic individuals, inter-eye differences in refractive error were not significantly correlated with inter-eye differences in neuroretinal rim area and mean visual field defect nor were the neuroretinal rim area, the horizontal and vertical cup/disk diameter ratios and the mean visual field loss correlated with refractive error in an interindividual statistical analysis [65].

A previous study revealed that at a given IOP in patients with chronic open-angle glaucoma, the amount of optic nerve damage was more marked in highly myopic eyes with large optic discs than in non-highly myopic eyes [68]. This observation was supported by a hospital-based study in which Nagaoka and colleagues examined 172 patients with a mean axial length of 30.1 ± 2.3 mm (range: 24.7–39.1 mm) and in which the prevalence of GON (overall: 28%) was 3.2 times higher ($P < 0.001$) in large optic discs (>3.79 mm^2) than in normal-sized discs or small discs (<1.51 mm^2) after adjusting for older age. Interestingly, axial length was not significantly ($P = 0.38$) associated with glaucoma prevalence in that model [70]. It suggested that the axial elongation-associated enlargement of the optic disc as compared to the axial elongation itself was one of the main factors for the increased glaucoma susceptibility in the highly myopic eyes. In a following study, it was additionally detected that an enlarged parapapillary delta zone, together with an enlarged optic disc, was associated with the increased glaucoma prevalence in highly myopic eyes, while in the multivariate analysis, parapapillary gamma zone was not related with the glaucoma prevalence [71]. In that study on 519 eyes with a mean axial length of 29.5 ± 2.2 mm, prevalence of GON increased from 12.2% in the group with an axial length of <26.5 mm to 28.5% (24.4, 32.5) in the group with an axial length of ≥26.5 mm, to 32.6% in the group with an axial length of ≥28 mm, to 36.0% in the group with an axial length of ≥29 mm, and to 42.1% in eyes with an axial length of ≥30 mm.

11.4 Potential Reasons for the Association Between Glaucoma and High Myopia

The main factors associated with the increased prevalence of GON in the highly myopic eyes were the size of the optic disc and the prevalence and size of parapapillary delta zone. Histomorphometric studies have revealed that the axial elongation-associated enlargement of the optic disc is associated with an elongation and thinning of the lamina cribrosa. Since the lamina cribrosa is the functional border tissue between the intraocular compartment with the IOP and the retrobulbar compartment with the orbital cerebrospinal fluid pressure, a thinning of the lamina cribrosa leads to a decreased distance between both compartments and to a steepening of the trans-lamina cribrosa pressure gradient between both compartments [17, 18]. An elevated the trans-lamina cribrosa pressure difference or a steepening of the trans-lamina cribrosa pressure gradient have been discussed to be associated with the glaucomatous damage to the retinal ganglion cell axons when passing through the lamina cribrosa [72–76]. The thinning of the lamina cribrosa may thus be one of the reasons for the association between an enlargement of the optic disc size and a higher prevalence of GON. Additional potential reasons for the increased glaucoma susceptibility in highly myopic optic disc may be a rearrangement of the lamina cribrosa pores and the whole lamina cribrosa architecture by the axial elongation-associated stretching of the lamina cribrosa. Theoretically, it may have a similar effect as the scarring of the lamina cribrosa due to the glaucomatous process itself, what may also lead to increased glaucoma susceptibility at a given IOP [77].

Histological studies have additionally shown that the myopic enlargement of the posterior surface of the lamina cribrosa leads to an exposure of a peripheral annular-like region of the lamina directly to the orbital cerebrospinal fluid space [18]. Since the cerebrospinal fluid in contrast to the solid optic nerve tissue cannot resist a local backward bowing of the lamina cribrosa, the exposure of the posterior lamina cribrosa surface to the cerebrospinal fluid space may allow the development of acquired pits of the optic nerve head which are typically located at the optic disc border.

The peripapillary scleral flange is the biomechanical anchor of the lamina cribrosa to the posterior sclera, with both tissues being partially separated from each other by the peripapillary border tissue of Elschnig the scleral flange [38]. In the process of axial elongation, the length of the peripapillary scleral flange can increase by a factor of 10×, and its thickness can get reduced to 10% of its original value [19, 78]. These marked anatomical changes may have an effect on the biomechanical properties of the flange as the anchor of the lamina cribrosa and may be one of the reasons for the increased glaucoma susceptibility in high myopia. This notion fits with the observation that the size of parapapillary gamma zone, after adjusting for axial length was not significantly associated with the glaucoma prevalence. Gamma is the zone free of Bruch's membrane, and Bruch's membrane, connected with the lamina cribrosa by the thin peripapillary choroidal border tissue of Jacoby may not directly be involved in the biomechanics of the lamina cribrosa in glaucoma.

The lamina cribrosa is nourished by vessels originating from the peripapillary arterial circle of Zinn-Haller, which is located approximately at the merging point of the posterior sclera with the dura mater of the optic nerve [40, 41, 79]. The longer the peripapillary scleral flange, the larger is the distance between the arterial circle and the optic nerve head. The axial elongation-associated elongation of the peripapillary scleral flange may thus potentially have importance for the blood supply of the lamina cribrosa and be another factor for an increased susceptibility of a highly myopic disc for optic nerve damage.

It has remained unclear whether the axial elongation-associated enlargement of the optic disc is an independent risk factor for an increased GON susceptibility in high myopia. In non-highly myopic eyes, the optic disc size was not associated with the prevalence and amount of GON [77, 80, 81]. Since the elongation and thinning of the lamina cribrosa and of the peripapillary scleral flange are strongly associated with the optic disc enlargement, one may assume that the disc enlargement is secondarily, and not causally, associated with the increased prevalence of GON in high myopia. It has also remained elusive whether the axial elongation-associated thinning of the peripapillary choroid has an influence on the GON susceptibility [82].

11.5 Intraocular Pressure and Glaucoma in High Myopia

In a recent pilot study on 517 eyes with a mean axial length of 29.5 ± 2.2 mm, the IOP did not differ significantly (P = 0.53) between the glaucoma group (n = 141 (27.3%) eyes) and the non-glaucomatous group (n = 376 (72.7%)) (14.5 ± 3.3 mmHg versus 14.7 ± 2.5 mmHg) [83]. Only in the eyes with an axial length of equal to or less than 27.4 mm, the prevalence of GON was correlated with higher IOP (P = 0.037; odds ratio (OR): 1.35; 95% confidence interval (CI):1.02, 1.80), while in the eyes with a longer axial length, the prevalence of GON was not significantly (P = 0.97) associated with IOP in a multivariate analysis adjusting for age, axial length, shorter vertical diameter of the temporal arterial arcade and longer minimal optic disc diameter. There were major limitations of the study as follows: the diagnosis of GON was based on the ophthalmoscopic appearance of the optic nerve head, without taking into account results of visual field examinations or findings obtained by optical coherence tomography; and the glaucomatous group as compared to the non-glaucomatous group had a significantly higher prevalence of anti-glaucomatous therapy. It could suggest that the lack of a difference in IOP between both groups was due to the higher prevalence of IOP-lowering therapy in the glaucomatous group. In the multivariate analysis with adjustment for the prevalence of anti-glaucomatous treatment however, the IOP was not significantly associated with the glaucomatous versus non-glaucoma group.

If the results of the study are valid, it may not indicate that there is no association between IOP and glaucoma in high myopia, but that highly myopic glaucomatous eyes as compared with non-highly myopic glaucomatous eyes may have a markedly lower IOP threshold to develop optic nerve damage. It could indicate that an IOP of perhaps lower than 10 mmHg might be necessary to prevent the development of GON in these highly myopic eyes, and that in highly myopic eyes with axial elongation associated enlargement and stretching of the optic disc and parapapillary region as the main risk factors for GON in high myopia a normal IOP may be sufficient to lead to GON.

11.6 Therapy of Glaucoma in High Myopia

Although it has not yet been firmly proven that GON in high myopia is dependent on IOP, and although a randomized trial on the effect of lowering of IOP as therapy of glaucoma in highly myopic eyes has not been performed yet, most researchers recommend lowering IOP in highly myopic patients with glaucoma. Based on the morphological findings described above, the target pressure in highly myopic glaucoma may be lower than in non-highly myopic glaucoma. A factor markedly complicating the clinical situation is the difficulty in detecting the presence of GON and, in particular, in detecting the progression of optic nerve damage in highly myopic glaucoma. Due to the peculiar anatomy of the optic nerve head in highly myopic eyes, most diagnostic procedures fail in precisely assessing the status of the optic nerve in highly myopic eyes with glaucoma. It includes factors such as:

- a decreased spatial and color contrast between the neuroretinal rim and the optic cup making a delineation of both structures more difficult;
- a peripapillary retinoschisis leading to an incorrect segmentation of the retinal nerve fiber layer upon optical coherence tomography;
- a large gamma zone (and delta zone) which makes using the end of Bruch's membrane as reference point for the measurement of the neuroretinal rim useless;
- a large gamma zone also markedly further reduces the anyway relatively low value of parapapillary beta zone as indicator for GON; and
- macular Bruch's membrane defects and other reasons for non-glaucomatous visual field defects which reduces the diagnostic precision of perimetry for the detection of presence and progression of GON.

The mode of therapy of lowering IOP in highly myopic glaucoma is similar to the therapy of open-angle glaucoma in non-highly myopic eyes and includes topically applied drugs reducing the production of aqueous humor and/or increasing the outflow of aqueous humor, laser procedures aimed at the trabecular meshwork to increase aqueous humor outflow, and surgical procedures for increase of aqueous humor outflow or reduction of aqueous humor production. If fistulating procedures, such as trabeculectomy, are performed, one may have to take into account a potentially increased risk of postoperative choroidal swelling and detachment and even expulsive hemorrhage. Potential reasons might be the marked thinning (compression) of the choroid in highly myopic eyes and an oblique course of the short posterior ciliary arteries (and potentially vortex veins) through the sclera in highly myopic eyes, while in emmetropic eyes the short posterior ciliary arteries run almost perpendicularly through the sclera (Fig. 11.2).

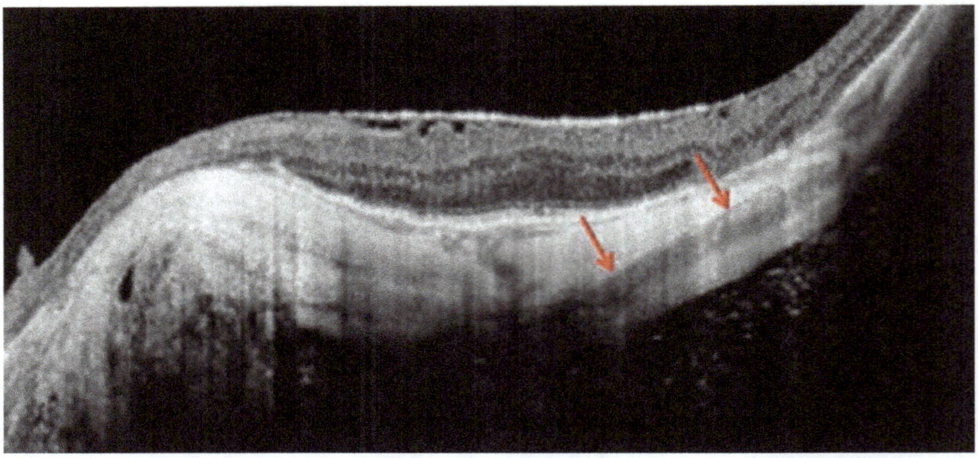

Fig. 11.2 Optical coherence tomographic image of the posterior sclera in a highly myopic eye showing the oblique course of a short posterior ciliary artery (red arrows) through the sclera

References

1. Heine L. Beiträge zur Anatomie des myopischen Auges. Arch Augenheilk. 1899;38:277–90.
2. Vurgese S, Panda-Jonas S, Jonas JB. Sclera thickness in human globes and its relations to age, axial length and glaucoma. PLoS One. 2012;7:e29692.
3. Jonas JB, Holbach L, Panda-Jonas S. Scleral cross section area and volume and axial length. PLoS One. 2014;9:e93551.
4. Shen L, Xu X, You QS, Gao F, Zhang Z, Li B, Jonas JB. Scleral thickness in Chinese eyes. Invest Ophthalmol Vis Sci. 2015;56:2720–7.
5. Shen L, You QS, Xu X, Gao F, Zhang Z, Li B, Jonas JB. Scleral and choroidal volume in relation to axial length in infants with retinoblastoma versus adults with malignant melanomas or end-stage glaucoma. Graefes Arch Clin Exp Ophthalmol. 2016;254:1779–86.
6. Wei WB, Xu L, Jonas JB, Shao L, Du KF, Wang S, Chen CX, Xu J, Wang YX, Zhou JQ, You QS. Subfoveal choroidal thickness: the Beijing Eye Study. Ophthalmology. 2013;120:175–80.
7. Jonas JB, Ohno-Matsui K, Jiang WJ, Panda-Jonas S. Bruch membrane and the mechanism of myopization. A new theory. Retina. 2017;37:1428–40.
8. Jonas JB, Holbach L, Panda-Jonas S. Bruch's membrane thickness in high myopia. Acta Ophthalmol. 2014;92:e470–4.
9. Wang X, Teoh CKG, Chan ASY, Thangarajoo S, Jonas JB, Girard MJA. Biomechanical properties of Bruch's membrane-choroid complex and their influence on optic nerve head biomechanics. Invest Ophthalmol Vis Sci. 2018;59:2808–17.
10. Jonas JB, Ohno-Matsui K, Holbach L, Panda-Jonas S. Retinal pigment epithelium cell density in relationship to axial length in human eyes. Acta Ophthalmol. 2017;95:e22–8.
11. Jonas JB, Xu L, Wei WB, Pan Z, Yang H, Holbach L, Panda-Jonas S, Wang YX. Retinal thickness and axial length. Invest Ophthalmol Vis Sci. 2016;57:1791–7.
12. Jonas RA, Wang YX, Yang H, Li JJ, Xu L, Panda-Jonas S, Jonas JB. Optic disc - fovea distance, axial length and parapapillary zones. The Beijing Eye Study 2011. PLoS One. 2015;10:e0138701.
13. Guo Y, Liu LJ, Tang P, Feng Y, Wu M, Lv YY, Xu L, Jonas JB. Optic disc-fovea distance and myopia progression in school children: the Beijing Children Eye Study. Acta Ophthalmol. 2018. https://doi.org/10.1111/aos.13728.

14. Jonas JB, Wang YX, Zhang Q, Liu Y, Xu L, Wei WB. Macular Bruch's membrane length and axial length. The Beijing Eye Study. PLoS ONE. 2015;10:e0136833.
15. Jonas JB, Dichtl A. Optic disc morphology in myopic primary open-angle glaucoma. Graefes Arch Clin Exp Ophthalmol. 1997;235:627–33.
16. Xu L, Li Y, Wang S, et al. Characteristics of highly myopic eyes. The Beijing Eye Study. Ophthalmology. 2007;114:121–6.
17. Jonas JB, Berenshtein E, Holbach L. Lamina cribrosa thickness and spatial relationships between intraocular space and cerebrospinal fluid space in highly myopic eyes. Invest Ophthalmol Vis Sci. 2004;45:2660–5.
18. Jonas JB, Berenshtein E, Holbach L. Anatomic relationship between lamina cribrosa, intraocular space, and cerebrospinal fluid space. Invest Ophthalmol Vis Sci. 2003;44:5189–95.
19. Jonas JB, Jonas SB, Jonas RA, Holbach L, Dai Y, Sun X, Panda-Jonas S. Parapapillary atrophy: histological gamma zone and delta zone. PLoS One. 2012;7(10):e47237.
20. Dai Y, Jonas JB, Huang H, et al. Microstructure of parapapillary atrophy: beta zone and gamma zone. Invest Ophthalmol Vis Sci. 2013;54:2013–8.
21. Jonas JB, Wang YX, Zhang Q, Fan YY, Xu L, Wei WB, Jonas RA. Parapapillary gamma zone and axial elongation-associated optic disc rotation: The Beijing Eye Study. Invest Ophthalmol Vis Sci. 2016;57:396–402.
22. Fan YY, Jonas JB, Wang YX, Chen CX, Wei WB. Horizontal and vertical optic disc rotation. The Beijing Eye Study. PLoS One. 2017;12:e0175749.
23. Jonas JB, Ohno-Matsui K, Holbach L, Panda-Jonas S. Association between axial length and horizontal and vertical globe diameters. Graefes Arch Clin Exp Ophthalmol. 2017;255:237–42.
24. Jonas JB, Ohno-Matsui K, Spaide RF, et al. Macular Bruch's membrane holes in high myopia: associated with gamma zone and delta zone of parapapillary region. Invest Ophthalmol Vis Sci. 2013;54:1295–30.
25. You QS, Peng XY, Xu L, Chen CX, Wei WB, Wang YX, Jonas JB. Macular Bruch's membrane defects in highly myopic eyes. The Beijing Eye Study. Retina. 2016;36:517–23.
26. Ohno-Matsui K, Jonas JB, Spaide RF. Macular Bruch's membrane holes in choroidal neovascularization-related myopic macular atrophy by swept-source optical coherence tomography. Am J Ophthalmol. 2015;162:133–9.
27. Shinohara K, Tanaka N, Jonas JB, Shimada N, Moriyama M, Yoshida T, Ohno-Matsui K. Ultrawide-field OCT to investigate relationships between myopic macular retinoschisis and posterior staphyloma. Ophthalmology. 2018. https://doi.org/10.1016/j.ophtha.2018.03.053.
28. Jonas JB, Gusek GC, Naumann GO. Optic disc, cup and neuroretinal rim size, configuration and correlations in normal eyes. Invest Ophthalmol Vis Sci. 1988;29:1151–8.
29. Na JH, Moon BG, Sung KR, Lee Y, Kook MS. Characterization of peripapillary atrophy using spectral domain optical coherence tomography. Korean J Ophthalmol. 2010;24:353–9.
30. Lee KY, Tomidokoro A, Sakata R, Konno S, Mayama C, Saito H, Hayashi K, Iwase A, Araie M. Cross-sectional anatomic configurations of peripapillary atrophy evaluated with spectral domain-optical coherence tomography. Invest Ophthalmol Vis Sci. 2010;51:666–71.
31. Park SC, De Moraes CG, Tello C, Liebmann JM, Ritch R. In-vivo microstructural anatomy of beta-zone parapapillary atrophy in glaucoma. Invest Ophthalmol Vis Sci. 2010;51:6408–13.
32. Manjunath V, Shah H, Fujimoto JG, Duker JS. Analysis of peripapillary atrophy using spectral domain optical coherence tomography. Ophthalmology. 2011;118:531–6.
33. Nonaka A, Hangai M, Akagi T, Mori S, Nukada M, Nakano N, Yoshimura N. Biometric features of peripapillary atrophy beta in eyes with high myopia. Invest Ophthalmol Vis Sci. 2011;52:6706–13.
34. Park SC, De Moraes CG, Teng CC, Tello C, Liebmann JM, Ritch R. Enhanced depth imaging optical coherence tomography of deep optic nerve complex structures in glaucoma. Ophthalmology. 2012;119:3–9.
35. Hayashi K, Tomidokoro A, Lee KY, Konno S, Saito H, Mayama C, Aihara M, Iwase A, Araie M. Spectral-domain optical coherence tomography of β-zone peripapillary atrophy: influence of myopia and glaucoma. Invest Ophthalmol Vis Sci. 2012;53:1499–505.

36. Reis AS, Sharpe GP, Yang H, Nicolela MT, Burgoyne CF, Chauhan BC. Optic disc margin anatomy in patients with glaucoma and normal controls with spectral domain optical coherence tomography. Ophthalmology. 2012;119:738–47.
37. Jonas JB, Jonas SB, Jonas RA, Holbach L, Panda-Jonas S. Histology of the parapapillary region in high myopia. Am J Ophthalmol. 2011;152:1021–9.
38. Jonas JB, Holbach L, Panda-Jonas S. Peripapillary ring: histology and correlations. Acta Ophthalmol. 2014;92:e273–9.
39. Jonas JB, Jonas RA, Jonas SB, Panda-Jonas S. Lamina cribrosa thickness correlated with peripapillary sclera thickness. Acta Ophthalmol. 2012;90:e248–50.
40. Jonas JB, Jonas SB. Histomorphometry of the circular arterial ring of Zinn-Haller in normal and glaucomatous eyes. Acta Ophthalmol. 2010;88:e317–22.
41. Jonas JB, Holbach L, Panda-Jonas S. Peripapillary arterial circle of Zinn-Haller: location and spatial relationships. PLoS One. 2013;8:e78867.
42. Jonas JB, Papastathopoulos KI. Optic disc shape in glaucoma. Graefes Arch Clin Exp Ophthalmol. 1996;234:S167–73.
43. Guo Y, Liu LJ, Xu L, Lv YY, Tang P, Feng Y, Zhou JQ, Meng M, Jonas JB. Optic disc ovality in primary school children in Beijing. Invest Ophthalmol Vis Sci. 2015;56:4547–53.
44. Dai Y, Jonas JB, Ling Z, Sun X. Ophthalmoscopic-perspectively distorted optic disc diameters and real disc diameters. Invest Ophthalmol Vis Sci. 2015;56:7076–83.
45. Demer JL. Optic nerve sheath as a novel mechanical load on the globe in ocular ductionoptic nerve sheath constrains duction. Invest Ophthalmol Vis Sci. 2016;57:1826–38.
46. Wang X, Rumpel H, Lim WE, Baskaran M, Perera SA, Nongpiur ME, Aung T, Milea D, Girard MJ. Finite element analysis predicts large optic nerve head strains during horizontal eye movements. Invest Ophthalmol Vis Sci. 2016;57:2452–62.
47. Jonas JB, Dai Y, Panda-Jonas S. Peripapillary suprachoroidal cavitation, parapapillary gamma zone and optic disc rotation due to the biomechanics of the optic nerve dura mater. Invest Ophthalmol Vis Sci. 2016;57:4373.
48. Wang X, Rumpel H, Lim WE, Baskaran M, Perera SA, Nongpiur ME, Aung T, Milea D, Girard MJ. Author Response: Peripapillary suprachoroidal cavitation, parapapillary gamma zone and optic disc rotation due to the biomechanics of the optic nerve dura mater. Invest Ophthalmol Vis Sci. 2016;57:4374–5.
49. Ohno-Matsui K, Shimada N, Akiba M, Moriyama M, Ishibashi T, Tokoro T. Characteristics of intrachoroidal cavitation located temporal to optic disc in highly myopic eyes. Eye. 2013;27:630–8.
50. Dai Y, Jonas JB, Ling Z, Wang X, Sun X. Unilateral peripapillary intrachoroidal cavitation and optic disc rotation. Retina. 2015;35:655–9.
51. Jonas JB. Optic disc size correlated with refractive error. Am J Ophthalmol. 2005;139:346–8.
52. Xu L, Wang YX, Wang S, Jonas JB. Definition of high myopia by parapapillary atrophy. The Beijing Eye Study. Acta Ohthalmol. 2010;88:e350–1.
53. Xu L, Wang Y, Wang S, Wang Y, Jonas JB. High myopia and glaucoma susceptibility. The Beijing Eye Study. Ophthalmology. 2007;114:216–20.
54. Liu HH, Xu L, Wang YX, Wang S, You QS, Jonas JB. Prevalence and progression of myopic retinopathy in Chinese adults: The Beijing Eye Study. Ophthalmology. 2010;117:1763–8.
55. Nakazawa M, Kurotaki J, Ruike H. Longterm findings in peripapillary crescent formation in eyes with mild or moderate myopia. Acta Ophthalmol. 2008;86:626–9.
56. Podos S, Becker B, Mortion W. High myopia and primary open-angle glaucoma. Am J Ophthalmol. 1966;62:1039–43.
57. Greve EL, Furuno F. Myopia and glaucoma. Graefes Arch Clin Exp Ophthalmol. 1980;213:33–41.
58. Daubs JG, Crick RP. Effect of refractive error on the risk of ocular hypertension and open angle glaucoma. Trans Ophthalmol Soc Aust. 1981;101:121–6.
59. Phelps CD. Effect of myopia on prognosis in treated primary open-angle glaucoma. Am J Ophthalmol. 1982;93:622–8.

60. Perkins ES, Phelps CD. Open angle glaucoma, ocular hypertension, low-tension glaucoma, and refraction. Arch Ophthalmol. 1982;100:1464–7.
61. Leske MC, Connell AM, Wu SY, Hyman LG, Schachat AP. Risk factors for open-angle glaucoma. The Barbados Eye Study. Arch Ophthalmol. 1995;113:918–24.
62. Chihara E, Liu X, Dong J, Takashima Y, Akimoto M, Hangai M, Kuriyama S, Tanihara H, Hosoda M, Tsukahara S. Severe myopia as a risk factor for progressive visual field loss in primary open-angle glaucoma. Ophthalmologica. 1997;211:66–71.
63. Mitchell P, Hourihan F, Sandbach J, Wang JJ. The relationship between glaucoma and myopia: the Blue Mountains Eye Study. Ophthalmology. 1999;106:2010–5.
64. Grodum K, Heijl A, Bengtsson B. Refractive error and glaucoma. Acta Ophthalmol Scand. 2001;79:560–6.
65. Jonas JB, Martus P, Budde WM. Anisometropia and degree of optic nerve damage in chronic open-angle glaucoma. Am J Ophthalmol. 2002;134:547–51.
66. Wong TY, Klein BE, Klein R, Knudtson M, Lee KE. Refractive errors, intraocular pressure, and glaucoma in a white population. Ophthalmology. 2003;110:211–7.
67. Leske MC, Heijl A, Hussein M, Bengtsson B, Hyman L, Komaroff E, Early Manifest Glaucoma Trial Group. Factors for glaucoma progression and the effect of treatment: the early manifest glaucoma trial. Arch Ophthalmol. 2003;121:48–56.
68. Jonas JB, Budde WM. Optic nerve damage in highly myopic eyes with chronic open-angle glaucoma. Eur J Ophthalmol. 2005;15:41–7.
69. Kuzin AA, Varma R, Reddy HS, Torres M, Azen SP, Los Angeles Latino Eye Study Group. Ocular biometry and open-angle glaucoma: the Los Angeles Latino Eye Study. Ophthalmology. 2010;117:1713–9.
70. Nagaoka N, Jonas JB, Morohoshi K, Moriyama M, Shimada N, Yoshida T, Ohno-Matsui K. Glaucomatous-type optic discs in high myopia. PLoS One. 2015;10:e0138825.
71. Jonas JB, Weber P, Nagaoka N, Ohno-Matsui K. Glaucoma in high myopia and parapapillary delta zone. PLoS One. 2017;12:e0175120.
72. Balaratnasingam C, Morgan WH, Johnstone V, et al. Histomorphometric measurements in human and dog optic nerve and an estimation of optic nerve pressure gradients in human. Exp Eye Res. 2009;89:618–28.
73. Morgan WH, Yu DY, Balaratnasingam CX. The role of cerebrospinal fluid pressure in glaucoma pathophysiology: the dark side of the optic disc. J Glaucoma. 1998;17:408–13.
74. Berdahl JP, Allingham RR, Johnson DH. Cerebrospinal fluid pressure is decreased in primary open-angle glaucoma. Ophthalmology. 2008;115:763–8.
75. Ren R, Jonas JB, Tian G, Zhen Y, Ma K, Li S, Wang H, Li B, Zhang X, Wang N. Cerebrospinal fluid pressure in glaucoma. A prospective study. Ophthalmology. 2010;117:259–66.
76. Jonas JB, Wang N, Yang D, Ritch R, Panda-Jonas S. Facts and myths of cerebrospinal fluid pressure for the physiology of the eye. Prog Retin Eye Res. 2015;46:67–83.
77. Burgoyne CF, Morrison JC. The anatomy and pathophysiology of the optic nerve head in glaucoma. J Glaucoma. 2001;10:S16–8.
78. Dichtl A, Jonas JB, Naumann GO. Histomorphometry of the optic disc in highly myopic eyes with absolute secondary angle closure glaucoma. Br J Ophthalmol. 1998;82:286–9.
79. Hayreh SS. Blood supply of the optic nerve head and its role in optic atrophy, glaucoma, and oedema of the optic nerve. Br J Ophthalmol. 1969;53:721–48.
80. Jonas JB, Xu L, Zhang L, Wang Y, Wang Y. Optic disk size in chronic glaucoma. The Beijing Eye Study. Am J Ophthalmol. 2006;142:168–70.
81. Wang YX, Hu LN, Yang H, Jonas JB, Xu L. Frequency and associated factors of structural progression of open-angle glaucoma in the Beijing Eye Study. Br J Ophthalmol. 2012;96:811–5.
82. Jiang R, Wang YX, Wei WB, Xu L, Jonas JB. Peripapillary choroidal thickness in adult Chinese: The Beijing Eye Study. Invest Ophthalmol Vis Sci. 2015;56:4045–52.
83. Jonas JB, Nagaoka N, Fang YX, Weber P, Ohno-Matsui K. Intraocular pressure and glaucomatous optic neuropathy in high myopia. Invest Ophthalmol Vis Sci. 2017;58:5897–906.

12

Clinical Interventions for MTM

Jerry K. H. Lok, Raymond L. M. Wong, Lawrence P. L. Iu, and Ian Y. H. Wong

Key Points

- MTM is an important treatable cause of visual loss among individuals with high myopia.
- A certain proportion of cases of MTM do not progress. Treatment should be offered to patients with more advanced disease with progressive visual loss.
- Fovea-sparing instead of complete peeling of the ILM and avoidance of gas tamponade could prevent the formation of secondary macular hole in MTM.
- Surgical adjuncts should be considered for macular hole especially in high-risk cases (persistent macular hole despite initial surgery, large and chronic macular hole, atrophic macula, etc.)

J. K. H. Lok
Department of Ophthalmology, Hong Kong Eye Hospital, Kowloon, Hong Kong

R. L. M. Wong
Department of Ophthalmology, Hong Kong Eye Hospital, Kowloon, Hong Kong

Department of Ophthalmology, LKS Faculty of Medicine, University of Hong Kong, Pok Fu Lam, Hong Kong

L. P. L. Iu
Department of Ophthalmology, LKS Faculty of Medicine, University of Hong Kong, Pok Fu Lam, Hong Kong

Department of Ophthalmology, Prince of Wales Hospital, Sha Tin, Hong Kong

I. Y. H. Wong (✉)
Department of Ophthalmology, LKS Faculty of Medicine, University of Hong Kong, Pok Fu Lam, Hong Kong

Department of Ophthalmology, Hong Kong Sanatorium and Hospital, Happy Valley, Hong Kong

12.1 Introduction

As described in the previous chapter, myopic foveal retinoschisis was first described in 1958 [1], then by Takano and Kishi in 1999 through the advent of optical coherence tomography (OCT) [2]. Subsequently, the various pathological effects of traction on the macula in patients with high myopia were collectively termed *myopic traction maculopathy* (MTM) by Panozzo and Mercanti in 2004 [3]. It was estimated to occur in approximately 8–34% in individuals with high myopia [4–6]. The term MTM originally encompassed retinal thickening, macular retinoschisis, foveal detachment, and lamellar macular hole with or without epiretinal membrane and/or vitreomacular traction [3]. The spectrum was extended to include full-thickness macular hole (HM) with or without retinal detachment.

Central to the pathogenesis of MTM is traction, which was postulated to arise from one or more of the following mechanisms [7]: vitreomacular traction associated with perifoveal posterior vitreous detachment (PVD) [8–10]; relative incompliance of inner retinal structures (e.g., internal limiting membrane [ILM] [11–15], epiretinal membrane [ERM] [6, 8, 16–18], and cortical vitreous remnant after PVD [19]) to the outer retina which conforms to the shape of the posterior staphyloma; and traction exerted by retinal arterioles [14, 20, 21].

Not all patients with MTM require interventions [10, 22, 23]. A study on the natural history of MTM with 207 eyes found that while 12% of cases progressed during a mean follow-up period of 36 months, the majority (84%) remained stable and a small proportion (4%) even had improvement or complete resolution of the disease [24]. The extent of macular retinoschisis was identified as a predictor of progression, with stage 4 disease (i.e., involving the entire macula) having the higher chance of progression than any other stages [24]. It is generally accepted that eyes with complications such as foveal detachment or full-thickness MH with or without retinal detachment, or eyes with significant progression in the extent of macular retinoschisis on OCT should undergo intervention early. On the other hand, an early macular retinoschisis involving only a limited area of the macula with preserved vision should be monitored with OCT for any progression.

There are numerous reported interventions for MTM. The principles of the treatment are: (1) to relieve traction, mainly achieved through pars plana vitrectomy (PPV) with or without ILM peeling; (2) to minimize surgical damage to the weakened macula through technique modifications in order to prevent the formation of postoperative MH; and (3) in the presence of full-thickness MH to maximize the chance of hole closure through the use of various surgical adjuncts.

12.2 Surgical Procedures

12.2.1 Pars Plana Vitrectomy

PPV serves several purposes in the treatment of MTM. It allows removal of all premacular tractional forces, including posterior vitreous cortex and ERM. It also creates a potential space in the posterior segment for gas tamponade to be performed.

12.2.1.1 Microincision Vitrectomy Surgery

With the advent of microincision vitrectomy system, PPV can be performed with small sclerotomy wounds and instruments in the size of 23 gauge, 25 gauge, or 27 gauge. Small sclerotomy wounds tend to be self-sealing and do not require sutures. It has the advantages of reduced ocular trauma, reduced inflammation, less conjunctival scarring, shorter operation time, better patient comfort, and faster postoperative recovery [25]. The design of closer opening near the tip of vitreous cutter probe also facilitates engagement and induction of PVD.

12.2.1.2 Induction of Posterior Vitreous Detachment

Since the pathogenesis of MTM involves abnormal vitreoretinal traction at the macula, induction of PVD is crucial to a successful operation. After core vitrectomy, induction of PVD is performed by using an aspiration port, usually the vitreous cutter probe, to engage the posterior hyaloid just anterior to optic disc. Once the posterior hyaloid is engaged by applying aspiration, the port is lifted upward to detach the posterior hyaloid from the retinal surface.

Induction of PVD can be difficult in MTM due to tight vitreoretinal adhesion and presence of vitreoschisis. Vitreoschisis refers to splitting of posterior vitreous cortex which occurs when there is vitreous gel liquefaction but without dehiscence at the vitreoretinal interface [26]. Vitreoschisis is common in MTM and is present in around half of the patients with MH [27]. To facilitate induction of PVD, triamcinolone acetonide [28] or trypan blue can be injected to stain the posterior hyaloid to improve visualization. If PVD cannot be induced by aspiration, intraocular forceps or diamond-dusted membrane scraper can be used to lift and assist detachment of the posterior hyaloid [29, 30].

12.2.1.3 Epiretinal Membrane Peeling

It is necessary to remove all ERM if any present on the macula. Removal of ERM allows removal of tractional forces on the macula, and allows access and identification of the underlying ILM with vital dyes.

Trypan blue is useful to stain the ERM to enhance visualization [31, 32]. Trypan blue is often injected after fluid-air exchange [33], or it can be mixed with 10% glucose isovolumetrically to create a heavy dye denser than balanced salt solution so that it will fall onto the macula with less dispersion in vitreous cavity [34]. There are also products combining trypan blue, brilliant blue, and polyethylene glycol with increased molecular weight so that the dye falls onto the macula to enhance tissue staining.

12.2.1.4 Internal Limiting Membrane Peeling

ILM is the innermost layer of a normal retina. It has significant contribution to retinal rigidity [35]. ILM peeling therefore improves retinal compliance and allows the retina to restore its normal anatomy [35]. The potential complications of ILM peeling include iatrogenic damage to retinal nerve fiber layer, retinal hemorrhage, and retinal defect formation, especially at sites of ILM flap creation and grasping points [35]. Due to the thinner retina and longer distance required to reach the posterior pole, ILM peeling is more technically challenging in highly myopic eyes than normal eyes and complications may be more common.

ILM is barely visible and requires staining with vital dyes for identification. Triamcinolone acetonide and trypan blue do not stain ILM well. The better dyes for ILM staining are brilliant blue and indocyanine green (ICG) [31, 32]. ICG adheres well to the extracellular matrix of ILM such as collagen type 4 and laminin and allows good visualization of ILM [31]. However, there are concerns of potential retinal toxicity, especially when ICG is in direct contact with the photoreceptors and retinal pigment epithelium through a MH [31]. ICG retinal toxicity has been shown with electrophysiology and histological studies in animal models [36, 37]. The risk increases with endoillumination light exposure [32]. In comparison, brilliant blue is a much safer alternative. A recent meta-analysis showed that postoperative visual acuity was better with brilliant blue than ICG in MH surgeries [38].

After ILM staining, an ILM flap can be created at the extrafoveal region using intraocular forceps by direct pinch method [35]. Alternatively, a pick, diamond-dusted membrane scraper or flexible nitinol loop can be used to create an ILM flap by scrapping [11]. The ILM flap is then lifted with intraocular forceps and moved in a circular fashion so that the whole ILM is peeled off from the macula.

Full-Thickness Macular Hole

In full-thickness MH, ILM peeling helps to reduce retinal rigidity and improve retinal compliance and thus the chance of MH closure [35]. It also helps to reduce postoperative ERM formation and risk of MH reopening [35]. A meta-analysis of four randomized controlled trials showed that ILM peeling for stages 2, 3, and 4 full-thickness MH has a significantly higher closure rate than without ILM peeling [39]. Another meta-analysis showed that MH reopening rate reduced from 7 to 1% when ILM peeling was performed.

Concerning the extent of ILM peeling, there is no consensus on the optimal size required [35]. Extended ILM peeling up to arcade is often performed for large MH to ensure traction has been sufficiently removed. Extended ILM peeling, however, is performed at the expense of longer operation time and higher risk of iatrogenic retinal trauma due to repeated ILM grasping [35]. Dissociated optic nerve fiber layer (DONFL) and swelling of arcuate retinal nerve fiber layer (SANFL), which can be shown on imaging modalities such as OCT scan and infrared fundus photographs, are two known structural changes secondary to ILM peeling [40, 41]. ILM flap initiation techniques might affect the chance of these structural complications, with pinch technique shown to be less damaging than diamond dust membrane scraping [40].

Myopic Foveoschisis

For myopic foveoschisis, ILM peeling helps to ensure that all tractional forces from premacular glial cells and vitreous cortex are completely removed [42]. It increases retinal compliance and allows the retina to better conform to the posterior staphyloma [42].

Favorable anatomical and visual outcomes have been reported for combined PPV, ILM peeling, and gas tamponade. However, development of postoperative full-thickness MH is not uncommon and occurs in around 13–28% of patients [43].

Shimada et al. [44] and Ho et al. [45] introduced the technique of *fovea-sparing ILM peel* in 2012. Instead of complete ILM removal, this technique involves removal of the perifoveal ILM only and leaving the ILM over the central foveola intact. It is believed that preservation of foveolar ILM would preserve foveolar Muller cells integrity and therefore reduce the risk of postoperative MH development [46]. Although studies suggested this technique might be useful to reduce the risk of MH development and foveolar thinning [46], leaving ILM on the fovea could result in late ILM contraction and retinal thickening [44]. This technique is also more technically demanding and requires more tissue manipulation than conventional complete ILM peeling.

In view of the risk of secondary macular hole development in foveoschisis patients undergone ILM peeling, conservative treatment can be considered in foveoschisis patients without foveal detachment.

12.2.1.5 Gas Tamponade

The commonly used gases for tamponade include air, sulfur hexafluoride (SF_6), and perfluoropropane (C_3F_8). Gas tamponade is commonly performed for MTM, particularly in cases with FTMH. For myopic foveoschisis without FTMH, it is still controversial whether gas tamponade is necessary. Gas tamponade may help the retina to adhere better to the posterior staphyloma and tamponade against unnoticeable macular holes [47]. In the presence of outer retinal detachment, the subretinal fluid (SRF) could be displaced toward areas with healthier retinal pigment epithelial (RPE) cells, which can facilitate SRF absorption [48–50]. More rapid resolution of foveoschisis was also reported by a study [51]. However, the study showed that the chance of successful resolution was similar between the group with gas tamponade and that without gas tamponade [51]. Indeed, a meta-analysis showed that for eyes undergoing vitrectomy for myopic foveoschisis, gas tamponade did not have significant impact on visual acuity or the rate of resolution of foveoschisis, yet it was associated with more complications [42]. Several studies also reported the paradoxical occurrence of FTHM from the use of gas tamponade, which could squeeze SRF within the limited space through the weak point of fovea [52–54]. The use of gas tamponade as an adjunct for FTMH would be discussed below.

12.2.2 Additional Measures (Adjuncts) to Improve Outcome of Macular Hole Surgery

12.2.2.1 Endotamponade

PPV with endotamponade agents is the most commonly employed technique for the management of myopic macular hole with or without retinal detachment. Gas tamponade with long-acting gases, commonly SF_6 and C_3F_8, has the advantages of high surface tension and buoyancy compared to silicone oil. A study comparing C_3F_8 and silicone oil as a tamponade agent for myopic MH retinal detachment (MHRD) showed higher initial success rate for C_3F_8 than silicone oil [55]. Due to lower buoyancy, silicone oil is less conforming to posterior staphyloma, rendering it less effective for MHRD. However, silicone oil still has advantages over gases for longer duration of tamponade, shorter duration of face down posturing, earlier visual recovery as well as allowing immediate air travel.

12.2.2.2 Inverted Internal Limiting Membrane Flap

Even with extended ILM peeling, a proportion of large chronic MH remains open after operation. Michalewska et al. introduced the *inverted ILM flap technique* in 2009 and reported closure rate of large MH reached 98% [56]. Instead of complete ILM removal, this technique involves leaving a hinge of ILM flap at the edge of MH during ILM peeling. This ILM flap is then inverted upside-down to cover or fill the MH. Some surgeons would inject an ophthalmic viscosurgical device on the inverted ILM flap in order to keep it in place. It is postulated that this technique facilitates MH closure by (1) providing a flap which contains Muller cell fragments to induce glial cells proliferation, and (2) providing a scaffold for retinal tissue to approximate [56]. Despite an apparently promising closure rate for large or persistent MH, it has been reported that the visual recovery and recovery of retinal microstructures such as external limiting membrane and the ellipsoid zone are worse among cases managed with inverted ILM flap when compared to conventional complete ILM peeling [57]. This can possibly be due to mechanical obstruction of functional recovery of retinal layers by the presence of an ILM plug in the MH.

12.2.2.3 Autologous Internal Limiting Membrane Transplantation

Although the inverted ILM flap technique proposed by Michalewska and associates seems to be a good surgical adjunct for anatomical closure of large MH, this method cannot be applied to patients who suffer from persistent macular hole after vitrectomy and conventional ILM peeling, since ILM surrounding MH has already been removed in the previous procedure. In view of this limitation, Morizane et al. introduced a new method of ILM flap, which is the autologous ILM transplantation (free ILM flap) [58]. Brilliant Blue G solution is used to stain the remaining ILM in those refractory MH cases. Subsequently appropriately sized ILM is peeled off, which is supposed to match the size of the macular hole, and is placed as a free flap onto the persistent MH. Infusion should be turned off during the procedure in order to avoid accidental loss of the ILM flap. In order to stabilize the flap, an ophthalmic viscosurgical device is injected on the top of the flap before fluid-air exchange is performed. It has been demonstrated that with this method of autologous ILM transplantation, up to 90% of refractory MH (with previous vitrectomy and ILM peeled) could achieve MH closure [58, 59].

12.2.2.4 Autologous Blood

In order to prevent subretinal migration of dye and the resultant retinal toxicity associated with vital stains, it was proposed to use autologous blood to cover the MH before injection of brilliant blue dye. Ghosh et al. collected autologous heparinized whole blood from patients' antecubital vein and injected to MH before injection of brilliant blue dye assisted ILM peeling. It has been demonstrated that compared to conventional method, the use of prestaining autologous blood led to better visual acuity outcomes and continuity of ellipsoid zone at all postoperative time points; and the outer retinal layer is thicker as well [60].

Apart from being used in the prevention of subretinal migration of dye, the therapeutic effect of autologous blood in persistent and refractory MH has also been investigated. It has been shown that injection of autologous blood or platelet concentrate into MH after ILM peeling can improve closure rate of macular hole and visual recovery [61–63]; and the efficacy of autologous platelet concentrate might even be better than whole blood. In one study in which 75 subjects were included, MH closure rate after revitrectomy plus autologous platelet concentrate was 85.2% versus 7.1% in the group using autologous whole blood instead [64].

12.2.2.5 Lens Capsular Flap Transplantation

Due to the possible lack of residual accessible ILM in reoperative cases of persistent MH, transplantation of lens capsules to MH have been proposed to increase the surgical success rate. In patients with cataract, phacoemulsification would be performed in the same setting and capsular flap would be harvested during continuous curvilinear capsulorhexis and stained with indocyanine green solution or brilliant blue solution for better visualization. In aphakic or pseudophakic patients with insufficient anterior capsule, capsular flap can be harvested from their fellow eyes requiring cataract operations. Alternatively, posterior capsular flap can be used instead. Since capsular flaps are more rigid than ILM flap, it is easier to manipulate during the operation. Moreover, due to the higher specific gravity of capsular flap, it will sink in balanced salt solution, therefore shall fall nicely onto the preretinal surface, unlike ILM flap that is tended to float inside the vitreous cavity. Chen et al. demonstrated a 100% MH closure rate with anterior capsular transplantation among patients with refractory MH, whereas the complete closure rate of MH after posterior capsular transplantation was only 50% and with another 30% enjoyed partial MH closure [65]. Similarly, Peng et al. reported a 90% MH closure rate after transplantation of anterior capsule to refractory MH [66].

12.2.2.6 Macular Buckle

One of the major etiological factors of MTM is the elongation of axial length of the globe leading to tension and traction on retinal layers. The aim of vitrectomy is to remove vitreous traction and ILM peeling to reduce the rigidity and improve the compliance of retina. Nevertheless, none of these procedures tackle the primary pathology, which is the long axial length in high myopes.

Macula buckles have been used to shorten the axial length of myopic eyeballs in conditions such as MHRD, myopic foveoschisis with or without foveal detachment and MH with foveoschisis. There are many types of macular buckle, including scleral sponge, T-shaped or L-shaped buckle, Ando Plombe, wire-strengthened sponge exoplant, and even donor sclera and suprachoroidal injectable long-acting hyaluronic acid. Chandelier light is attached to the indenting head of macular buckle when necessary for better localization and positioning of the buckle. The purpose of all the aforementioned macular buckles is to shape the globe back to normal length along the visual axis, thereby reducing the anteroposterior traction on retina and the tension within retinal layers [67].

Studies have been carried out to compare the efficacy of vitrectomy and macular buckle in inducing retinal reattachment and MH closure in patients suffering from MHRD. Fifty to seventy-nine percent of patients with previous vitrectomy had their retina successfully reattached whereas 93.3–100% of the patients managed with macular buckles enjoyed flattening of the retina [68–70]. The differences in MH closure rates between the two treatment modalities are even higher. Similarly, comparing to less than 50% MH closure rate by vitrectomy, macular buckle surgeries achieved a 100% closure rate in patients with MH and concomitant foveoschisis, and more than 80% of these patients had improvement in final visual acuity [67]. In patients with very poor MTM, combined vitrectomy and macular buckle surgeries can be considered.

Despite the high success rate in the latest macular buckle surgeries, these procedures are technically demanding and are not without risks. Complications of macular buckles include globe perforation, problems with extraocular movement, squint, choroidal effusion, changes in retinal pigment epithelium and the need for removal of buckle.

12.2.2.7 Autologous Neurosensory Retinal Transplantation

In 2016, Grewal and Mahmoud reported the technique of autologous neurosensory retinal free flap transplantation for the closure of refractory macular hole after initial PPV with peeling of ILM [71].

The technique involves bimanually harvesting a free flap of neurosensory retina superior to the superotemporal arcade, with the harvest site first secured by endolaser barricade and endodiathermy. The free flap was translocated in its correct orientation over the macular hole and perfluoro-*n*-octane heavy liquid (PFC) was instilled over it, followed by direct PFC-silicone oil exchange.

In order to prevent flap dislocation intraoperatively and postoperatively, the intraocular pressure should be lowered to reduce fluid turbulence [72]. The edge of the flap could be tucked underneath the edge of MH [72]. A technique combining autologous blood and autologous retinal free flap transplantation was described to secure the flap with blood clot [72].

There were small case series using similar techniques with good results, in terms of both anatomical closure rate and visual recovery [73–75]. The recovery of vision was postulated to be in part due to integration of the free flap to the surrounding retinal tissue with partial recovery of the ellipsoid zone and external limiting membrane, as observed postoperatively using OCT. It was hypothesized that the flap served more than a scaffold, providing glial cells and growth factors for structural and functional restoration. The implications of this observation to other macular diseases are yet to be determined.

12.3 Conclusion

The pathological changes associated with high myopia lead to a range of retinal complications, including MTM. An understanding of the pathogenesis and natural history of the disease sheds light on its management. Advances in surgical instruments and skills have shown promises in the management of this challenging condition.

References

1. Philips C. Retinal detachment at the posterior pole. Br J Ophthalmol. 1958;42(12):749–53.
2. Takano M, Kishi S. Foveal retinoschisis and retinal detachment in severely myopic eyes with posterior staphyloma. Am J Ophthalmol. 1999;128(4):472–6. https://doi.org/10.1016/S0002-9394(99)00186-5.
3. Panozzo G, Mercanti A. Optical coherence tomography findings in myopic traction maculopathy. Arch Ophthalmol. 2004;122(10):1455–60. https://doi.org/10.1001/archopht.122.10.1455.
4. Wu PC, Chen YJ, Chen YH, et al. Factors associated with foveoschisis and foveal detachment without macular hole in high myopia. Eye. 2009;23(2):356–61. https://doi.org/10.1038/sj.eye.6703038.
5. Baba T, Ohno-Matsui K, Futagami S, et al. Prevalence and characteristics of foveal retinal detachment without macular hole in high myopia. Am J Ophthalmol. 2003;135(3):338–42. https://doi.org/10.1016/S0002-9394(02)01937-2.
6. Fang X, Weng Y, Xu S, et al. Optical coherence tomographic characteristics and surgical outcome of eyes with myopic foveoschisis. Eye. 2009;23(6):1336–42. https://doi.org/10.1038/eye.2008.291.
7. Vanderbeek BL, Johnson MW. The diversity of traction mechanisms in myopic traction maculopathy. Am J Ophthalmol. 2012;153(1):93–102. https://doi.org/10.1016/j.ajo.2011.06.016.
8. Yeh S-I, Chang W-C, Chen L-J. Vitrectomy without internal limiting membrane peeling for macular retinoschisis and foveal detachment in highly myopic eyes. Acta Ophthalmol. 2008;86(2):219–24. https://doi.org/10.1111/j.1600-0420.2007.00974.x.
9. Smiddy WE, Kim SS, Lujan BJ, Gregori G. Myopic traction maculopathy: spectral domain optical coherence tomographic imaging and a hypothesized mechanism. Ophthalmic Surg Lasers Imaging. 2009;40(2):169–73. https://doi.org/10.3928/15428877-20090301-21.
10. Gaucher D, Haouchine B, Tadayoni R, et al. Long-term follow-up of high myopic foveoschisis: natural course and surgical outcome. Am J Ophthalmol. 2007;143(3):455–62. https://doi.org/10.1016/j.ajo.2006.10.053.
11. Ikuno Y, Sayanagi K, Soga K, Oshima Y, Ohji M, Tano Y. Foveal anatomical status and surgical results in vitrectomy for myopic foveoschisis. Jpn J Ophthalmol. 2008;52(4):269–76. https://doi.org/10.1007/s10384-008-0544-8.
12. Ikuno Y, Sayanagi K, Ohji M, et al. Vitrectomy and internal limiting membrane peeling for myopic foveoschisis. Am J Ophthalmol. 2004;137(4):719–24. https://doi.org/10.1016/j.ajo.2003.10.019.
13. Kuhn F. Internal limiting membrane removal for macular detachment in highly myopic eyes. Am J Ophthalmol. 2003;135(4):547–9. https://doi.org/10.1016/S0002-9394(02)02057-3.
14. Panozzo G, Mercanti A. Vitrectomy for myopic traction maculopathy. Arch Ophthalmol. 2007;125(6):767–72. https://doi.org/10.1001/archopht.125.6.767.
15. Kumagai K, Furukawa M, Ogino N, Larson E. Factors correlated with postoperative visual acuity after vitrectomy and internal limiting membrane peeling for myopic foveoschisis. Retina. 2010. https://doi.org/10.1097/IAE.0b013e3181c703fc.
16. Kwok AKH, Lai TYY, Yip WWK. Vitrectomy and gas tamponade without internal limiting membrane peeling for myopic foveoschisis. Br J Ophthalmol. 2005. https://doi.org/10.1136/bjo.2005.069427.
17. Tang J, Rivers MB, Moshfeghi AA, Flynn HW, Chan C-C. Pathology of macular foveoschisis associated with degenerative myopia. J Ophthalmol. 2010. https://doi.org/10.1155/2010/175613.
18. Sayanagi K, Morimoto Y, Ikuno Y, Tano Y. Spectral-domain optical coherence tomographic findings in myopic foveoschisis. Retina. 2010. https://doi.org/10.1097/IAE.0b013e3181ca4e7c.
19. Spaide RF, Fisher Y. Removal of adherent cortical vitreous plaques without removing the internal limiting membrane in the repair of macular detachments in highly myopic eyes. Retina. 2005. https://doi.org/10.1097/00006982-200504000-00007.

20. Sayanagi K, Ikuno Y, Gomi F, Tano Y. Retinal vascular microfolds in highly myopic eyes. Am J Ophthalmol. 2005. https://doi.org/10.1016/j.ajo.2004.11.025.
21. Ikuno Y, Gomi F, Tano Y. Potent retinal arteriolar traction as a possible cause of myopic foveoschisis. Am J Ophthalmol. 2005. https://doi.org/10.1016/j.ajo.2004.09.078.
22. Ripandelli G, Rossi T, Scarinci F, Scassa C, Parisi V, Stirpe M. Macular vitreoretinal interface abnormalities in highly myopic eyes with posterior staphyloma: 5-year follow-up. Retina. 2012. https://doi.org/10.1097/IAE.0b013e318255062c.
23. Benhamou N, Massin P, Haouchine B, Erginay A, Gaudric A. Macular retinoschisis in highly myopic eyes. Am J Ophthalmol. 2002. https://doi.org/10.1016/S0002-9394(02)01394-6.
24. Shimada N, Tanaka Y, Tokoro T, Ohno-Matsui K. Natural course of myopic traction maculopathy and factors associated with progression or resolution. Am J Ophthalmol. 2013. https://doi.org/10.1016/j.ajo.2013.06.031.
25. Mohamed S, Claes C, Tsang CW. Review of Small Gauge Vitrectomy: Progress and Innovations. J Ophthalmol. 2017. https://doi.org/10.1155/2017/6285869.
26. Sebag J. Vitreoschisis. Graefe's Arch Clin Exp Ophthalmol. 2008. https://doi.org/10.1007/s00417-007-0743-x.
27. Gupta P, Yee KMP, Garcia P, et al. Vitreoschisis in macular diseases. Br J Ophthalmol. 2011. https://doi.org/10.1136/bjo.2009.175109.
28. Peyman GA, Cheema R, Conway MD, Fang T. Triamcinolone acetonide as an aid to visualization of the vitreous and the posterior hyaloid during pars plana vitrectomy. Retina. 2000. https://doi.org/10.1097/00006982-200005000-00024.
29. Takeuchi M, Takayama K, Sato T, Ishikawa S, Fujii S, Sakurai Y. Non-aspiration technique to induce posterior vitreous detachment in minimum incision vitrectomy system. Br J Ophthalmol. 2012. https://doi.org/10.1136/bjophthalmol-2012-301628.
30. Gómez-Resa M, Burés-Jelstrup A, Mateo C. Myopic traction maculopathy. Dev Ophthalmol. 2014. https://doi.org/10.1159/000360468.
31. Rodrigues EB, Costa EF, Penha FM, et al. The use of vital dyes in ocular surgery. Surv Ophthalmol. 2009. https://doi.org/10.1016/j.survophthal.2009.04.011.
32. Farah M, Maia M, Rodrigues E. Dyes in ocular surgery: principles for use in chromovitrectomy. Am J Ophthalmol. 2009;148(3):332–40.
33. Badaro E, Novais EA, Penha FM, Maia M, Farah ME, Rodrigues EB. Vital dyes in ophthalmology: a chemical perspective. Curr Eye Res. 2014. https://doi.org/10.3109/02713683.2013.865759.
34. Lesnik Oberstein SY, De Smet MD. Use of heavy trypan blue in macular hole surgery. Eye. 2010. https://doi.org/10.1038/eye.2010.3.
35. Chatziralli I, Theodossiadis P, Steel D. Internal limiting membrane peeling in macular hole surgery; why, when and how? Retina. 2018;38(5):870–82.
36. Enaida H, Sakamoto T, Hisatomi T, Goto Y, Ishibashi T. Morphological and functional damage of the retina caused by intravitreous indocyanine green in rat eyes. Graefe's Arch Clin Exp Ophthalmol. 2002. https://doi.org/10.1007/s00417-002-0433-7.
37. Penha FM, Maia M, Farah ME, et al. Effects of subretinal injections of indocyanine green, trypan blue, and glucose in rabbit eyes. Ophthalmology. 2007. https://doi.org/10.1016/j.ophtha.2006.09.028.
38. Azuma K, Noda Y, Hirasawa K, Ueta T. Brilliant blue G-assisted internal limiting membrane peeling for macular hole: a systematic review of literature and meta-analysis. Retina. 2016. https://doi.org/10.1097/IAE.0000000000000968.
39. Spiteri Cornish K, Lois N, Scott N, et al. Vitrectomy with internal limiting membrane (ILM) peeling versus vitrectomy with no peeling for idiopathic full-thickness macular hole (FTMH). Cochrane Database Syst Rev. 2013. https://doi.org/10.1002/14651858.CD009306.pub2.
40. Steel DHW, Dinah C, Habib M, White K. ILM peeling technique influences the degree of a dissociated optic nerve fibre layer appearance after macular hole surgery. Graefe's Arch Clin Exp Ophthalmol. 2015. https://doi.org/10.1007/s00417-014-2734-z.

41. A S, G G, E A, et al. Arcuate nerve fiber layer changes after internal limiting membrane peeling in idiopathic epiretinal membrane. Retina. 2018;38(9):1777–85.
42. Meng B, Zhao L, Yin Y, et al. Internal limiting membrane peeling and gas tamponade for myopic foveoschisis: a systematic review and meta-analysis. BMC Ophthalmol. 2017. https://doi.org/10.1186/s12886-017-0562-8.
43. Lee C, Wu W, Chen K, Chiu L, Wu K, Chang Y. Modified internal limiting membrane peeling technique (maculorrhexis) for myopic foveoschisis surgery. Acta Ophthalmol. 2017;95(2):e128–31.
44. Shimada N, Sugamoto Y, Ogawa M, Takase H, Ohno-Matsui K. Fovea-sparing internal limiting membrane peeling for myopic traction maculopathy. Am J Ophthalmol. 2012. https://doi.org/10.1016/j.ajo.2012.04.013.
45. Ho TC, Chen MS, Huang JS, Shih YF, Ho H, Huang YH. Foveola nonpeeling technique in internal limiting membrane peeling of myopic foveoschisis surgery. Retina. 2012. https://doi.org/10.1097/IAE.0B013E31824D0A4B.
46. Ho TC, Yang CM, Huang JS, et al. Long-term outcome of foveolar internal limiting membrane nonpeeling for myopic traction maculopathy. Retina. 2014. https://doi.org/10.1097/IAE.0000000000000149.
47. Rizzo S, Giansanti F, Finocchio L, et al. Vitrectomy with internal limiting membrane peeling and air tamponade for myopic foveoschisis. Retina. 2018. https://doi.org/10.1097/IAE.0000000000002265.
48. Wu TY, Yang CH, Yang CM. Gas tamponade for myopic foveoschisis with foveal detachment. Graefe's Arch Clin Exp Ophthalmol. 2013. https://doi.org/10.1007/s00417-012-2192-4.
49. Li X, Wang W, Tang S, Zhao J. Gas injection versus vitrectomy with gas for treating retinal detachment owing to macular hole in high myopes. Ophthalmology. 2009. https://doi.org/10.1016/j.ophtha.2009.01.003.
50. Chen FT, Yeh PT, Lin CP, Chen MS, Yang CH, Yang CM. Intravitreal gas injection for macular hole with localized retinal detachment in highly myopic patients. Acta Ophthalmol. 2011. https://doi.org/10.1111/j.1755-3768.2009.01649.x.
51. Kim K, Lee S, Lee W. Vitrectomy and internal limiting membrane peeling with and without gas tamponade for myopic foveoschisis. Am J Ophthalmol. 2012;153(2):320–6.
52. Hirakata A, Hida T. Vitrectomy for myopic posterior retinoschisis or foveal detachment. Jpn J Ophthalmol. 2006. https://doi.org/10.1007/s10384-005-0270-4.
53. Zheng B, Chen Y, Zhao Z, et al. Vitrectomy and internal limiting membrane peeling with perfluoropropane tamponade or balanced saline solution for myopic foveoschisis. Retina. 2011. https://doi.org/10.1097/IAE.0b013e3181f84fc1.
54. Lim SJ, Kwon YH, Kim SH, You YS, Kwon OW. Vitrectomy and internal limiting membrane peeling without gas tamponade for myopic foveoschisis. Graefe's Arch Clin Exp Ophthalmol. 2012. https://doi.org/10.1007/s00417-012-1983-y.
55. Mancino R, Ciuffoletti E, Martucci A, et al. Anatomical and functional results of macular hole retinal detachment surgery in patients with high myopia and posterior staphyloma treated with perfluoropropane gas or silicone oil. Retina. 2013. https://doi.org/10.1097/IAE.0b013e3182670fd7.
56. Michalewska Z, Michalewski J, Adelman RA, Nawrocki J. Inverted internal limiting membrane flap technique for large macular holes. Ophthalmology. 2010. https://doi.org/10.1016/j.ophtha.2010.02.011.
57. Iwasaki M, Kinoshita T, Miyamoto H, Imaizumi H. Influence of inverted internal limiting membrane flap technique on the outer retinal layer structures after a large macular hole surgery. Retina. 2018. https://doi.org/10.1097/IAE.0000000000002209.
58. Morizane Y, Shiraga F, Kimura S, et al. Autologous transplantation of the internal limiting membrane for refractory macular holes. Am J Ophthalmol. 2014. https://doi.org/10.1016/j.ajo.2013.12.028.

59. Leisser C, Hirnschall N, Döller B, et al. Internal limiting membrane flap transposition for surgical repair of macular holes in primary surgery and in persistent macular holes. Eur J Ophthalmol. 2018. https://doi.org/10.5301/ejo.5001037.
60. Ghosh B, Arora S, Goel N, et al. Comparative evaluation of sequential intraoperative use of whole blood followed by brilliant blue versus conventional brilliant blue staining of internal limiting membrane in macular hole surgery. Retina. 2016. https://doi.org/10.1097/IAE.0000000000000948.
61. Lyu W-J, Ji L-B, Xiao Y, Fan Y-B, Cai X-H. Treatment of refractory giant macular hole by vitrectomy with internal limiting membrane transplantation and autologous blood. Int J Ophthalmol. 2018;11(5):818–22.
62. Dimopoulos S, William A, Voykov B, Ziemssen F, Bartz-Schmidt KU, Spitzer MS. Anatomical and visual outcomes of autologous thrombocyte serum concentrate in the treatment of persistent full-thickness idiopathic macular hole after ILM peeling with brilliant blue G and membrane blue dual. Acta Ophthalmol. 2017. https://doi.org/10.1111/aos.12971.
63. Figueroa MS, Govetto A, De Arriba-Palomero P. Short-term results of platelet-rich plasma as adjuvant to 23-G vitrectomy in the treatment of high myopic macular holes. Eur J Ophthalmol. 2015. https://doi.org/10.5301/ejo.5000729.
64. Purtskhvanidze K, Frühsorger B, Bartsch S, Hedderich J, Roider J, Treumer F. Persistent full-thickness idiopathic macular hole: anatomical and functional outcome of revitrectomy with autologous platelet concentrate or autologous whole blood. Ophthalmologica. 2017. https://doi.org/10.1159/000481268.
65. Chen SN, Yang CM. Lens capsular flap transplantation in the management of refractory macular hole from multiple etiologies. Retina. 2016. https://doi.org/10.1097/IAE.0000000000000674.
66. Peng J, Chen C, Jin H, Zhang H, Zhao P. Autologous lens capsular flap transplantation combined with autologous blood application in the management of refractory macular hole. Retina. 2017;38(11):2177–83. https://doi.org/10.1097/IAE.0000000000001830.
67. Alkabes M, Mateo C. Macular buckle technique in myopic traction maculopathy: a 16-year review of the literature and a comparison with vitreous surgery. Graefes Arch Clin Exp Ophthalmol. 2018;256(5):863–77. https://doi.org/10.1007/s00417-018-3947-3.
68. Ripandelli G, Coppe AM. Evaluation of Primary Surgical Procedures for Retinal Detachment with Macular Hole in highly myopic eyes. Ophthalmology. 2001;108(12):2258–64.
69. Ando F, Ohba N, Touura K, Hirose H. Anatomical and visual outcomes after episcleral macular buckling compared with those after pars plana vitrectomy for retinal detachment caused by macular hole in highly myopic eyes. Retina. 2007;27(1):37–44. https://doi.org/10.1097/01.iae.0000256660.48993.9e.
70. Qi Y, Duan AL, You QS, Jonas JB, Wang N. Posterior scleral reinforcement and vitrectomy for myopic foveoschisis in extreme myopia. Retina. 2015;35(2):351–7. https://doi.org/10.1097/IAE.0000000000000313.
71. Grewal DS, Mahmoud TH. Autologous neurosensory retinal free flap for closure of refractory myopic macular holes. JAMA Ophthalmol. 2016;134(2):229–30. https://doi.org/10.1001/jamaophthalmol.2015.5237.
72. Wu A-L, Chuang L-H, Wang N-K, et al. Refractory macular hole repaired by autologous retinal graft and blood clot. BMC Ophthalmol. 2018;18:213.
73. Thomas AS, Mahmoud TH. Subretinal transplantation of an autologous retinal free flap for chronic retinal detachment with proliferative vitreoretinopathy with and without macular hole. Retina. 2017;38(Suppl 1):S121–4. https://doi.org/10.1097/IAE.0000000000002026.
74. Ding C, Li S, Zeng J. Autologous neurosensory retinal transplantation for unclosed and large macular holes. Ophthalmic Res. 2018;61(2):88–93.
75. de Giacinto C, D'Aloisio R, Cirigliano G, Pastore MR, Tognetto D. Autologous neurosensory retinal free patch transplantation for persistent full-thickness macular hole. Int Ophthalmol. 2018;39(5):1147–50.

13

Myopic Choroidal Neovascularization in Adults and its Treatment

Shaun Sim, Chee Wai Wong, and Gemmy C. M. Cheung

Key Points

- The prevalence of myopic choroidal neovascularization (CNV) was between 5.2% and 11.3% in individuals with pathological myopia and was more common in females.
- Fundus fluorescein angiography (FFA) and optical coherence tomography are the imaging modalities of choice to diagnose myopic CNV and assess activity.
- Current evidence supports the use of intravitreal anti-vascular endothelial growth factor as the gold standard of treatment for myopic CNV, following a pro re nata (PRN) treatment regimen without a loading phase.
- Long-term visual outcomes remain less favorable, largely due to the devel opment of chorioretinal atrophy around the regressed CNV.

13.1 Disease Overview

Myopic choroidal neovascularization (myopic CNV), a subtype of CNV associated with pathological myopia, is the second most common cause of CNV after age-related macular degeneration (AMD) [1, 2]. Compared to CNV secondary to AMD, key differences include occurrence in a younger age group, less prominent exudative and hemorrhagic changes, generally smaller choroidal

S. Sim · C. W. Wong · G. C. M. Cheung (✉)
Singapore National Eye Centre, Singapore, Singapore

Singapore Eye Research Institute, Singapore, Singapore
e-mail: gemmy.cheung.c.m@singhealth.com.sg

neovascular membranes, excellent response to anti-vascular endothelial growth factor treatment and better long-term visual prognosis [3–5]. It is one of the most sight-threatening complications of pathological myopia [6, 7], with individuals typically reporting acute loss of central vision. Estimated to develop in 5–10% of eyes with pathological myopia, myopic CNV is the most common cause of CNV in people aged 50 years or younger [1], with significant social and economic burden.

13.2 Incidence and Prevalence

Owing to a lack of uniform diagnostic criteria, the reported incidence and the prevalence of myopic CNV have varied widely and may be well underestimated. A recent systematic review reported that the prevalence of myopic CNV was between 5.2% and 11.3% in individuals with pathological myopia [8], with female preponderance seen in most studies [1, 2, 6, 9]. Myopic CNV was also bilateral in approximately 15% of individuals [1, 9]. Table 13.1 shows the prevalence as reported in population-based studies and in individuals with pathological myopia.

Table 13.1 Prevalence of myopic CNV

Reference	Definition of PM	Definition of CNV-type lesion	Age	Subjects (eyes)	Prevalence of CNV
Pathological myopia studies					
Curtin et al. (1970) [9]	AL >26.5 mm	Fuchs' spot	All ages	(538)	5.2%, bilateral in 16.7%
Grossniklaus et al. (1992) [10]	AL 25.5–26.5 mm, refractive error −5.0 to −7.5 D	Subretinal neovascularization, Fuchs' spot	All ages	202 (308)	5.2%—subretinal neovascularization 3.2%—Fuchs' spot
Hayashi et al. (2010) [11]	AL ≥26.5 mm or refractive error ≥−8 D	CNV	All ages	429 (806)	11.3%
General population studies					
The Blue Mountains Eye Study	"Myopic retinopathy"	CNV or Fuchs' spot	≥49 years	44 (67)	6.0%—CNV 1.5%—Fuchs' spot
The Beijing Eye Study	"Myopic retinopathy"	Fuchs' spot	≥40 years	132 (198)	1.5%

PM pathological myopia, *AL* axial length, *CNV* choroidal neovascularization

13.3 Natural History

The long-term outcome of CNV is poor if left untreated. In a 10-year follow-up study of 25 patients with myopic CNV, visual acuity deteriorated to 20/200 or worse in 89% and 96% of eyes in 5 and 10 years respectively [2]. Approximately 35% of individuals with myopic CNV in one eye developed CNV in the fellow eye, with a mean period of 8 years between eyes [12].

In the late twentieth century, Tokoro et al. classified myopic CNV into three stages; active, scar, and atrophic stages [13]. Several other authors subsequently examined longitudinally the natural course of CNV and the three stages associated with visual loss [14, 15]. In the active phase, myopic CNV is characterized by hemorrhage with or without serous retinal detachment. In the scar phase, there is absorption of hemorrhage with development of fibrotic scars, some of which can become hyperpigmented, known classically as Fuchs' spots. Finally, in the atrophic phase, as the myopic CNV regresses, the development of macular chorioretinal atrophy ensues. Recent studies using swept source optical coherence tomography have revealed the presence of macular Bruch's membrane defect associated with myopic CNV. The expansion of these defects was found to be related to the enlargement of chorioretinal atrophy surrounding a regressed CNV [16]. In a small proportion of patients, poor visual outcome might be due to formation of myopic macular hole, particularly in eyes where chorioretinal atrophy is greater than one disc area [17].

13.4 Risk Factors

Compared to systemic risk factors, ocular risk factors have a much stronger influence on the development of myopic CNV. A prospective study found that eyes with myopic CNV had higher grade myopic maculopathy (with patchy retinal atrophy or worse) than eyes without myopic CNV. In the same series, eyes with higher grade myopic maculopathy were also 3.55 times more likely to develop myopic CNV than those with lower grade myopic maculopathy [18]. Higher grade lacquer cracks defined as crisscrossing lacquer cracks with or without linear cracks were also found in a significantly higher proportion of eyes with myopic CNV as compared to the fellow uninvolved eye [19, 20]. Choroidal thinning, in particular the subfoveal and inferior choroid, was found to be significantly thinner in eyes with myopic CNV than in the fellow uninvolved eyes [19, 21]. Furthermore, in patients with newly diagnosed myopic CNV, it was reported that the incidence of myopic CNV development in the fellow eye was 34.8% compared to 6.1% in those with no previous CNV [12]. Other studies have also established an association between highly myopic eyes with higher aqueous humor levels of the inflammatory cytokines interleukin 6 and 8 [22, 23]. Systemic risk factors implicated in the development of myopic CNV include higher levels of C-reactive protein and complement factors C3 and CH50 [24]. Older age (>40 years), subfoveal CNV location, larger baseline lesion size

(>400 μm), and lower best corrected visual acuity (BCVA) at baseline have been identified as factors leading to poorer visual outcomes [8, 25].

13.5 Pathogenesis

The pathogenesis of myopic CNV has not been clarified although several theories have been proposed. The mechanical theory postulates that progressive elongation of the anteroposterior axis leads to breaks in the retinal pigment epithelium (RPE)–Bruch's membrane–choriocapillaris complex with formation of lacquer cracks, which in turn facilitates neovascularization from choriocapillaris [26–28]. Lacquer cracks have been more frequently observed in fellow eyes of patients with unilateral myopic CNV, hence the suggestion that breaks in Bruch's membrane as the predisposing factor for development of CNV in pathological myopia [12]. It has also been reported that in vitro, progressive elongation of the posterior pole results in mechanical stress of the RPE cell layer, thus upregulating the expression and secretion of angiogenic factors [29]. The increased expression of vascular endothelial growth factor (VEGF) in aqueous humor of eyes with myopic CNV compared to cataract controls has also been reported in a comparative study [22]. Notably, VEGF levels in myopic CNV were lower than those in CNV secondary to AMD and can be explained by the smaller size of CNV membranes in myopic CNV. It is the imbalance between pro-angiogenic and anti-angiogenic factors that results in the development of myopic CNV.

The heredo-degenerative theory has been supported by genetic factors associated with myopic CNV based on twin and familial aggregation studies of pathologic myopia [30]. In a recent study that analyzed 15 genes associated with age-related macular degeneration, it was found that a single nucleotide polymorphism in the complement factor I (*CFI*) gene was significantly associated with myopic CNV [31]. Complement factor I is a regulatory protein involved in three complement pathways and is expressed by macrophages, lymphocytes, and fibroblasts, suggesting that inflammation via the complement pathway may be involved in the development of myopic CNV.

The hemodynamic theory suggests that alterations in choroidal perfusion of myopic eyes with choroidal filling delay may result in choroidal ischemia [32]. This leads to subsequent upregulation of angiogenic factors and the subsequent development of myopic CNV [7]. Doppler ultrasound imaging of the retrobulbar vessels revealed significantly higher vascular flow resistance in the posterior ciliary artery in eyes with myopic CNV as compared to the fellow eye, thus further implicating dysfunction of choroidal circulation in the development of myopic CNV [33].

13.6 Diagnosis and Monitoring

On slit-lamp biomicroscopy, myopic CNV manifests as a small, flat, grayish subretinal lesion adjacent to or beneath the fovea [2, 6, 34, 35]. There may be associated macular hemorrhage with or without exudation or subretinal fluid. Spectral

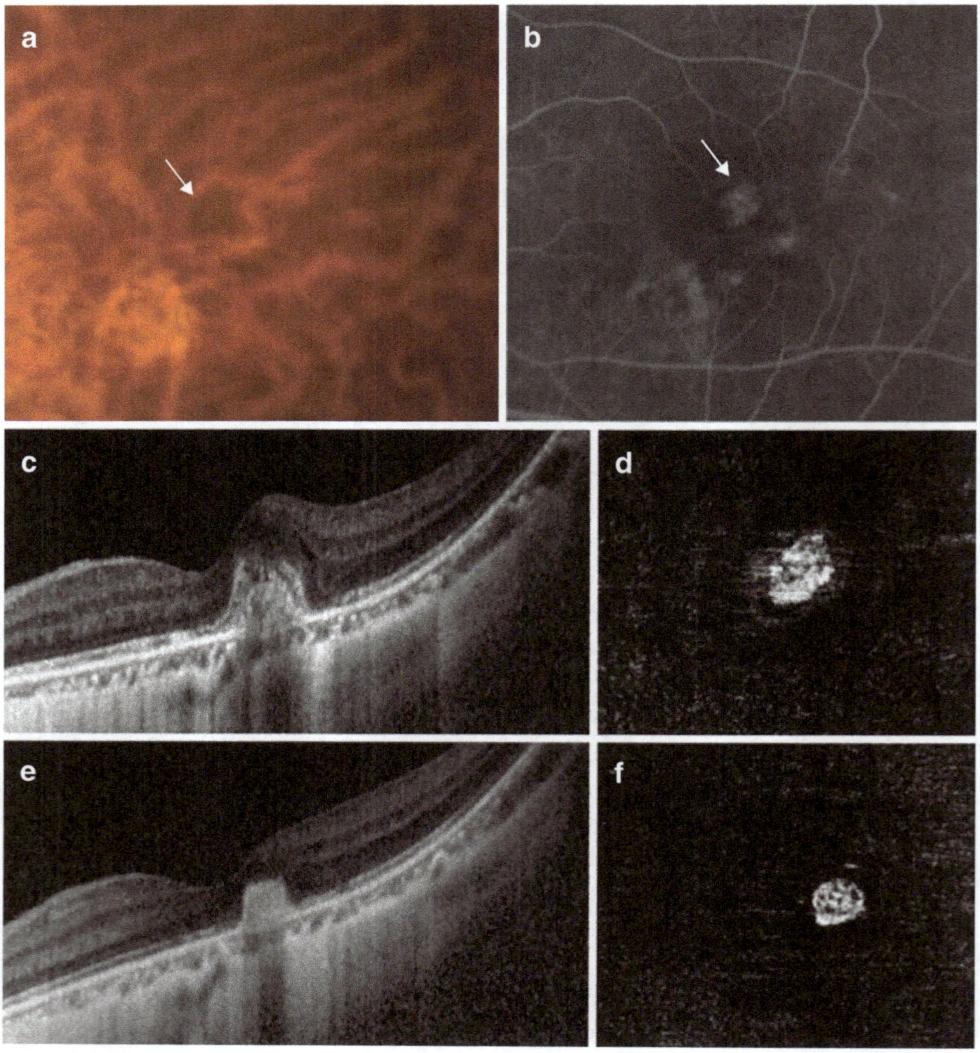

Fig. 13.1 Myopic CNV in a 57-year-old female. (**a**) Fundus photo shows a spot of subretinal hemorrhage (white arrow). (**b**) Fundus fluorescein angiogram shows early hyperfluorescence (white arrow) with a halo of hypofluoresence. (**c**) Optical coherence tomography (OCT) B scan shows a subretinal hyper-reflective lesion with indistinct margins, representing a type 2 CNV. (**d**) OCT angiography shows flow signals representing the choroidal neovascular membrane in the outer retina slab. (**e**) OCT B scan after treatment with a single intravitreal injection of anti-vascular endothelial growth factor. The subretinal hyper-reflective lesion is now inactive and has acquired well-demarcated margins. (**f**) OCT angiography shows persistence of flow signals despite inactivity

domain optical coherence tomography (SD-OCT) is a useful non-invasive screening tool that can be performed rapidly. On SD-OCT, myopic CNV presents as a hyper-reflective material above the RPE band (type 2 CNV), with a variable amount of subretinal fluid (Fig. 13.1). OCT appearance is helpful to assess the activity of mCNV: signs of activity include ill-defined margins and disruption of the external limiting membrane, with a variable amount of intraretinal or subretinal fluid. As the lesion becomes inactive, it consolidates and acquires a distinct border.

Clinical diagnosis is confirmed by fundus fluorescein angiography (FFA). Most myopic CNVs are type 2 neovascularization and present with a "classic" pattern on fluorescein angiography (FA). The amount of leakage may vary, depending on the level of the activity, the size of the lesion and the health of the RPE. FA has been shown to have higher sensitivity for detecting the activity than OCT. In some eyes, subtle late leakage on FA may be the only sign of myopic CNV activity [35]. Myopic CNV with dense macular hemorrhage may result in masking of both early hyperfluorescence and late leakage. Indocyanine green angiography (ICGA) is useful in these cases to detect CNV. In addition, imaging also provides important prognostic indications. The size and location of the lesion can be better evaluated on FFA, while lacquer cracks and chorio-retinal atrophy are best seen with ICGA [3]. ICGA also aids in exclusion of polypoidal choroidal vasculopathy (PCV) in those with macular hemorrhage, particularly important amongst Asian patients with the higher prevalence of PCV [36].

OCT angiography (OCTA) allows non-invasive imaging of the retinal and choroidal microvasculature. It is able to detect type 2 CNV with high sensitivity and specificity when compared against FFA and ICGA [37]. OCTA is able to detect flow within myopic CNV vascular complexes and hence delineates vascular networks in these myopic neovascular membranes that lie above the RPE where flow signals are spared from attenuation [38]. On OCTA, CNV shape could be described as circular or irregular, margins could be well defined or poorly defined and appearance could be interlacing or tangled/disorganized vascular loops. In eyes with active myopic CNV lesions, the OCTA appearance is primarily interlacing, while inactive CNV neovascular networks appear primarily tangled [39–41]. OCTA is also able to clearly visualize the choriocapillaris in myopic eyes, with varying loss of choriocapillaris depending on the extent of myopic maculopathy and the presence of lacquer cracks [42, 43]. Although sensitivity and specificity compared to FFA as gold standard have not been fully evaluated for the diagnosis of myopic CNV, it is felt that OCTA may reduce the need for FFA if CNV is clearly visualized on OCTA at the commencement of anti-VEGF therapy. However, there remain limitations concerning OCTA: It is currently still unable to provide information on the disease activity as flow signals can persist in an inactive myopic CNV [39–41]. Therefore, activity assessment should be evaluated with clinical examination and multi-modal imaging, including structural OCT with or without FA. Motion or image artifacts and segmentation errors may further complicate its interpretation. Therefore, it is still recommended to complement SD-OCT and FFA to increase diagnostic accuracy and monitoring of the disease activity.

The imaging features of various stages of myopic CNV are summarized in Table 13.2.

Table 13.2 Imaging characteristics of the different phases of myopic choroidal neovascularization

Phase	Fundus appearance	Fluorescein angiography	Indocyanine green angiography	Optical coherence tomography
Active	Small grayish subretinal lesion at or near the fovea, with or without hemorrhage	Early hyperfluorescence increasing in size and intensity with time	Late hyperflu-orescence	Ill-defined subretinal hyper-reflective lesion with or without subretinal fluid
Scar	Grayish white, sometimes pigmented spot. Absence of hemorrhage	Early hyperfluorescence decreasing in intensity with time, indicating fluorescein staining of subretinal scar	Hypoflu-orescence	Subretinal hyper-reflective lesion with well-demarcated margins
Atrophic	Well-demarcated whitish lesion centered on fovea. Absence of hemorrhage	Hypofluorescence	Hypoflu-orescence	Absence of RPE–Bruch's membrane–choriocapillaris complex with hypertransmission of signal into the underlying sclera and retro-orbital fat

13.7 Differential Diagnosis

There are several differential diagnoses that must be excluded from myopic CNV.

13.7.1 Macular Hemorrhage Secondary to Lacquer Cracks (Fig. 13.2)

In individuals with macular hemorrhage, it is critical to differentiate eyes with myopic CNV from those with simple hemorrhage associated with lacquer cracks (Fuch's hemorrhage). Eyes with Fuch's hemorrhage secondary to lacquer cracks tend to have better prognosis than myopic CNV and do not require anti-VEGF therapy [44]. In cases with thick blood, the myopic CNV may not be visible even in FA or OCTA due to masking. In these cases, late phases of ICGA will be able to visualize the myopic CNV if it is present [20].

13.7.2 Inflammatory CNV

Punctate inner choroidopathy (PIC) with or without secondary CNV may present with OCT appearance similar to that of myopic CNV. The clinical manifestation

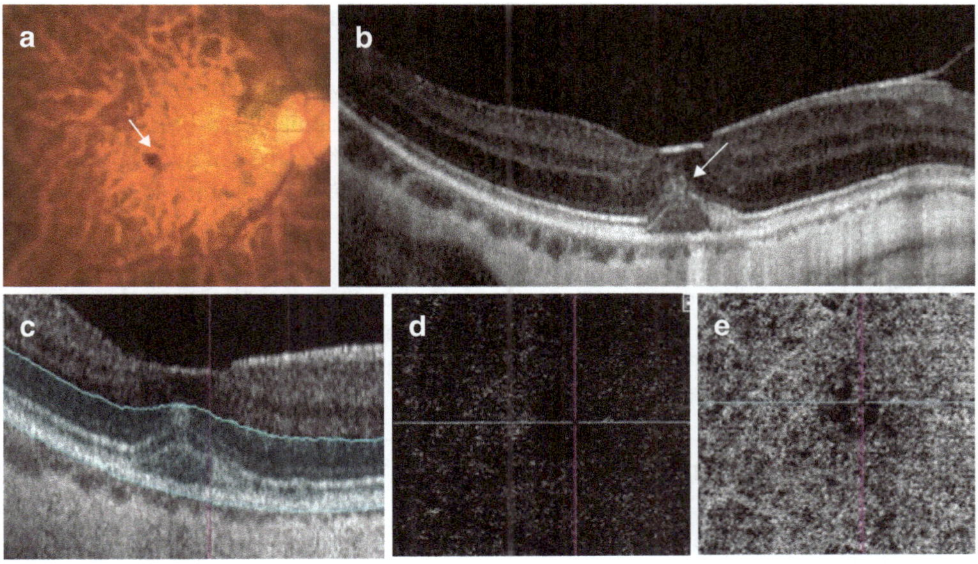

Fig. 13.2 A 51-year-old highly myopic male with lacquer crack hemorrhage. (**a**) Fundus photo shows a red spot suggestive of subretinal hemorrhage (white arrow). (**b**) Optical coherence tomographic scan shows a separation between the RPE and the underlying Bruch's membrane in the subfoveal position (white arrow head), with hyper-reflectivity in the subretinal space (white arrow) corresponding to the area of subretinal hemorrhage. Optical coherence tomographic angiography of the region of interest (**c**) shows no flow signals suggestive of choroidal neovascularization in the outer retinal slab (**d**) or the choriocapillaris slab (**e**)

of punctate inner choroidopathy differs from myopic CNV, with characteristic creamy yellow-white lesions located at the RPE and inner choroid. A prospective series revealed that PIC lesions go through a five-stage evolution process with differing SD-OCT findings at each stage: choroidal infiltration (stage I: mostly normal but can present with hyper-reflective fine spots within the outer nuclear layer), formation of sub-RPE nodules (stage II: focal elevation of RPE with corresponding ellipsoid zone disruption), chorioretinal nodules (stage III: nodule that breaks through the RPE and progresses towards and replaces the photoreceptor layer that eventually domes the outer plexiform layer (OPL)), regression (stage IV: noted to begin from the apex towards the choroid and with herniation of the OPL and inner retina through the RPE break) and retinal herniation (stage V: sagging of the OPL and inner retina with loss of photoreceptor layer and RPE proliferation that relieves the retinal hernia) [45]. Of these various stages, only stage III may ostensibly be misdiagnosed as myopic CNV. The use of OCTA and its ability to identify vascular network can be particularly useful in this instance to distinguish myopic CNV from PIC as inflammatory lesions do not manifest vascular flow signals [46]. Unlike myopic CNV, the late phases of ICGA would reveal multiple areas of hypercyanescence in punctate inner choroidopathy [47].

13.7.3 Dome-Shaped Maculopathy with Serous Detachment

Dome-shaped maculopathy (DSM) is characterized by an inward bulge within the chorioretinal posterior concavity of the eye in the macular area [48, 49]. Serous foveal detachment is a complication of DSM that has been postulated to be related to the abnormal curvature of the macula [50]. On FFA, DSM with serous retinal detachment can be distinguished from myopic CNV where it may be associated with pinpoint leakage. On ICGA, it presents as punctate hypercyanescent spots [51]. The absence of macular hemorrhage, with the characteristic dome-shaped profile of the macula visualized on OCT, and the leakage of dye in later frames help differentiate this entity from myopic CNV.

13.8 Management

13.8.1 Anti-Vascular Endothelial Growth Factor Drugs

Prior to the advent of anti-VEGF therapy, the main treatment options for myopic CNV were limited to thermal laser photocoagulation [52] and photodynamic therapy with verteporfin (vPDT) [53, 54]. These treatments had limited efficacy in improving vision significantly and have now largely been relegated to the annals of history by the anti-vascular endothelial growth factor (anti-VEGF) therapy [55].

13.9 Ranibizumab

Ranibizumab is a Fab fragment of humanized monoclonal antibody against all isoforms of VEGF-A, and it was the first anti-VEGF agent to be FDA approved for the treatment of myopic CNV. The strongest evidence of anti-VEGF use for myopic CNV comes from two large multi-centered, double-masked, randomized, controlled clinical trials [56, 57]. The RADIANCE study ($n = 277$) was a 12-month, phase III, randomized, double-masked, multicenter study comparing the efficacy and safety of intravitreal ranibizumab 0.5 mg versus vPDT in patients with myopic CNV [56]. This trial demonstrated the superiority of ranibizumab 0.5 mg, with a mean visual acuity gain of 10.5–10.6 letters compared to 2.2 letters with vPDT at 3 months and maintained through 12 months. The study further compared two retreatment protocols and showed that the disease activity guided retreatment based on OCT could achieve similar visual outcomes with a lower median number of injections (2.0) compared to retreatment according to visual acuity stabilization (4.0 injections). The RADIANCE study confirmed the results of the REPAIR trial, a phase II prospective, open-label, multicenter study of intravitreal ranibizumab 0.5 mg in myopic CNV in 65 eyes. In this study, a mean visual gain of 13.8 letters was achieved with a mean of 3.6 ranibizumab injections over 12 months in a cohort of treatment-naïve patients with myopic CNV [58]. These trials were performed in predominantly Caucasian populations. To support the use of ranibizumab for Asian patients with myopic CNV, the BRILLIANCE study was conducted with a design similar to the RADIANCE study. This was a 12-month, double-masked trial in which study participants with myopic CNV were randomized into one of three treatment groups: ranibizumab guided by visual acuity stabilization criteria (group 1, $n = 182$), ranibizumab guided by disease activity (group 2, $n = 184$) and vPDT followed by ranibizumab/vPDT/both treatments at month 3, guided by the disease activity (group 3, $n = 91$) [55]. Findings from the BRILLIANCE study corroborated with those from the RADIANCE study. Both ranibizumab arms experienced significantly better visual acuity gains at 3 months compared to the vPDT arm (Group I/II: +9.5/+9.8 letters vs. Group III: +4.5 letters; both $P < 0.001$), and ranibizumab treatment guided by disease activity was noninferior to treatment guided by visual acuity stabilization, achieving similar visual acuity outcomes with a median of three and four injections over 12 months, respectively. These results confirmed the efficacy of ranibizumab for the treatment of myopic CNV in Asian patients.

In a large post-marketing surveillance study of ranibizumab for the treatment of Japanese patients with myopic CNV ($n = 318$) over a 12-month observation period, ranibizumab was found to be safe (incidence of 0.6% and 0.3% of adverse drug reactions and serious adverse events, respectively) and effective with a low number of injections needed for the therapeutic effect (median injection number of 1 and 52.2% requiring only 1 injection) [59].

13.10 Aflibercept

Aflibercept is a recombinant human fusion protein that acts as a soluble decoy receptor for VEGF family members VEGF-A, VEGF-B and placental growth factor, preventing these ligands from binding to, and activating, their receptors. The MYRROR trial was a 48-week, phase III, multicenter, randomized, double-masked, sham-controlled study investigating the efficacy and safety of intravitreal aflibercept 2 mg for the treatment of myopic CNV [57]. Patients treated with intravitreal aflibercept ($n = 91$) achieved a mean visual gain of 12 letters compared to a 2-letter loss in the sham group ($n = 31$). The mean number of injections was low in this study (4.2 injections over 48 weeks). Significant improvement in the quality of life (National Eye Institute Visual Function Questionnaire 25 and EuroQol-5 Dimension score) was also demonstrated in patients treated with aflibercept.

13.11 Bevacizumab

Bevacizumab was the first angiogenesis inhibitor to be approved for clinical use, initially for the treatment of metastatic colorectal cancer. Since then, it has been used as an open-label drug and a lower cost option for the treatment of choroidal neovascularization, including myopic CNV. There is a lack of randomized controlled trials assessing the efficacy of bevacizumab in the treatment of myopic CNV, but many clinical case series have reported significant visual gains ranging from 5 to 20 letters with the open-label use of bevacizumab [60–64]. Long-term studies have also demonstrated maintenance of visual gains for up to 4 years after the initial treatment [52, 65].

13.12 Conbercept

Conbercept is a recombinant fusion protein containing the second Ig-like domain of VEGFR-1, the third and fourth Ig-like domains of VEGFR-2 and a human IgG Fc fragment, with binding affinity to VEGF and placental growth factor (PIGF) [66]. There are no prospective interventional trials on the use of conbercept for myopic CNV. Yan et al. performed a retrospective analysis of 42 consecutive eyes with myopic CNV treated with three loading doses of conbercept at monthly intervals, followed by as-needed injections based on monthly follow-up visits till month 12. BCVA improved from 0.67 logMAR at baseline to 0.32 at 12 months, with 71.4% achieving three lines or more improvement at final follow-up with a mean of 3.76 injections [67].

13.13 Factors Related to Treatment Outcomes

As previously mentioned, older age, subfoveal location of CNV, larger lesion size and poorer presenting visual acuity are poor prognostic factors for myopic CNV [8, 25, 68]. In addition, subretinal hemorrhage, duration of CNV and previous photodynamic therapy were found to confer a poorer prognosis after treatment [68]. Similarly, older age, larger CNV size and greater central macular thickness were factors associated with the need for retreatment [69–71]. Thinner choroid and lacquer cracks were also found to be associated with the need for a higher number of intravitreal injections [71].

The presence of vitreomacular abnormalities, in particular epiretinal membrane (ERM), is common in high myopes. ERM often coexists with myopic CNV. The presence of ERM has been shown to hamper visual gains after treatment of myopic CNV with ranibizumab compared to eyes without ERM (visual stabilization from a baseline of 0.3–0.4 compared to improvement from 0.3 to 0.1, $p = 0.008$). The coexistence of ERM with myopic CNV neither influenced the median number of injections (3) nor the reduction in central foveal thickness [72]. As regards the myopic macular retinoschisis (MRS), a post hoc analysis of the RADIANCE trial showed that eyes with MRS received more injections (5.8 ± 2.1 vs 4.0 ± 2.9; $P = 0.0001$), had slower visual gain at 3 months (+2.8 letters vs +12.3 letters) and poorer visual outcomes at 12 months (+7.1 letters vs +14.4 letters) than eyes without MRS [73]. Post hoc analysis further evaluated whether baseline myopic macular degeneration (MMD) influenced the treatment outcomes in 115 eyes. Change in BCVA from baseline to week 48 was not significantly different between eyes with mild MMD

(META-PM category 1–2) and eyes with severe MMD (META-PM category 1–2) (+13.5 letters vs +12.4 letters, $p = 0.83$), and were achieved with a similar number of injections (3.9 vs 5.4, $p = 0.23$) [74].

13.14 Recurrence

The recurrence rate of myopic CNV is generally low, with most recurrences occurring during the first year. Yang et al. reported a recurrence rate of 23.3% in a retrospective series of 103 eyes of 89 consecutive patients with subfoveal myopic CNV, followed over 2 years. 72.7% of recurrences occurred in the first year of treatment. Baseline CNV size was found to be a significant prognostic factor for recurrence on multivariate analysis [71]. In the post-RADIANCE observation study (12–48 months), only 10% of eyes experienced a recurrence [75]. These findings reinforce the importance of monitoring for recurrences in the first year of treatment.

13.15 Treatment Regimen and Follow-Up

Once active myopic CNV is diagnosed, prompt treatment with intravitreal anti-VEGF therapy should be administered as soon as possible [56, 58]. Current evidence suggests that a pro re nata (PRN) regimen without a loading phase can be considered in most patients. Patients should be monitored monthly with OCT and treatment administered until cessation of the disease activity on OCT or visual stabilization. FA may be performed to confirm inactive disease before stopping treatment, especially if there are uncertainties regarding activity based on OCT. Thereafter, review can be progressively lengthened on an individualized basis if no further activity is observed in the first year to monitor for recurrence or development of myopic CNV in the fellow eye. After the first year of treatment, patients without recurrence can have their visit interval prolonged to 6 months. Patients should be advised to return if vision drops or metamorphopsia recurs [3].

13.16 Long-Term Outcomes

Although anti-VEGF therapy for myopic CNV has demonstrated remarkable short- and mid-term efficacy, longer term visual outcomes are generally less favorable, with most studies reporting a gradual decline back to baseline visual acuity [60, 61, 75–79]. Onishi et al. reported the 5-year outcomes of 51 patients who received treatment with ranibizumab for myopic CNV. Mean baseline BCVA (0.38 logMAR) was significantly improved at 1 year (0.27 logMAR) but not in the subsequent years (0.31, 0.35 and 0.32 logMAR at 2, 4 and 5 years, respectively). Sarao et al. reported similar findings in a prospective interventional study with mean BCVA improvement of −0.13 at 24 months in 101 eyes with myopic CNV treated with bevacizumab and an increase in the area of chorioretinal atrophy in the same period [61]. In contrast, the long-term visual outcomes of 41 patients who had completed the RADIANCE trial were shown to be sustained up to 48 months post initiation of treatment. Mean visual gain from baseline (56.5 ± 12.1 letters) was significant up to 48 months (+16.3 ± 18.7, $n = 16$, $p = 0.0034$). Of the 16 patients who completed 48 months of follow-up, 63% gained ≥10 letters and 13% lost ≥10 letters. Over the post-RADIANCE observation period (months 12–48), 83% of patients required no further treatment and 10% experienced recurrences [75].

Similar results were reported in Caucasian patients with myopic CNV ($n = 40$) treated with intravitreal ranibizumab: baseline visual acuity improved from 55.4 letters to 63.4 letters at 3 years ($p = 0.039$) and 35% gained 15 letters or more at the final follow-up, achieved with a mean of 4.1 injections in the first year, 2.4 in the second year and 1.1 in the third year [76]. A longer term follow-up study in Caucasian eyes treated with bevacizumab or ranibizumab found that visual gains could be maintained at 3 (+9.0 letters, $n = 52$), 4 (+9.0 letters, $n = 28$) and 5 years (+9.8 letters, $n = 13$) [77]. A 5-year outcome study by the PAN-American Collaborative Retina Study Group with intravitreal bevacizumab ($n = 33$) reported a significant decline in visual acuity from 0.65 ± 0.33 logMAR at baseline to 0.73 ± 0.50 logMAR units at final follow-up ($p = 0.003$) [80].

In the longest follow-up study to date, Pastore et al. reported on the visual outcomes of 17 eyes with myopic CNV, treated with ranibizumab according to a strict pro re nata regimen over 9 years. Mean visual acuity was significantly improved from baseline (56.2 ± 13.5 letters) at 1 (69.7 ± 12.2 letters) and 2 years (69.9 ± 12.8 letters) post treatment initiation, but gradually receded towards baseline at 9 years (57.4 ± 17.7 letters). Only 11.8% of eyes lost 3 lines or more, while 17.7% maintained 3 lines or more gain in vision at 9 years, achieved with a mean of 1.24 ± 1.70 injections per year (range 2–25) [78]. Despite a loss of visual gains, these results demonstrate a considerably superior visual prognosis for patients with myopic CNV than patients with CNV secondary to age-related macular degeneration over the long term [81, 82].

Myopic CNV-related chorioretinal atrophy (CRA) is the major culprit for the loss of visual gain over the long term. Ohno Matsui et al. found that the macular atrophy developing after myopic CNV may be related to rupture of Bruch's membrane. This defect in Bruch's membrane may continue to expand in spite of adequate treatment of myopic CNV, leading to macular atrophy and loss of vision [16]. This point was demonstrated in a 5-year outcome study of eyes with myopic CNV treated with intravitreal ranibizumab ($n = 51$), in which visual stability was achieved (baseline best corrected visual acuity 20/49 compared to 20/42) at 5 years, where good visual outcome was shown to be significantly associated with a lack of enlargement of CNV-related macular atrophy, in addition to better baseline visual acuity and a lower number of injections [79]. These outcomes were achieved with a mean of 1.6 injections over 5 years, and two-thirds received only 1 injection. Another study by Ohno Matsui's group observed similar findings in patients treated with bevacizumab ($n = 36$). Visual acuity improved significantly from a baseline of 0.5 logMAR to 0.31 and 0.39 at years 2 and 4, respectively, but not at 6 years (0.45), achieved with a mean of 1.78 injections. Again, visual outcomes at 6 years were correlated with the size of CNV-related macular atrophy, as well as baseline visual acuity and CNV size. Further, in a long-term (mean follow-up 80.6 ± 28.0 months) retrospective review of 54 eyes with myopic CNV treated with photodynamic therapy and/or intravitreal ranibizumab and eyes with myopic maculopathy alone, the progression of macular atrophy was significantly greater in myopic CNV eyes compared to the eyes with only myopic maculopathy. The risk of progression was related to age, degree of myopia and presence of staphyloma, but not the type of treatment [83].

13.17 Conclusions

Myopic CNV is a sight-threatening complication of pathologic myopia that, fortunately, has an effective treatment in the form of anti-VEGF injections. Early detection, accurate diagnosis with multimodal imaging, early initiation of treatment, and careful post-treatment monitoring are key to achieving good treatment outcomes. Although FFA and OCT remain the gold standard for diagnosis, OCTA is emerging as a good adjunct imaging modality to screen for the presence of neovascular networks in patients with suspected myopic CNV. Anti-VEGF therapy has been shown to be efficacious and safe with a low treatment burden. Finally, long-term visual outcomes remain less favorable, largely due to the development of chorioretinal atrophy around the regressed CNV. Therapeutic strategies to prevent the enlargement of CNV-related atrophy should form the focus of future research for the treatment of myopic CNV.

References

1. Cohen SY, Laroche A, Leguen Y, Soubrane G, Coscas GJ. Etiology of choroidal neovascularization in young patients. Ophthalmology. 1996;103(8):1241–4.
2. Yoshida T, Ohno-Matsui K, Yasuzumi K, et al. Myopic choroidal neovascularization: a 10-year follow-up. Ophthalmology. 2003;110(7):1297–305.
3. Ohno-Matsui K, Ikuno Y, Lai TYY, Gemmy Cheung CM. Diagnosis and treatment guideline for myopic choroidal neovascularization due to pathologic myopia. Prog Retin Eye Res. 2018;63:92–106.
4. Cheung CMG, Arnold JJ, Holz FG, et al. Myopic choroidal neovascularization: review, guidance, and consensus statement on management. Ophthalmology. 2017;124(11): 1690–711.
5. Ohno-Matsui K, Lai TY, Lai CC, Cheung CM. Updates of pathologic myopia. Prog Retin Eye Res. 2016;52:156–87.
6. Avila MP, Weiter JJ, Jalkh AE, Trempe CL, Pruett RC, Schepens CL. Natural history of choroidal neovascularization in degenerative myopia. Ophthalmology. 1984;91(12): 1573–81.
7. Neelam K, Cheung CM, Ohno-Matsui K, Lai TY, Wong TY. Choroidal neovascularization in pathological myopia. Prog Retin Eye Res. 2012;31(5):495–525.
8. Wong TY, Ferreira A, Hughes R, Carter G, Mitchell P. Epidemiology and disease burden of pathologic myopia and myopic choroidal neovascularization: an evidence-based systematic review. Am J Ophthalmol. 2014;157(1):9–25.e12.
9. Curtin BJ, Karlin DB. Axial length measurements and fundus changes of the myopic eye. I. The posterior fundus. Trans Am Ophthalmol Soc. 1970;68:312–34.

10. Grossniklaus HE, Green WR. Pathologic findings in pathologic myopia. Retina. 1992;12(2):127–33.
11. Hayashi K, Ohno-Matsui K, Shimada N, Moriyama M, Kojima A, Hayashi W, Yasuzumi K, Nagaoka N, Saka N, Yoshida T, Tokoro T, Mochizuki M. Long-term pattern of progression of myopic maculopathy: a natural history study. Ophthalmology. 2010;117(8):1595–611. 1611.e1–4.
12. Ohno-Matsui K, Yoshida T, Futagami S, et al. Patchy atrophy and lacquer cracks predispose to the development of choroidal neovascularisation in pathological myopia. Br J Ophthalmol. 2003;87(5):570–3.
13. Tokoro T. Atlas of posterior fundus changes in pathologic myopia. Tokyo: Springer; 1998.
14. Ohno-Matsui K. What is the fundamental nature of pathologic myopia? Retina. 2017;37(6):1043–8.
15. Ohno-Matsui K, Yoshida T. Myopic choroidal neovascularization: natural course and treatment. Curr Opin Ophthalmol. 2004;15(3):197–202.
16. Ohno-Matsui K, Jonas JB, Spaide RF. Macular Bruch membrane holes in choroidal neovascularization-related myopic macular atrophy by swept-source optical coherence tomography. Am J Ophthalmol. 2016;162:133–139.e131.
17. Shimada N, Ohno-Matsui K, Yoshida T, Futagami S, Tokoro T, Mochizuki M. Development of macular hole and macular retinoschisis in eyes with myopic choroidal neovascularization. Am J Ophthalmol. 2008;145(1):155–61.
18. Cheung CM, Loh BK, Li X, et al. Choroidal thickness and risk characteristics of eyes with myopic choroidal neovascularization. Acta Ophthalmol. 2013;91(7):e580–1.
19. Ikuno Y, Jo Y, Hamasaki T, Tano Y. Ocular risk factors for choroidal neovascularization in pathologic myopia. Invest Ophthalmol Vis Sci. 2010;51(7):3721–5.
20. Kim YM, Yoon JU, Koh HJ. The analysis of lacquer crack in the assessment of myopic choroidal neovascularization. Eye. 2011;25(7):937–46.
21. Ng WY, Ting DS, Agrawal R, et al. Choroidal structural changes in myopic choroidal neovascularization after treatment with antivascular endothelial growth factor over 1 year. Invest Ophthalmol Vis Sci. 2016;57(11):4933–9.
22. Tong JP, Chan WM, Liu DT, et al. Aqueous humor levels of vascular endothelial growth factor and pigment epithelium-derived factor in polypoidal choroidal vasculopathy and choroidal neovascularization. Am J Ophthalmol. 2006;141(3):456–62.
23. Yamamoto Y, Miyazaki D, Sasaki S, et al. Associations of inflammatory cytokines with choroidal neovascularization in highly myopic eyes. Retina. 2015;35(2):344–50.
24. Long Q, Ye J, Li Y, Wang S, Jiang Y. C-reactive protein and complement components in patients with pathological myopia. Optom Vis Sci. 2013;90(5):501–6.
25. Wong TY, Ohno-Matsui K, Leveziel N, et al. Myopic choroidal neovascularisation: current concepts and update on clinical management. Br J Ophthalmol. 2015;99(3):289–96.
26. Curtin BJ, Karlin DB. Axial length measurements and fundus changes of the myopic eye. Am J Ophthalmol. 1971;71(1 Pt 1):42–53.
27. Noble KG, Carr RE. Pathologic myopia. Ophthalmology. 1982;89(9):1099–100.
28. Lloyd RI. Clinical studies of the myopic macula. Trans Am Ophthalmol Soc. 1953;51:273–84.
29. Seko Y, Fujikura H, Pang J, Tokoro T, Shimokawa H. Induction of vascular endothelial growth factor after application of mechanical stress to retinal pigment epithelium of the rat in vitro. Invest Ophthalmol Vis Sci. 1999;40(13):3287–91.
30. Young TL. Dissecting the genetics of human high myopia: a molecular biologic approach. Trans Am Ophthalmol Soc. 2004;102:423–45.
31. Leveziel N, Yu Y, Reynolds R, et al. Genetic factors for choroidal neovascularization associated with high myopia. Invest Ophthalmol Vis Sci. 2012;53(8):5004–9.
32. Wakabayashi T, Ikuno Y. Choroidal filling delay in choroidal neovascularisation due to pathological myopia. Br J Ophthalmol. 2010;94(5):611–5.
33. Dimitrova G, Tamaki Y, Kato S, Nagahara M. Retrobulbar circulation in myopic patients with or without myopic choroidal neovascularisation. Br J Ophthalmol. 2002;86(7):771–3.
34. Ohno-Matsui K, Kawasaki R, Jonas JB, et al. International photographic classification and grading system for myopic maculopathy. Am J Ophthalmol. 2015;159(5):877–883.e877.
35. Lai TY, Cheung CM. Myopic choroidal neovascularization: diagnosis and treatment. Retina. 2016;36(9):1614–21.

36. Cheung CMG, Lai TYY, Ruamviboonsuk P, et al. Polypoidal choroidal vasculopathy: definition, pathogenesis, diagnosis, and management. Ophthalmology. 2018;125(5):708–24.
37. Soomro T, Talks J, Medscape. The use of optical coherence tomography angiography for detecting choroidal neovascularization, compared to standard multimodal imaging. Eye. 2018;32(4):661–72.
38. Jia Y, Bailey ST, Wilson DJ, et al. Quantitative optical coherence tomography angiography of choroidal neovascularization in age-related macular degeneration. Ophthalmology. 2014;121(7):1435–44.
39. Bruyere E, Miere A, Cohen SY, et al. Neovascularization secondary to high myopia imaged by optical coherence tomography angiography. Retina. 2017;37(11):2095–101.
40. Miyata M, Ooto S, Hata M, et al. Detection of myopic choroidal neovascularization using optical coherence tomography angiography. Am J Ophthalmol. 2016;165:108–14.
41. Querques L, Giuffre C, Corvi F, et al. Optical coherence tomography angiography of myopic choroidal neovascularisation. Br J Ophthalmol. 2017;101(5):609–15.
42. Sayanagi K, Ikuno Y, Uematsu S, Nishida K. Features of the choriocapillaris in myopic maculopathy identified by optical coherence tomography angiography. Br J Ophthalmol. 2017;101(11):1524–9.
43. Wong CW, Teo YCK, Tsai STA, et al. Characterization of the choroidal vasculature in myopic maculopathy with optical coherence tomographic angiography. Retina. 2018. https://doi.org/10.1097/IAE.0000000000002233.
44. Moriyama M, Ohno-Matsui K, Shimada N, et al. Correlation between visual prognosis and fundus autofluorescence and optical coherence tomographic findings in highly myopic eyes with submacular hemorrhage and without choroidal neovascularization. Retina. 2011;31(1):74–80.
45. Zhang X, Zuo C, Li M, Chen H, Huang S, Wen F. Spectral-domain optical coherence tomographic findings at each stage of punctate inner choroidopathy. Ophthalmology. 2013;120(12):2678–83.
46. Tan ACS, Tan GS, Denniston AK, et al. An overview of the clinical applications of optical coherence tomography angiography. Eye. 2018;32(2):262–86.
47. Spaide RF, Goldberg N, Freund KB. Redefining multifocal choroiditis and panuveitis and punctate inner choroidopathy through multimodal imaging. Retina. 2013;33(7):1315–24.
48. Gaucher D, Erginay A, Lecleire-Collet A, et al. Dome-shaped macula in eyes with myopic posterior staphyloma. Am J Ophthalmol. 2008;145(5):909–14.
49. Caillaux V, Gaucher D, Gualino V, Massin P, Tadayoni R, Gaudric A. Morphologic characterization of dome-shaped macula in myopic eyes with serous macular detachment. Am J Ophthalmol. 2013;156(5):958–967.e951.
50. Ellabban AA, Tsujikawa A, Matsumoto A, et al. Three-dimensional tomographic features of dome-shaped macula by swept-source optical coherence tomography. Am J Ophthalmol. 2013;155(2):320–328.e322.
51. Viola F, Dell'Arti L, Benatti E, et al. Choroidal findings in dome-shaped macula in highly myopic eyes: a longitudinal study. Am J Ophthalmol. 2015;159(1):44–52.
52. Virgili G, Menchini F. Laser photocoagulation for choroidal neovascularisation in pathologic myopia. Cochrane Database Syst Rev. 2005;4:CD004765.
53. Blinder KJ, Blumenkranz MS, Bressler NM, et al. Verteporfin therapy of subfoveal choroidal neovascularization in pathologic myopia: 2-year results of a randomized clinical trial--VIP report no. 3. Ophthalmology. 2003;110(4):667–73.
54. Verteporfin in Photodynamic Therapy Study G. Photodynamic therapy of subfoveal choroidal neovascularization in pathologic myopia with verteporfin. 1-year results of a randomized clinical trial--VIP report no. 1. Ophthalmology. 2001;108(5):841–52.
55. Chen Y, Sharma T, Li X, et al. Ranibizumab versus verteporfin photodynamic therapy in asian patients with myopic choroidal neovascularization: brilliance, a 12-month, randomized, double-masked study. Retina. 2018. https://doi.org/10.1097/IAE.0000000000002292.
56. Wolf S, Balciuniene VJ, Laganovska G, et al. RADIANCE: a randomized controlled study of ranibizumab in patients with choroidal neovascularization secondary to pathologic myopia. Ophthalmology. 2014;121(3):682–692.e682.

57. Ikuno Y, Ohno-Matsui K, Wong TY, et al. Intravitreal aflibercept injection in patients with myopic choroidal neovascularization: the MYRROR study. Ophthalmology. 2015;122(6):1220–7.
58. Tufail A, Narendran N, Patel PJ, et al. Ranibizumab in myopic choroidal neovascularization: the 12-month results from the REPAIR study. Ophthalmology. 2013;120(9):1944–1945.e1941.
59. Ohno-Matsui K, Suzaki M, Teshima R, Okami N. Real-world data on ranibizumab for myopic choroidal neovascularization due to pathologic myopia: results from a post-marketing surveillance in Japan. Eye. 2018;32(12):1871–8.
60. Kasahara K, Moriyama M, Morohoshi K, et al. Six-year outcomes of intravitreal bevacizumab for choroidal neovascularization in patients with pathologic myopia. Retina. 2017;37(6):1055–64.
61. Sarao V, Veritti D, Macor S, Lanzetta P. Intravitreal bevacizumab for choroidal neovascularization due to pathologic myopia: long-term outcomes. Graefes Arch Clin Exp Ophthalmol. 2016;254(3):445–54.
62. Baba T, Kubota-Taniai M, Kitahashi M, Okada K, Mitamura Y, Yamamoto S. Two-year comparison of photodynamic therapy and intravitreal bevacizumab for treatment of myopic choroidal neovascularisation. Br J Ophthalmol. 2010;94(7):864–70.
63. Ikuno Y, Nagai Y, Matsuda S, et al. Two-year visual results for older Asian women treated with photodynamic therapy or bevacizumab for myopic choroidal neovascularization. Am J Ophthalmol. 2010;149(1):140–6.
64. Gharbiya M, Cruciani F, Parisi F, Cuozzo G, Altimari S, Abdolrahimzadeh S. Long-term results of intravitreal bevacizumab for choroidal neovascularisation in pathological myopia. Br J Ophthalmol. 2012;96(8):1068–72.
65. Peiretti E, Vinci M, Fossarello M. Intravitreal bevacizumab as a treatment for choroidal neovascularisation secondary to myopia: 4-year study results. Can J Ophthalmol. 2012; 47(1):28–33.
66. Wu Z, Zhou P, Li X, et al. Structural characterization of a recombinant fusion protein by instrumental analysis and molecular modeling. PLoS One. 2013;8(3):e57642.
67. Yan M, Huang Z, Lian HY, Song YP, Chen X. Conbercept for treatment of choroidal neovascularization secondary to pathologic myopia. Acta Ophthalmol. 2018. https://doi.org/10.1111/aos.13632.
68. Wang J, Kang Z. Summary of prognostic factors for choroidal neovascularization due to pathological myopia treated by intravitreal bevacizumab injection. Graefes Arch Clin Exp Ophthalmol. 2012;250(12):1717–23.
69. Iacono P, Battaglia Parodi M, Selvi F, et al. Factors influencing visual acuity in patients receiving anti-vascular endothelial growth factor for myopic choroidal neovascularization. Retina. 2017;37(10):1931–41.
70. Ng DS, Kwok AK, Tong JM, Chan CW, Li WW. Factors influencing need for retreatment and long-term visual outcome after intravitreal bevacizumab for myopic choroidal neovascularization. Retina. 2015;35(12):2457–68.
71. Yang HS, Kim JG, Kim JT, Joe SG. Prognostic factors of eyes with naive subfoveal myopic choroidal neovascularization after intravitreal bevacizumab. Am J Ophthalmol. 2013;156(6):1201–1210.e1202.
72. Iacono P, Battaglia Parodi M, Iuliano L, Bandello F. How vitreomacular interface modifies the efficacy of anti-Vegf therapy for myopic choroidal neovascularization. Retina. 2018;38(1):84–90.
73. Ceklic L, Munk MR, Wolf-Schnurrbusch U, Gekkieva M, Wolf S. Visual acuity outcomes of ranibizumab treatment in pathologic myopic eyes with macular retinoschisis and choroidal neovascularization. Retina. 2017;37(4):687–93.
74. Gemmy Chui Ming Cheung KO-M, Tien Yin Wong, Tummy Li, Friedrich Asmus, Sergio L, et al. Influence of myopic macular degeneration (MMD) severity on treatment outcomes of myopic choroidal neovascularization (mCNV) in the MYRROR Study. In: Presented at the American Academy of Ophthalmology (AAO) Congress Chicago, IL 2016.

75. Tan NW, Ohno-Matsui K, Koh HJ, et al. Long-term outcomes of ranibizumab treatment of myopic choroidal neovascularization in East-Asian patients from the radiance study. Retina. 2017;38(11):2228–38.
76. Franqueira N, Cachulo ML, Pires I, et al. Long-term follow-up of myopic choroidal neovascularization treated with ranibizumab. Ophthalmologica. 2012;227(1):39–44.
77. Freitas-da-Costa P, Pinheiro-Costa J, Carvalho B, et al. Anti-VEGF therapy in myopic choroidal neovascularization: long-term results. Ophthalmologica. 2014;232(1):57–63.
78. Pastore MR, Capuano V, Bruyere E, et al. Nine-year outcome of ranibizumab monotherapy for choroidal neovascularization secondary to pathologic myopia. Ophthalmologica. 2018;239(2-3):133–42.
79. Onishi Y, Yokoi T, Kasahara K, et al. Five-year outcomes of intravitreal ranibizumab for choroidal neovascularization in patients with pathologic myopia. Retina. 2018. https://doi.org/10.1097/IAE.0000000000002164.
80. Chhablani J, Paulose RM, Lasave AF, et al. Intravitreal bevacizumab monotherapy in myopic choroidal neovascularisation: 5-year outcomes for the PAN-American Collaborative Retina Study Group. Br J Ophthalmol. 2018;102(4):455–9.
81. Rofagha S, Bhisitkul RB, Boyer DS, Sadda SR, Zhang K, Group S-US. Seven-year outcomes in ranibizumab-treated patients in anchor, marina, and horizon: a multicenter cohort study (SEVEN-UP). Ophthalmology. 2013;120(11):2292–9.
82. Maguire MG, Martin DF, Comparison of Age-related Macular Degeneration Treatments Trials Research G, et al. Five-year outcomes with anti-vascular endothelial growth factor treatment of neovascular age-related macular degeneration: the comparison of age-related macular degeneration treatments trials. Ophthalmology. 2016;123(8):1751–61.
83. Farinha CL, Baltar AS, Nunes SG, et al. Progression of myopic maculopathy after treatment of choroidal neovascularization. Ophthalmologica. 2014;231(4):211–20.

14

Myopia Control Methods: Optical Interventions

Wing Chun Tang, Myra Leung, Angel C. K. Wong, Chi-ho To, and Carly S. Y. Lam

Key Points

- Optical intervention for myopia control can slow down myopia progression by 50–60%.
- Simultaneous myopic defocus and refractive error correction have been proved to be effective in myopia control.
- Different myopia control methods and their pros and cons aid clinicians to select the best treatment for patients.

14.1 Introduction

A variety of clinical methods are currently utilized for retarding myopia progression. However, none of the methods have been proven to cease the development or progression of myopia completely and they may not work for some individuals. As described in previous chapters, the main clinical interventions for myopia control currently include optical lenses, pharmaceutical agents and outdoor activities. This chapter provides an overview of the various types of optical interventions for slowing down myopia progression. The findings of the clinical trials of these methods are summarized and the relative effectiveness of these methods in myopia control is compared. In general, the optical methods for myopia control in children can be summarized into two categories: spectacle lenses and contact lenses.

The original version of this chapter was revised. A correction to this chapter can be found at https://doi.org/10.1007/978-981-13-8491-2_15.

W. C. Tang · M. Leung · A. C. K. Wong · C.-h. To · C. S. Y. Lam (✉)
Centre for Myopia Research, School of Optometry, The Hong Kong Polytechnic University, Kowloon, Hong Kong
e-mail: Carly.lam@polyu.edu.hk

14.2 Spectacle Lenses

14.2.1 Under-Correction of Myopia

Studies using animals, such as chicks and mammals, have shown that the use of optical lenses to impose myopic defocus inhibits myopic eye growth in developing eyes [1–5]. These studies have led to the hypothesis that under-correction of myopia, that is, prescribing spectacles for distance vision that does not fully correct the myopic refraction, may be a viable method for slowing myopia progression in humans. As near work and accommodation were proposed as key factors for the development and progression of myopia, in theory, under-correction could reduce accommodative demand during near viewing, thereby halting the myopia progression of myopia.

Contrary to the animal studies, two clinical trial studies showed that under-correction actually accelerates myopia development and progression in myopic humans [6, 7]. In a randomized study by Chung et al. [6], children in the experimental group were assigned to wear spectacle lenses that were under corrected by 0.50–0.75 D to achieve distance visual acuity of 6/12, while children in the control group were prescribed their full correction. After 2 years, the under-correction group had greater myopia progression of −1.00 D as compared to the control group who progressed by −0.77 D. A retrospective study investigating clinical data from a private optometric practice also found that under-correction resulted in greater myopia progression compared to full correction [7].

One recent study in Beijing reported that children with no spectacle correction had slower myopia progression and less axial elongation than those given a full spectacle correction over 2 years [8]. In this study, myopia progression decreased significantly with an increasing amount of under-correction, but the effect on slowing myopia progression was slowed by only 0.27 D over 2 years, which is not clinically meaningful. In view of these conflicting results, there is no convincing evidence to indicate that under-correction should be used for slowing myopia progression in children.

14.2.2 Bifocal or Multifocal Spectacles

Over the past decades, numerous studies have assessed the effect of bifocal, multifocal, and progressive addition lens (PALs) spectacles on myopia progression. Table 14.1 summarizes the clinical trials of using the different spectacle lens types. Bifocals and PALs allow the wearers to clearly see objects in the distance through the upper part of the glasses by providing correction of distance refractive error. The bottom part of the lens consists of an addition power that may retard myopia progression by reducing accommodative effort and lag at near in a similar way as under-correction.

The majority of these studies have shown that PALs have an insignificant effect on slowing myopia progression rate (less than 0.2 D per year) overall (Table 14.1)

Table 14.1 Myopia control studies using PALs, bifocal and multifocal spectacles

Authors and years	Study duration (years)	Design	Age (years), ethnicity	Subject Rx range, diopters (D)	Interventions and sample size (*n*)	Treatment effect in slowing myopia progression during study period, D (%)
Fulk et al. (2000) [15]	2.5	Randomized, masked	6–13	−0.50 to −6.00 (under 9 years old) or −8.00 (9 years old or older)	SV, $n = 40$ Bifocals with 1.50 D add, $n = 42$	0.25 (20%)
Edward et al. (2002) [9]	2	Randomized, double masked	7–10.5, Chinese	−1.25 to −4.50	SV, $n = 132$ PAL (1.5 D add), $n = 121$	0.14 (11%)
Gwiazda et al. (2003) [10]	3	Randomized, masked	6–11, diverse ethnicity	−1.25 to −4.50	SV, $n = 233$ PAL (2 D add), $n = 229$	0.20 (14%)
Yang et al. (2009) [11]	2	Randomized, masked	7–13, Chinese	−0.50 to −3.00	SV, $n = 75$ PAL (1.5 D add), $n = 74$	0.26 (17%)
COMET2 (2011) [12]	3	Randomized, masked, multicenter	8–12, diverse ethnicity	−0.75 to −2.50	SV, $n = 58$ PAL (2 D add), $n = 52$	0.28 (24%)
Sankaridurg et al. (2011) [17]	1	Randomized	6–16, Chinese	−0.75 to −3.50	Type I, III lenses, SV, $n = 50$ each group Type II, $n = 60$	Type III lens: 0.29 (30% only in a subgroup of children with myopic parents)
Berntsen et al. (2012) [13]	1	Randomized, masked, all subjects worn SV in 2nd year	6–11	−0.75 to −4.50	SV, $n = 42$ PAL (2 D add), $n = 41$	0.18 (35%)
Hasbe et al. (2014) [14]	1.5	Randomized, masked, cross-over	6–12, Japanese	−1.25 to −6.00	SV, $n = 44$ PAL (1.5 D add), $n = 42$	1st period: 0.31 (18%) 2nd period: 0.02 (2%)
Cheng et al. (2014) [16]	3	Randomized, masked	8–13, Chinese	−1 to −5.50	SV, $n = 41$ BF (1.5 D add), $n = 48$ PBF (1.5 D add, 3ΔBI), $n = 46$	BF: 0.81 (39%) PBF: 1.05 (51%)
Lam et al. (2019) [19]	2	Randomized, masked	8–13, Chinese	−1.00 to −5.00	SV = 90 DIMS = 93	0.44 (52%)

COMET2 and PEDIG Correction of Myopia Evaluation Trial 2 Study Group and the Paediatric Eye Disease Investigator Group, *SV* single vision spectacle lens, *PAL* progressive addition lens, *BF* bifocal spectacle lens, *PBF* prismatic bifocal lens, *DIMS* defocus incorporated multiple segments spectacle lens

[9–14]. Some myopic children with esophoria and accommodative lag may benefit from PALs, but the retardation effect is not clinically significant.

For bifocal spectacles, an early randomized trial performed by Fulk et al. [15] found that bifocals with +1.5 D add slowed myopia progression by 20% in the children with esophoria. The clinical trial by Cheng et al. [16] found that both executive top bifocals with and without 3Δ base-in prism have shown a more meaningful myopia control effect in a selected group of fast progressing myopic children when compared with single vision spectacles. The myopia progression rate was reduced by approximately 40–50% over 3 years, with the effect being more prominent among those with low accommodative lag. The inclusion of base-in prism in the experimental lenses was an attempt to reduce fusional vergence demand to enhance the treatment effects of the bifocals. A positive effect of myopia control was exhibited as changes in spherical equivalent refraction in the study. Axial length changes were similar between those with and without base-in prism in their bifocals; it is rather unclear whether there is a benefit in having base-in prism in the bifocal lens. This option may also not be preferable for some children having anisometropia, and it results in poor cosmesis.

Another hypothesis is that the correction or reduction of relative peripheral hyperopia may have an effect on myopia progression [17, 18]. Sankaridurg et al. [17] performed a clinical trial to test this hypothesis by using three custom-designed spectacle lenses that reduced peripheral hyperopic defocus while maintaining clear central vision. After 12 months of lens wear, no significant reduction in myopia progression was found between the treatment groups and the control group. Only one type of the treatment lenses showed 30% reduction of myopia progression in a subgroup of the children whose parents were myopes. A similar clinical trial in soft contact lens [18], based on the same hypothesis, exhibited meaningful effects and will be discussed later in the section on soft multifocal contact lenses.

More recently, a specially designed bifocal spectacle lens, called Defocus Incorporated Multiple Segments (DIMS) spectacle lens (also known as multisegment of myopic defocus (MSMD) spectacle lens), has been used for myopia control in a randomized trial by Lam et al. [19]. DIMS lens design is based on the principle of simultaneous vision with myopia defocus for myopia control where it comprises a central optical zone for correcting refractive error and multiple segments of constant myopic defocus (+3.50 D) surrounding the central zone. This enables the lens to provide clear vision and myopic defocus simultaneously for wearers regardless of whether they are looking at distance, intermediate or near objects. The results from the clinical trial showed that the children wearing DIMS lenses had 52% less myopia progression and 62% less axial elongation when compared with children wearing single vision spectacle lenses over 2 years. Moreover, about 20% of the DIMS lens wearers had no myopia progression during the study period. Further studies in other study populations are required to validate these promising results.

Figure 14.1 presents a comparison of the percentage myopia progression that slowed down from PALs, bifocals, and prismatic bifocals use as well as other types of multiple spectacle lenses [9–16].

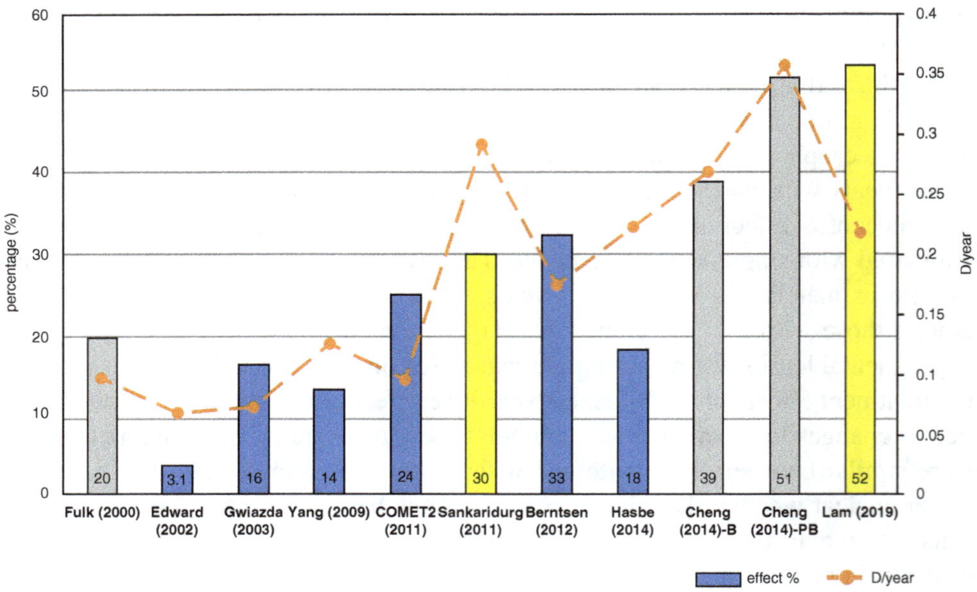

Fig. 14.1 The effect on slowing of myopia progression, in terms of percentage within the study period (effect %) and diopter per year (D/year), reported by various controlled clinical studies using bifocal or multifocal spectacles. The bars represent effect % using bifocals (gray), progressive addition lenses (blue) and other types of multifocal spectacle lenses (yellow). The value of effect % is indicated in the bar. The dotted line represents treatment effect in D/year (*B* bifocals, *PB* prismatic bifocals)

14.3 Contact Lenses

14.3.1 Rigid Gas Permeable Contact Lenses

Several studies in the later part of the twentieth century investigated whether daytime wear of rigid gas permeable (RGP) contact lenses slowed myopia progression, but all those studies had various limitations in their study designs, such as subject criteria outside the expected age of progression, lack of randomization, and unequal loss to follow-up [20–22]. Two randomized clinical trials [23, 24] showed that RGP contact lenses did not retard axial eye growth. However, Walline et al. [23] reported significant slower myopia progression in the group of RGP lenses compared with soft contact lenses. Despite that no differences were found in axial elongation between the groups. The proposed reason for a treatment effect on the refractions may be due to the changes in corneal curvature. As wear of RGP contact lenses is likely to induce only temporary changes in corneal curvature, the retardation of myopia progression may be transient. Therefore, the authors concluded that RGP lens wear does not slow myopia progression.

14.3.2 Orthokeratology

Orthokeratology (Ortho-K) lenses are specially designed RGP contact lenses that are worn overnight to reshape the cornea and thereby temporarily correct low to moderate myopia. It has become a popular modality for controlling myopia in children in the last few decades. In addition to the enhancement of unaided vision at daytime, Ortho-K is also able to control myopia progression.

Modern Ortho-K lens designs include four zones, namely the central optic zone, the reverse zone, the alignment zone and the peripheral zone [25, 26]. The central optic zone helps to flatten the central cornea and is used for refractive correction. The reverse zone, which has a steeper curvature than the central zone, enhances the corneal reshaping to maximize the myopic reduction. The alignment zone, usually aspherical or tangent, plays a very important role in optimizing the lens centration, while the peripheral curve promotes tear exchange. Apart from spherical designs, toric lenses are also available commercially and are recommended for use in patients with more than 1.50 D astigmatism. Fitting of Ortho-K is simple nowadays with manufacturers providing trial lens sets or computer software that directly calculates the most suitable and precise parameters based on the corneal topography. Although many different Ortho-K lens designs are available on the market, Tahhan et al. [27] found no significant variation on the clinical efficacy between the different lens designs.

The main hypothesis of myopia control using Ortho-K is the introduction of myopic defocus on the peripheral retina [27]. It is proposed that after Ortho-K treatment, the corneal shape changes to an oblate shape, which results in a peripheral refraction that has less hyperopic defocus [28]. Another hypothesis of the mechanism behind the myopia control effect of Ortho-K is that the changes in lag of accommodation may be due to increasing positive spherical aberration and changes in choroidal thickness [29, 30]. It seems that further investigation is required in order to determine the actual mechanism for the efficacy of Ortho-K.

Various clinical studies have demonstrated the effectiveness of inhibiting myopic progression with Ortho-K. Table 14.2 summarizes recent clinical trials using Ortho-K for myopia control in children. The effect of slowing axial length elongation ranges from 32% to 63% [31–38]. The overall treatment effect is around 50%. Figure 14.2 shows a comparison of the effect on retarding axial elongation using Ortho-K among different studies [31–37].

A recent study by Swabrick et al. [39] used a contralateral eye cross-over study design to investigate the effects of Ortho-K on axial length growth over 1 year. The results revealed that there were no changes in axial length at each 6-month phase of Ortho-K wear, while significant increases in axial length were found in the control group who wore daytime gas permeable lenses.

To the best of our knowledge, there is no research investigating the maximum power of myopia reduction with overnight Ortho-K, and most studies use −4.00 D as the exclusion criteria. Charm et al. investigated the myopic control effect of Ortho-K by partial reduction to the power of −4.00 D as the target in children with high myopia (spherical equivalent refraction at least −5.75 D and myopia ≥−5.00 D). The remaining refractive error was corrected by single vision spectacles. The myopia control effect was comparable to other studies of Ortho-K in low–moderate myopic subjects over 2 years [37]. As the risk of having corneal staining and lens decentration increases with the amount of myopia correction [39], partial reduction of myopia might be a better option in high myopes instead of the full correction.

Table 14.2 Myopia control studies using Ortho-K lenses

Authors and years	Study design	Study duration (years)	Control group	Mean change in AL (mm)		Treatment effect in retarding axial length elongation, mean difference in mm (%)
				Ortho-K	Control	
Cho et al. (2005) [31]	Self-selected prospective	2	SV	0.29	0.54	0.25 (46)
Walline et al. (2009) [32]	Prospective, historical controls	2	SVCL	0.25	0.57	0.32 (56)
Kakita et al. (2011) [33]	Self-selected retrospective	2	SV	0.39	0.61	0.22 (36)
Cho and Cheung (2012) [34]	Randomized, single-masked	2	SV	0.36	0.63	0.27 (43)
Hiraoka et al. (2012) [35]	Self-selected retrospective	5	SV	0.99	1.41	0.42 (30)
Santodomingo-Rubido et al. (2012) [36]	Self-selected prospective	2	SV	0.47	0.69	0.22 (32)
Charm and Cho (2013) [37]	Randomized, single-masked	2	SV	0.19	0.51	0.32 (63)
Chen et al. (2013) [38]	Self-selected prospective	2	SV	0.31	0.64	0.33 (52)

SV single vision spectacle lens, *SVCL* single vision soft contact lens

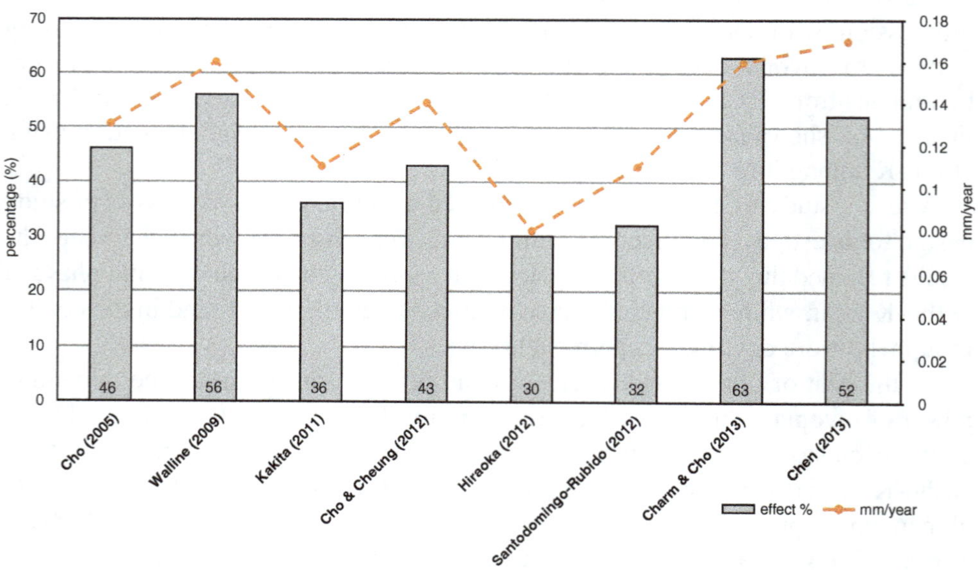

Fig. 14.2 Effect on slowing axial elongation reported by various studies using orthokeratology. The bar represents the treatment effect within the study period in terms of percentage (%) as compared to controls. The dotted line represents reduction in changes of axial length per year (mm/year)

Although Ortho-K is useful for myopic control in numerous studies, all the results were reported as an average value. Lipson et al [26] evaluated the axial length change over 3 years in children receiving Ortho-K treatment. Around 65% of the children had 0.5 mm or less axial elongation, while axial eye growth of more than 1.0 mm was seen in 15% of the children. Hence, the myopic control effect of Ortho-K lenses shows a large variation among individuals. Some researchers believed that the age at which Ortho-K is started, baseline myopia, cornea profile, and pupil size may be possible factors affecting the effectiveness of myopic control among Ortho-K wearers [26, 31, 34, 35, 40].

Interestingly, a recent study in Japan [41] showed that the combination of Ortho-K and low-concentration atropine (0.01%) eye drops was more effective in slowing axial elongation over 12 months than Ortho-K treatment alone in myopic children. More research is needed to show if this effect can be sustained in the longer term.

Although hypoxic reactions are rarely seen with Ortho-K wear due to the use of highly oxygen permeable materials, the need to wear contact lenses overnight may remain a concern for clinicians, as this type of lens wear pattern is associated with a higher risk of infectious keratitis [42–44]. A review of 50 cases of microbial keratitis done by Watt and Swarbrick [44] revealed that the majority of microbial keratitis cases are related to contamination of lenses due to patient non-compliance, such as improper lens handling or cleaning. A detailed systematic review on the safety of Ortho-K wear by Liu and Xie [45] also suggested that the training of practitioners and wearers, appropriate fitting procedures, compliance to lens care regimens and follow-up schedule are all factors affecting the incidence of microbial keratitis. A recent retrospective study compared the adverse events in Ortho-K wearers versus soft contact lens wearers over a 10-year period. The number of corneal complications such as keratitis and infiltrates were found to be significantly higher in the Ortho-K group, but no infectious keratitis was reported [46]. Bullimore et al. [47] found that there was no significant difference in the risk of getting microbial keratitis with Ortho-K wear compared to other overnight contact lens wear. This shows that with appropriate fitting and lens care, Ortho-K is a safe myopic control method. However, practitioners should always emphasize the importance of patient compliance, especially in lens care and follow-up visits, to reduce the risk of microbial keratitis [45].

Corneal staining is the most common complication in Ortho-K treatment. Studies confirmed the frequency and severity of staining associated with overnight lens wear [44]. Lens binding is one of the causes of creating central staining. Optimizing lens fitting, adding fenestration on lens and using artificial tears before lens removal could reduce the possibility of lens adhesion. Clinicians should be cautious if persistent or recurrent corneal staining is observed.

14.3.3 Soft Bifocal and Multifocal Contact Lenses

Soft contact lenses in the form of bifocal and multifocal have been designed to slow myopia progression in children, and there has been a rising interest in this area over the recent decade. These lenses are worn during the daytime. Compared to spectacles, contact lenses are more cosmetically acceptable and are more convenient for daily activities of some children, especially during sports activities [48, 49]. Also, they are generally able to be competently handled and worn by children [48]. For most of eye care practitioners, the fitting procedures of soft bifocal contact lenses are relatively simpler than those of Ortho-K.

Table 14.3 and Fig. 14.3 summarize recent clinical trials using soft bifocal contact lenses for myopia control [18, 50–56]. Generally, two main approaches are employed for the design of soft contact lenses for myopia control. Both lens designs incorporate a central distance zone to correct myopia. One design manipulates the peripheral lens curvature in order to lower peripheral hyperopic defocus. The other design uses concentric rings of alternating myopia defocus using addition (plus) powers and myopia correction powers in the periphery. This design is sometimes called 'dual power or dual focus' contact lenses in the literature. Both approaches allow the lens wearers to have good vision in their daily life and receive therapeutic optical defocus at the same time.

Several lens types, with a design to reduce peripheral hyperopia, have been reported to be promising in retarding myopia progression. Examples include a lens type used in a study by Sankaridurg et al. [18] and a multifocal contact lens used in a study by Walline et al. [50]. The former was reported to retard myopia progression by 34% over 1 year and the latter by 50% over 2 years. Paune et al. [51] carried out a study using 'soft radial refractive gradient' (SRRG) contact lens, which corrects the central refraction while producing peripheral myopic defocus that increases gradually from the central optical axis towards the periphery. After 2 years, children wearing the SRRG contact lens had retardation in myopia progression by 43%. Cheng et al. [52] developed a soft contact lens for myopia control that included a positive spherical aberration (+SA) in the optical design to shift retinal hyperopic defocus in the opposite direction, resulting in the reduction of relative peripheral hyperopia. The greatest effect of myopia control (56%) was observed during the first 6 months, and it decreased greatly to 20% by 12 months. The overall treatment effects of these contact lenses were better than ophthalmic lenses that used a similar approach [17]. This may be due to the soft contact lenses moving with the eye, and hence the optical correction remains centered for all viewing gazes.

Anstice and Phillips [53] investigated the use of a concentric bifocal power (also called dual-focus or dual power) soft contact lens with 2D of myopic defocus in retarding myopia progression in children. Children participating in their study were randomly assigned to wear the treatment lens in one eye and an ordinary single vision contact lens in the fellow eye for 10 months. The lens types were then switched between the eyes and the lenses were worn for another 10 months. On average, the eyes with the bifocal contact lenses showed about 45% less myopia progression than the eyes with single vision contact lenses. Several randomized clinical trials showed that concentric bifocal contact lenses exhibited meaningful effects on myopia control. Lam et al. [54] reported that the use of Defocus Incorporated Soft Contact (DISC) lens for at least 7 hours a day resulted in more effective myopia control, reaching nearly 60% reduction in myopia progression and

Table 14.3 Myopia control studies using soft bifocal and multifocal contact lenses

Authors and years	Study duration (months)	Study design	Age (years old), ethnicity	Subject Rx range (D)	Interventions and sample size (*n*)	Effect in slowing myopia progression in study period, D (%)
Anstice and Phillips (2011) [53]	20	Randomized, paired eye control, cross-over	11–14, diverse ethnicity	−1.25 to −4.50	DF (2 D add), $n = 40$ SVCL, $n = 40$	1st 10-month: 0.25 (37%) 2nd 10-month: 0.2 (54%)
Sankaridurg et al. (2011) [18]	12	Randomized	7–14, Chinese	−0.75 to −3.50	RPH CL, $n = 45$ SV, $n = 40$	0.29 (34%)
Walline et al. (2013) [50]	24	Matched study	8–11, diverse ethnicity	−1.00 to −6.00	Proclear multifocal D (2 D add), $n = 40$ Matched SVCL, $n = 40$	0.52 (50%)
Lam et al. (2014) [54]	24	Randomized, double-masked	8–13, Chinese	−1.00 to −5.00	DISC (2.5 D add), $n = 65$ SVCL, $n = 63$	0.21 (25%) 0.44 (50%) > 6 h 0.54 (58%) > 7 h 0.53 (60%) > 8 h
Paune et al. (2014) [51]	24	Prospective, nonrandomized	9–16, Caucasian	−0.75 to −7.00	SRRG, $n = 30$ OK, $n = 29$ SV, $n = 41$	0.42 (43%)
Aller et al. (2016) [57]	12	Randomized, masked	8–18,	−0.50 to −6.00	BFSCL, $n = 39$ SVCL, $n = -40$	0.57 (72% in children with eso fixation disparities)
Cheng et al. (2016) [52]	24 (only 12-month data)	Randomized, double-masked	8–11	−0.75 to −4.00	+SA, $n = 64$ SVCL, $n = 63$	6-month: 0.21 (56%) 12-month: 0.12 (20%)
Chamberlain et al. (2018) [55]	36	Randomized, double-masked	8–12	−0.75 to −4.00	DF (2 D add), $n = 70$ SVCL, $n = 74$	0.73 (59%)
Ruiz-Pomeda et al. (2018) [56]	24	Randomized, double-masked, multicenter	8–12	−0.75 to −4.00	DF (2 D add), $n = 46$ SVCL, $n = 33$	0.29 (39%)

DF dual focus contact lens, *SVCL* single vision contact lens, *RPH CL* contact lens designed to reduce relative peripheral hyperopia, *SV* single vision spectacle lens, *DISC* Defocus Incorporated Soft Contact lens, *SRRG* soft radial refractive gradient contact lens, *OK* Ortho-K, *BFSCL* bifocal soft contact lens, *+SA* soft contact lens with positive special aberration

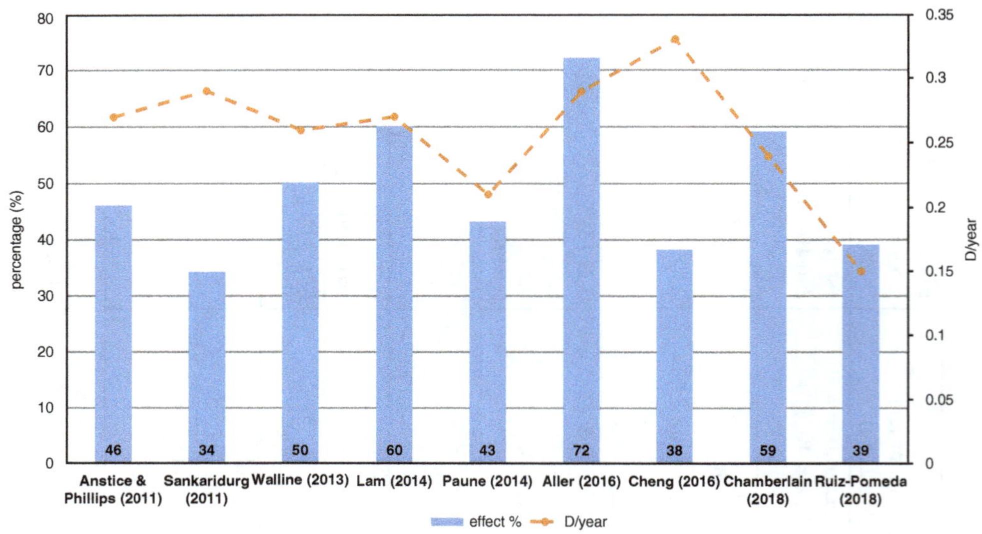

Fig. 14.3 Comparison of the treatment effect on slowing myopia progression among the studies using soft bifocal and multifocal contact lenses. The bar represents treatment effect within the study period in terms of percentage as compared with controls. The dotted line represents reduction of myopia progression per year (D/year)

axial length growth. The amount of myopic defocus used in the DISC lens was 2.50 D. Two more recent studies have indicated that a Dual-Focus 1-Day soft contact lens using 2D of myopic defocus also slows myopia progression in children. The multicenter study by Chamberlain et al. [55] has shown that the Dual-Focus 1-Day soft contact lens slows myopic progression and axial elongation in children by 59% and 52%, respectively, over 3 years. However, another study in Spain showed less myopia control effect, 39% and 36% in terms of refractive changes and axial growth, respectively [56]. A study by Aller et al. [57] reported the most promising effect of 70% with another type of bifocal soft contact lenses, but this was seen only for the children with eso fixation disparities at near.

Among the optical interventions for myopia control, Ortho-K lenses (45%), soft bifocal contact lenses (50%), prismatic bifocals (50%) and the very recent DIMS spectacle lenses (52%) have shown clinically significant treatment effects. However, the treatment effect of these methods is still inferior to that of pharmaceutical eye drops. The average reduction in myopia progression using regular dose (1%) of atropine is approximately 70% or above [58, 59]. Yet, the associated side effects, such as blurring of near vision, light sensitivity and possible allergic reactions and post-treatment rebound effects [58, 59], will be obstacles for the widespread application of atropine 1% in clinical practice. Lower doses of atropine (such as 0.5%, 0.02%, 0.01%) have been found to have minimal side effects, but long-term safety is unclear [60–62]. Atropine 0.01% has been found to have the least side effects with good myopia control and least rebound effects [61, 62]. However, optical treatment regimens are less invasive than those by pharmacological treatment and have been found to be more popular.

14.4 Others: Outdoor Activities and Violet Light Transmitting Lenses

Recent epidemiological studies have found that children who spend more time outdoors during daytime are less likely to become myopic and have less myopia progression, regardless of the amount of near work duration and parental history of myopia [63–65]. Some evidence for this relationship has been shown in young adults [63]. Outdoor time also appears to reduce the risk of myopia development in schoolchildren. A longitudinal study conducted in Taiwan found that children in a primary school who were encouraged to have outdoor activities during recess (outdoor group) were less likely to have myopia after a year compared to children in other schools who continued their normal recess routine (the control group) [64]. The proportion of children who had myopia onset after a year was significantly higher in the control group (18%) than in the intervention group (8%, $p < 0.001$).

The mechanism by which the outdoor activity could protect against myopia development is still unknown. However, there are a number of theories, such as relaxed accommodation for viewing distance receiving more myopic defocus in outdoor environments and higher light intensity in outdoor environments [65, 66]. The spectral composition of sunlight may also play a role in myopia control. Sunlight has a large portion of short-wavelength visible and non-visible light, such as blue light and ultraviolet light [67]. Animal studies have demonstrated that blue light has a suppressive effect against myopia [68, 69]. Recently, Torri et al. [70] proposed that violet light (VL) (which has a shorter wavelength than blue light), which is a missing light component in indoor environments, may play a role in the inhibition of myopia development and progression. They demonstrated that exposure to VL inhibited myopic shift and axial elongation in chicks. On the basis of the animal findings, they conducted a clinical trial in which myopic children were assigned to wear VL blocking eyeglasses, partially VL blocking contact lenses or VL transmitting contact lenses [70]. The results showed that children who wore VL transmitting contact lenses had significantly less axial length elongation compared to those wearing the other types of lenses over 1 year. These data provide evidence that VL may contribute to the protective effect against myopia progression. Further investigation is needed to determine whether VL transmitting lenses could slow myopia progression or prevent myopia in children.

14.5 Comparison of the Effectiveness on Myopia Control by Different Optical Interventions

Several studies have reviewed and compared the outcomes of the effect on myopia control using various treatments and methodologies [71–74]. In a review of nine randomized controlled trials that compared the effects of multifocal and single vision spectacle lenses, multifocals with add power ranging from +1.50 to +2.00 D were associated with a statistically significant decrease in myopia progression in school-age children compared with single vision lenses [74]. The effect was more prominent in children with a higher degree of myopia at baseline and could be sustained for a period of 24 months or more. Asian children were found to have greater benefit from the interventions than Caucasian children. A study comparing the treatment effect of atropine, soft bifocal and Ortho-K contact lens indicated that both atropine and Ortho-K showed treatment effects reaching over 75%, while soft bifocals had effects up to 48% [71].

In another study, a meta-analysis was performed to determine and compare 16 interventions for myopia control in children using pharmaceuticals or optical methods [73]. Among the optical methods, spectacle lens, contact lenses and Ortho-K were included. They concluded that atropine, pirenzepine, Ortho-K, soft contact lenses with myopia control features and progressive addition spectacle lenses are effective at reducing myopia progression in terms of refraction or axial length. For the pharmaceutical treatment, the average treatment effects reported in the literature are around 50%. For spectacle treatments, the effects range from minimal in the PAL trials to moderately effective in a study on executive bifocals. The investigators also compare different interventions with single vision spectacle lenses/placebo [73]. Atropine was found to be the most effective as it can retard myopia progression by around 0.50–0.60 D per year.

14.6 Conclusions

In summary, under-correction of myopia is not recommended for myopia control as it is likely to speed up myopia progression instead. Among spectacles, PALs and multifocal lenses do not yield clinically meaningful effects on slowing myopia progression in children. One single center study using prismatic bifocals in children with rapid progressing myopia showed a moderate treatment effect. Ortho-K, soft bifocal contact lenses and the very recent DIMS spectacle lenses have all shown clinically significant treatment effects ranging from 45% to 60% reduction in myopia progression. These methods demonstrated that myopic defocus as natural optical signals can inhibit refractive eye growth and control myopia progression through different optical designs. Although the effectiveness of myopia control with atropine is relatively better than those of optical methods, the associated side effects, such as sensitivity to light and near blur, hinder its widespread clinical application. Optical interventions are less invasive, which will make it likely to become more popular compared to pharmaceutical treatments.

Although there are a number of clinical methods currently available for myopia control for children, none of them have been proven to definitely halt the development or progression of myopia. The treatment effect also varies among individuals. Each therapy has its advantages and limitations. The suitable choice of treatment for each patient can vary and should be determined by the eye care professionals based on age, parental history, myopic progression rate, corneal health and lifestyle of the children. More research is needed to enhance the treatment effects of myopia control, particularly to prevent myopia before its onset through improved designs of optical lenses or pharmaceuticals. Several clinical trials are also testing the possibility of better myopia control with combined treatments, for example, optical lenses (soft bifocals, Ortho-K or DIMS spectacle lenses) with ophthalmic pharmaceutical (low-concentration atropine) or with other non-optical modalities (outdoor activities, intense bright light for near work). Also, there is still room for research on new myopia control methods, such as VL transmitting contact lenses or spectacles. When there is more evidence in the treatment effect, there is hope to reduce the prevalence of myopia and high myopia and its related ocular complications.

References

1. Siegwart JT, Norton TT. Binocular lens treatment in tree shrews: effect of age and comparison of plus lens wear with recovery from minus lens-induced myopia. Exp Eye Res. 2010;91:660–9. https://doi.org/10.1016/j.exer.2010.08.010.
2. Howlett MHC, McFadden SA. Spectacle lens compensation in the pigmented guinea pig. Vis Res. 2009;49:219–27. https://doi.org/10.1016/j.visres.2008.10.008.
3. Whatham AR, Judge SJ. Compensatory changes in eye growth and refraction induced by daily wear of soft contact lenses in young marmosets. Vis Res. 2001;41:267–73.
4. Smith EL, Hung L-F, Arumugam B. Visual regulation of refractive development: insights from animal studies. Eye (Lond). 2014;28:180–8. https://doi.org/10.1038/eye.2013.277.
5. Schaeffel F, Glasser A, Howland HC. Accommodation, refractive error and eye growth in chickens. Vis Res. 1988;28:639–57.
6. Chung K, Mohidin N, O'Leary DJ. Undercorrection of myopia enhances rather than inhibits myopia progression. Vis Res. 2002;42:2555–9.
7. Adler D, Millodot M. The possible effect of under correction on myopic progression in children. Clin Exp Optom. 2006;89:315–21. https://doi.org/10.1111/j.1444-0938.2006.00055.x.
8. Sun Y-Y, Li S-M, Li S-Y, et al. Effect of uncorrection versus full correction on myopia progression in 12-year-old children. Graefes Arch Clin Exp Ophthalmol. 2017;255:189–95. https://doi.org/10.1007/s00417-016-3529-1.
9. Edwards MH, Li RW-H, Lam CS-Y, et al. The Hong Kong progressive lens myopia control study: study design and main findings. Invest Ophthalmol Vis Sci. 2002;43:2852–8.
10. Gwiazda J, Hyman L, Hussein M, et al. A randomized clinical trial of progressive addition lenses versus single vision lenses on the progression of myopia in children. Invest Ophthalmol Vis Sci. 2003;44:1492–500.
11. Yang Z, Lan W, Ge J, et al. The effectiveness of progressive addition lenses on the progression of myopia in Chinese children. Ophthalmic Physiol Opt. 2009;29:41–8. https://doi.org/10.1111/j.1475-1313.2008.00608.x.
12. Correction of Myopia Evaluation Trial 2 Study Group for the Pediatric Eye Disease Investigator Group. Progressive-addition lenses versus single-vision lenses for slowing progression of myopia in children with high accommodative lag and near esophoria. Invest Ophthalmol Vis Sci. 2011;52:2749–57. https://doi.org/10.1167/iovs.10-6631.
13. Berntsen DA, Sinnott LT, Mutti DO, Zadnik K. A randomized trial using progressive addition lenses to evaluate theories of myopia progression in children with a high lag of accommodation. Invest Ophthalmol Vis Sci. 2012;53:640–9. https://doi.org/10.1167/iovs.11-7769.
14. Hasebe S, Jun J, Varnas SR. Myopia control with positively aspherized progressive addition lenses: a 2-year, multicenter, randomized, controlled trial. Invest Ophthalmol Vis Sci. 2014;55:7177–88. https://doi.org/10.1167/iovs.12-11462.
15. Fulk GW, Cyert LA, Parker DE. A randomized trial of the effect of single-vision vs. bifocal lenses on myopia progression in children with esophoria. Optom Vis Sci. 2000;77:395–401.
16. Cheng D, Woo GC, Drobe B, Schmid KL. Effect of bifocal and prismatic bifocal spectacles on myopia progression in children: three-year results of a randomized clinical trial. JAMA Ophthalmol. 2014;132:258–64. https://doi.org/10.1001/jamaophthalmol.2013.7623.
17. Sankaridurg P, Donovan L, Varnas S, et al. Spectacle lenses designed to reduce progression of myopia: 12-month results. Optom Vis Sci. 2010;87:631–41. https://doi.org/10.1097/OPX.0b013e3181ea19c7.

18. Sankaridurg P, Holden B, Smith E, et al. Decrease in rate of myopia progression with a contact lens designed to reduce relative peripheral hyperopia: one-year results. Invest Ophthalmol Vis Sci. 2011;52:9362–7. https://doi.org/10.1167/iovs.11-7260.
19. Lam CSY, Tang WC, Tse DY, et al. Defocus Incorporated Multiple Segments (DIMS) spectacle lenses slow myopia progression: a 2-year randomised clinical trial. Br J Ophthalmol. 2019 May 29. http://dx.doi.org/10.1136/bjophthalmol-2018-313739.
20. Khoo CY, Chong J, Rajan U. A 3-year study on the effect of RGP contact lenses on myopic children. Singap Med J. 1999;40:230–7.
21. Perrigin J, Perrigin D, Quintero S, Grosvenor T. Silicone-acrylate contact lenses for myopia control: 3-year results. Optom Vis Sci. 1990;67:764–9.
22. Stone J. The possible influence of contact lenses on myopia. Br J Physiol Opt. 1976;31:89–114.
23. Walline JJ, Jones LA, Mutti DO, Zadnik K. A randomized trial of the effects of rigid contact lenses on myopia progression. Arch Ophthalmol. 2004;122:1760–6. https://doi.org/10.1001/archopht.122.12.1760.
24. Katz J, Schein OD, Levy B, et al. A randomized trial of rigid gas permeable contact lenses to reduce progression of children's myopia. Am J Ophthalmol. 2003;136:82–90.
25. Swarbrick HA. Orthokeratology review and update. Clin Exp Optom. 2006;89:124–43. https://doi.org/10.1111/j.1444-0938.2006.00044.x.
26. Lipson MJ, Brooks MM, Koffler BH. The role of orthokeratology in myopia control: a review. Eye Contact Lens. 2018;44:224–30. https://doi.org/10.1097/ICL.0000000000000520.
27. Tahhan N, Du Toit R, Papas E, et al. Comparison of reverse-geometry lens designs for overnight orthokeratology. Optom Vis Sci. 2003;80:796–804.
28. Kang P, Swarbrick H. Peripheral refraction in myopic children wearing orthokeratology and gas-permeable lenses. Optom Vis Sci. 2011;88:476–82. https://doi.org/10.1097/OPX.0b013e31820f16fb.
29. Han X, Xu D, Ge W, et al. A comparison of the effects of orthokeratology lens, medcall lens, and ordinary frame glasses on the accommodative response in myopic children. Eye Contact Lens. 2018;44:268–71. https://doi.org/10.1097/ICL.0000000000000390.
30. Chen Z, Xue F, Zhou J, et al. Effects of orthokeratology on choroidal thickness and axial length. Optom Vis Sci. 2016;93:1064–71. https://doi.org/10.1097/OPX.0000000000000894.
31. Cho P, Cheung SW, Edwards M. The longitudinal orthokeratology research in children (LORIC) in Hong Kong: a pilot study on refractive changes and myopic control. Curr Eye Res. 2005;30:71–80.
32. Walline JJ, Jones LA, Sinnott LT. Corneal reshaping and myopia progression. Br J Ophthalmol. 2009;93:1181–5. https://doi.org/10.1136/bjo.2008.151365.
33. Kakita T, Hiraoka T, Oshika T. Influence of overnight orthokeratology on axial elongation in childhood myopia. Invest Ophthalmol Vis Sci. 2011;52:2170–4. https://doi.org/10.1167/iovs.10-5485.
34. Cho P, Cheung S-W. Retardation of myopia in Orthokeratology (ROMIO) study: a 2-year randomized clinical trial. Invest Ophthalmol Vis Sci. 2012;53:7077–85. https://doi.org/10.1167/iovs.12-10565.
35. Hiraoka T, Kakita T, Okamoto F, et al. Long-term effect of overnight orthokeratology on axial length elongation in childhood myopia: a 5-year follow-up study. Invest Ophthalmol Vis Sci. 2012;53:3913–9. https://doi.org/10.1167/iovs.11-8453.
36. Santodomingo-Rubido J, Villa-Collar C, Gilmartin B, Gutiérrez-Ortega R. Myopia control with orthokeratology contact lenses in Spain: refractive and biometric changes. Invest Ophthalmol Vis Sci. 2012;53:5060–5. https://doi.org/10.1167/iovs.11-8005.
37. Charm J, Cho P. High myopia-partial reduction ortho-k: a 2-year randomized study. Optom Vis Sci. 2013;90:530–9. https://doi.org/10.1097/OPX.0b013e318293657d.
38. Chen C, Cheung SW, Cho P. Myopia control using toric orthokeratology (TO-SEE study). Invest Ophthalmol Vis Sci. 2013;54:6510–7. https://doi.org/10.1167/iovs.13-12527.
39. Swarbrick HA, Alharbi A, Watt K, et al. Myopia control during orthokeratology lens wear in children using a novel study design. Ophthalmology. 2015;122:620–30. https://doi.org/10.1016/j.ophtha.2014.09.028.

40. Santodomingo-Rubido J, Villa-Collar C, Gilmartin B, Gutiérrez-Ortega R. Factors preventing myopia progression with orthokeratology correction. Optom Vis Sci. 2013;90:1225–36. https://doi.org/10.1097/OPX.0000000000000034.
41. Kinoshita N, Konno Y, Hamada N, et al. Additive effects of orthokeratology and atropine 0.01% ophthalmic solution in slowing axial elongation in children with myopia: first year results. Jpn J Ophthalmol. 2018;62:544–53. https://doi.org/10.1007/s10384-018-0608-3.
42. Dart JK, Stapleton F, Minassian D. Contact lenses and other risk factors in microbial keratitis. Lancet. 1991;338:650–3.
43. Cheng KH, Leung SL, Hoekman HW, et al. Incidence of contact-lens-associated microbial keratitis and its related morbidity. Lancet. 1999;354:181–5. https://doi.org/10.1016/S0140-6736(98)09385-4.
44. Watt K, Swarbrick HA. Microbial keratitis in overnight orthokeratology: review of the first 50 cases. Eye Contact Lens. 2005;31:201–8.
45. Liu YM, Xie P. The safety of orthokeratology--a systematic review. Eye Contact Lens. 2016;42:35–42. https://doi.org/10.1097/ICL.0000000000000219.
46. Hiraoka T, Sekine Y, Okamoto F, et al. Safety and efficacy following 10-years of overnight orthokeratology for myopia control. Ophthalmic Physiol Opt. 2018;38:281–9. https://doi.org/10.1111/opo.12460.
47. Bullimore MA, Sinnott LT, Jones-Jordan LA. The risk of microbial keratitis with overnight corneal reshaping lenses. Optom Vis Sci. 2013;90:937–44. https://doi.org/10.1097/OPX.0b013e31829cac92.
48. Walline JJ, Gaume A, Jones LA, et al. Benefits of contact lens wear for children and teens. Eye Contact Lens. 2007;33:317–21. https://doi.org/10.1097/ICL.0b013e31804f80fb.
49. Rah MJ, Walline JJ, Jones-Jordan LA, et al. Vision specific quality of life of pediatric contact lens wearers. Optom Vis Sci. 2010;87:560–6. https://doi.org/10.1097/OPX.0b013e3181e6a1c8.
50. Walline JJ, Greiner KL, McVey ME, Jones-Jordan LA. Multifocal contact lens myopia control. Optom Vis Sci. 2013;90:1207–14. https://doi.org/10.1097/OPX.0000000000000036.
51. Pauné J, Queiros A, Quevedo L, et al. Peripheral myopization and visual performance with experimental rigid gas permeable and soft contact lens design. Cont Lens Anterior Eye. 2014;37:455–60. https://doi.org/10.1016/j.clae.2014.08.001.
52. Cheng X, Xu J, Chehab K, et al. Soft contact lenses with positive spherical aberration for myopia control. Optom Vis Sci. 2016;93:353–66. https://doi.org/10.1097/OPX.0000000000000773.
53. Anstice NS, Phillips JR. Effect of dual-focus soft contact lens wear on axial myopia progression in children. Ophthalmology. 2011;118:1152–61. https://doi.org/10.1016/j.ophtha.2010.10.035.
54. Lam CSY, Tang WC, DY-Y T, et al. Defocus incorporated soft contact (DISC) lens slows myopia progression in Hong Kong Chinese schoolchildren: a 2-year randomised clinical trial. Br J Ophthalmol. 2014;98:40–5. https://doi.org/10.1136/bjophthalmol-2013-303914.
55. Chamberlain P, Back A, Lazon P, et al. 3 year effectiveness of a dual-focus 1 day soft contact lens for myopia control. Cont Lens Anterior Eye. 2018;41:S71–2. https://doi.org/10.1016/j.clae.2018.03.097.
56. Ruiz-Pomeda A, Pérez-Sánchez B, Valls I, et al. MiSight Assessment Study Spain (MASS). A 2-year randomized clinical trial. Graefes Arch Clin Exp Ophthalmol. 2018;256:1011–21. https://doi.org/10.1007/s00417-018-3906-z.
57. Aller TA, Liu M, Wildsoet CF. Myopia control with bifocal contact lenses: a randomized clinical trial. Optom Vis Sci. 2016;93:344–52. https://doi.org/10.1097/OPX.0000000000000808.
58. Chua W-H, Balakrishnan V, Chan Y-H, et al. Atropine for the treatment of childhood myopia. Ophthalmology. 2006;113:2285–91. https://doi.org/10.1016/j.ophtha.2006.05.062.
59. Tong L, Huang XL, Koh ALT, et al. Atropine for the treatment of childhood myopia: effect on myopia progression after cessation of atropine. Ophthalmology. 2009;116:572–9. https://doi.org/10.1016/j.ophtha.2008.10.020.
60. Wu P-C, Yang Y-H, Fang P-C. The long-term results of using low-concentration atropine eye drops for controlling myopia progression in schoolchildren. J Ocul Pharmacol Ther. 2011;27:461–6. https://doi.org/10.1089/jop.2011.0027.

61. Chia A, Chua W-H, Cheung Y-B, et al. Atropine for the treatment of childhood myopia: safety and efficacy of 0.5%, 0.1%, and 0.01% doses (atropine for the treatment of myopia 2). Ophthalmology. 2012;119:347–54. https://doi.org/10.1016/j.ophtha.2011.07.031.
62. Clark TY, Clark RA. Atropine 0.01% eyedrops significantly reduce the progression of childhood myopia. J Ocul Pharmacol Ther. 2015;31:541–5. https://doi.org/10.1089/jop.2015.0043.
63. Schmid KL, Leyden K, Chiu Y, et al. Assessment of daily light and ultraviolet exposure in young adults. Optom Vis Sci. 2013;90:148–55. https://doi.org/10.1097/OPX.0b013e31827cda5b.
64. Wu P-C, Tsai C-L, Wu H-L, et al. Outdoor activity during class recess reduces myopia onset and progression in school children. Ophthalmology. 2013;120:1080–5. https://doi.org/10.1016/j.ophtha.2012.11.009.
65. Karouta C, Ashby RS. Correlation between light levels and the development of deprivation myopia. Invest Ophthalmol Vis Sci. 2014;56:299–309. https://doi.org/10.1167/iovs.14-15499.
66. Li W, Lan W, Yang S, et al. The effect of spectral property and intensity of light on natural refractive development and compensation to negative lenses in guinea pigs. Invest Ophthalmol Vis Sci. 2014;55:6324–32. https://doi.org/10.1167/iovs.13-13802.
67. Thorne HC, Jones KH, Peters SP, et al. Daily and seasonal variation in the spectral composition of light exposure in humans. Chronobiol Int. 2009;26:854–66. https://doi.org/10.1080/07420520903044315.
68. Foulds WS, Barathi VA, Luu CD. Progressive myopia or hyperopia can be induced in chicks and reversed by manipulation of the chromaticity of ambient light. Invest Ophthalmol Vis Sci. 2013;54:8004–12. https://doi.org/10.1167/iovs.13-12476.
69. Rucker F, Britton S, Spatcher M, Hanowsky S. Blue light protects against temporal frequency sensitive refractive changes. Invest Ophthalmol Vis Sci. 2015;56:6121–31. https://doi.org/10.1167/iovs.15-17238.
70. Torii H, Kurihara T, Seko Y, et al. Violet light exposure can be a preventive strategy against myopia progression. EBioMedicine. 2017;15:210–9. https://doi.org/10.1016/j.ebiom.2016.12.007.
71. Smith MJ, Walline JJ. Controlling myopia progression in children and adolescents. Adolesc Health Med Ther. 2015;6:133–40. https://doi.org/10.2147/AHMT.S55834.
72. Walline JJ. Myopia control: a review. Eye Contact Lens. 2016;42:3–8. https://doi.org/10.1097/ICL.0000000000000207.
73. Huang J, Wen D, Wang Q, et al. Efficacy comparison of 16 interventions for myopia control in children: a network meta-analysis. Ophthalmology. 2016;123:697–708. https://doi.org/10.1016/j.ophtha.2015.11.010.
74. Li S-M, Ji Y-Z, Wu S-S, et al. Multifocal versus single vision lenses intervention to slow progression of myopia in school-age children: a meta-analysis. Surv Ophthalmol. 2011;56:451–60. https://doi.org/10.1016/j.survophthal.2011.06.002.

Permissions

All chapters in this book were first published by Springer; hereby published with permission under the Creative Commons Attribution License or equivalent. Every chapter published in this book has been scrutinized by our experts. Their significance has been extensively debated. The topics covered herein carry significant information for a comprehensive understanding. They may even be implemented as practical applications or may be referred to as a beginning point for further studies.

The contributors of this book come from diverse backgrounds, making this book a truly international effort. We would like to thank all the contributing authors for lending their expertise to make the book truly unique. They have played a crucial role in the development of this book. Without their invaluable contributions this book wouldn't have been possible. They have made vital efforts to compile up to date information on the varied aspects of this subject to make this book a valuable addition to the collection of many professionals and students.

This book was conceptualized with the vision of imparting up-to-date and integrated information in this field. To ensure the same, a matchless editorial board was set up. Every individual on the board went through rigorous rounds of assessment to prove their worth. After which they invested a large part of their time researching and compiling the most relevant data for our readers.

The editorial board has been involved in producing this book since its inception. They have spent rigorous hours researching and exploring the diverse topics which have resulted in the successful publishing of this book. They have passed on their knowledge of decades through this book. To expedite this challenging task, the publisher supported the team at every step. A small team of assistant editors was also appointed to further simplify the editing procedure and attain best results for the readers.

Apart from the editorial board, the designing team has also invested a significant amount of their time in understanding the subject and creating the most relevant covers. They scrutinized every image to scout for the most suitable representation of the subject and create an appropriate cover for the book.

The publishing team has been an ardent support to the editorial, designing and production team. Their endless efforts to recruit the best for this project, has resulted in the accomplishment of this book. They are a veteran in the field of academics and their pool of knowledge is as vast as their experience in printing. Their expertise and guidance has proved useful at every step. Their uncompromising quality standards have made this book an exceptional effort. Their encouragement from time to time has been an inspiration for everyone.

The publisher and the editorial board hope that this book will prove to be a valuable piece of knowledge for students, practitioners and scholars across the globe.

Index

www.ingramcontent.com/pod-product-compliance
Lightning Source LLC
LaVergne TN
LVHW062223200926
848484LV00006B/1465